Dermatoscopy A–Z

Dermatoscopy A–Z

Aimilios Lallas, MD, MSc, PhD
First Department of Dermatology
Aristotle University
Thessaloniki, Greece

Zoe Apalla, MD, PhD
Associate Professor, Dermatology & Venereology
Aristotle University
Head, State Dermatology Department
Hippokratio General Hospital
Thessaloniki, Greece

Elizabeth Lazaridou, MD, PhD
Associate Professor, Dermatology & Venereology
Head, Second Department of Dermatology
Aristotle University Medical School
Papageorgiou General Hospital
Thessaloniki, Greece

Dimitrios Ioannides, MD, PhD
Professor of Dermatology and Venereology
Head, 1st Department of Dermatology
Aristotle University
Hospital of Skin and Venereal Diseases
Thessaloniki, Greece

Co-authors

Theodosia Gkentsidi
Christina Fotiadou
Theocharis-Nektarios Kirtsios
Eirini Kyrmanidou
Konstantinos Lallas
Chryssoula Papageorgiou

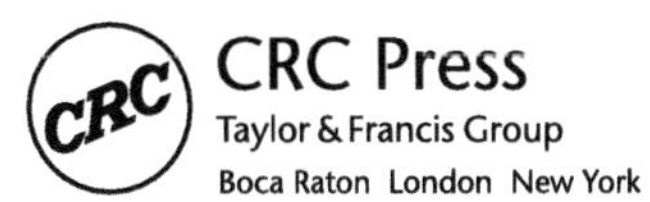

CRC Press is an imprint of the
Taylor & Francis Group, an **informa** business

CRC Press
Taylor & Francis Group
6000 Broken Sound Parkway NW, Suite 300
Boca Raton, FL 33487-2742

Printed on acid-free paper

International Standard Book Number-13: 978-0-367-19784-1 (Hardback)
978-0-367-19781-0 (Paperback)

Library of Congress Cataloging-in-Publication Data

Names: Lallas, Aimilios, author. | Apalla, Zoe, author. | Lazaridou, Elizabeth, author. | Ioannides, Dimitrios, author.
Title: Dermatoscopy A-Z / Aimilios Lallas, Zoe Apalla, Elizabeth Lazaridou, Dimitrios Ioannides.
Description: Boca Raton : CRC Press, [2020] | Includes bibliographical references and index. |
Identifiers: LCCN 2019034433 (print) | LCCN 2019034434 (ebook) | ISBN 9780367197810 (paperback ; alk. paper) | ISBN 9780367197841 (hardback ; alk. paper) | ISBN 9780429243240 (ebook)
Subjects: MESH: Skin Diseases--diagnosis | Dermoscopy--methods | Skin Pigmentation
Classification: LCC RL105 (print) | LCC RL105 (ebook) | NLM WR 141 | DDC 616.5/075--dc23
LC record available at https://lccn.loc.gov/2019034433
LC ebook record available at https://lccn.loc.gov/2019034434

Visit the Taylor & Francis Web site at
http://www.taylorandfrancis.com

and the CRC Press Web site at
http://www.crcpress.com

To the teachers who inspire us and the pupils who teach us

To the wonderful dermatoscopy family worldwide

Contents

Preface xi

1 Introduction to Dermatoscopy 1
1.1 Device 1
1.2 Basic Parameters 1
1.2.1 Colors 1
1.2.2 Basic Structures 5
1.3 Light Modes 13
Bibliography 15

2 Nevi 17
2.1 Common Nevi 19
2.1.1 Nevi of Trunk and Extremities 19
2.1.2 Scalp Nevi 24
2.1.3 Facial Nevi 24
2.1.4 Acral Nevi 24
2.1.5 Subungual Nevi 28
2.1.6 Mucosal Nevi 28
2.2 Spitz and Reed Nevi 29
2.2.1 Vessels and White Network (Nonpigmented Spitz Nevus) 29
2.2.2 Globules and White Network (Pigmented Spitz Nevus) 30
2.2.3 Starburst Pattern (Reed Nevus) 30
2.3 Blue Nevi 32
2.4 Special Nevus Types 33
2.4.1 Traumatized Nevus (Targetoid Hemosiderotic Nevus) 33
2.4.2 Eczematous Nevus (Meyerson Nevus) 33
2.4.3 Halo Nevus (Sutton Nevus) 33
2.4.4 Balloon Cell Nevus 35
2.4.5 Sclerosing Nevus (with Pseudomelanoma Features) 36
2.4.6 Recurrent Nevus 36
Bibliography 36

3 Melanoma 39
3.1 Conventional Melanoma 40
3.1.1 Melanoma of the Trunk and the Extremities 40
3.1.2 Facial Melanoma 48
3.1.3 Acral Melanoma 52
3.1.4 Subungual Melanoma 56
3.1.5 Mucosal Melanoma 60
3.2 Nodular Melanoma 63
3.3 Amelanotic Melanoma 66
Bibliography 70

4 Benign Nonmelanocytic Skin Tumors 75
4.1 Epithelial Skin Tumors 75
4.1.1 Solar Lentigo 75
4.1.2 Ink-Spot Lentigo 75
4.1.3 Seborrheic Keratosis 77
4.1.4 Lichen Planus–Like Keratosis 80
4.2 Vascular Tumors 80
4.2.1 Cherry Angioma 80
4.2.2 Angiokeratoma 81
4.2.3 Pyogenic Granuloma 81
4.2.4 Subcorneal and Subungual Hemorrhage 81
4.3 Tumors of the Fibrous Tissue 82
4.3.1 Dermatofibroma 82
4.4 Common Adnexal Tumors 84
4.4.1 Sebaceous Hyperplasia 84
4.4.2 Eccrine Poroma 84
4.5 Clear Cell Acanthoma 86
Bibliography 86

5 Malignant Nonmelanocytic Tumors 89
5.1 Basal Cell Carcinoma 89
5.1.1 Dermatoscopy and Histopathologic Subtype 90
5.1.2 Dermatoscopy and Response to Treatment 94
5.2 Keratinocyte Skin Cancer 96
5.2.1 Actinic Keratosis 96
5.2.2 Intraepidermal Carcinoma or Bowen's Disease 99
5.2.3 Squamous Cell Carcinoma 100
5.2.4 Dermatoscopic Model of the Progression from Actinic Keratosis into Squamous Cell Carcinoma 104
5.3 Basosquamous Carcinoma 105
5.4 Merkel Cell Carcinoma 106
5.5 Atypical Fibroxanthoma and Malignant Fibrous Histiocytoma 107
5.6 Malignant Vascular Tumors 107
5.6.1 Kaposi Sarcoma 107
5.6.2 Angiosarcoma 108
Bibliography 108

6 Inflammatory Skin Diseases 111
6.1 Psoriasis 111
6.2 Dermatitis 113
6.3 Lichen Planus 113
6.4 Pityriasis Rosea 115
6.5 Discoid Lupus Erythematosus 116
6.6 Lichen Sclerosus and Morphea 117
6.7 Granulomatous Skin Diseases 117
6.7.1 Sarcoidosis and Lupus Vulgaris 118
6.7.2 Necrobiosis Lipoidica and Granuloma Annulare 118
6.8 Rosacea 119

6.9 Porokeratosis 121
6.10 Urticaria and Urticarial Vasculitis 121
6.11 Mastocytosis 122
6.12 Pigmented Purpuric Dermatoses 122
6.13 Pityriasis Rubra Pilaris 122
6.14 Pityriasis Lichenoides et Varioliformis Acuta 123
6.15 Prurigo Nodularis 123
6.16 Acquired Perforating Dermatoses 124
6.17 Grover's Disease and Darier Disease 124
6.18 Mycosis Fungoides 125
6.19 Lymphomatoid Papulosis 126
Bibliography 126

7 Infectious Skin Diseases 131
7.1 Parasitoses 131
7.1.1 Scabies 131
7.1.2 Pediculosis 131
7.2 Viral Infections 134
7.2.1 Molluscum Contagiosum 134
7.2.2 Human Papillomavirus Infections 136
7.3 Other Infections 139
7.3.1 Tick Bites 139
7.3.2 Demodicosis 139
7.3.3 Leishmaniasis 140
7.3.4 Tinea Corporis 141
Bibliography 141

8 Trichoscopy 143
8.1 Noncicatricial Alopecias 144
8.1.1 Androgenetic Alopecia (Male and Female Pattern Hair Loss) 144
8.1.2 Alopecia Areata 147
8.1.3 Trichotillomania 151
8.1.4 Tinea Capitis 153
8.2 Primary Cicatricial Alopecias 154
8.2.1 Lichen Planopilaris 154
8.2.2 Discoid Lupus Erythematosus 156
8.2.3 Folliculitis Decalvans 158
8.2.4 Dissecting Cellulitis of the Scalp 159
8.3 Trichoscopy in Children 159
8.3.1 Temporal Triangular Alopecia 159
8.3.2 Loose Anagen Hair Syndrome 160
8.3.3 Aplasia Cutis 160
8.4 Hair Shaft Deformities 161
8.4.1 Monilethrix 161
8.4.2 Pseudomonilethrix or Pohl-Pinkus Constrictions 161
8.4.3 Trichorrhexis Nodosa 161
8.4.4 Trichorrhexis Invaginata 162
8.4.5 Trichoptilosis 163

8.4.6 Trichoschisis 163
8.4.7 Pili Torti 163
8.4.8 Pili Annulati 164
Bibliography 164

9 Special Clinical Scenarios 169
9.1 Pigmented Macules on the Face 169
9.2 Diagnosis and Management of Spitzoid-Looking Lesions 176
9.3 Management of Patients with Multiple Common Nevi and/or Clinically Atypical Nevi 182
9.4 Seven Rules to Not Miss Melanoma 186
Bibliography 190

Index 191

Preface

Approximately 30 years after the introduction of dermatoscopy, the reality justified the prediction that dermatoscopy would radically modify dermatology. In our opinion, this happened because dermatoscopy fulfills two prerequisites that are mandatory for any new technology to become really revolutionary: high efficacy and easy application.

It was never difficult to understand that by revealing structures invisible to the naked eye, dermatoscopy can enhance the morphological interpretation of skin tumors or eruptions. This seems reasonable for any kind of imaging device or technology that has the potential to expand the human visual limit. However, this was not enough to radically change the reality of dermatologic diagnosis.

Unlike other imaging tools, the dermatoscope is not a sophisticated device only available in specialized clinical settings. Dermatoscopes can be found anywhere the diagnosis of skin diseases takes place—in big hospitals but also in private offices, from the biggest city to the smallest village, and in research centers and purely clinical settings. It is used by experts and novices, by specialists and residents, in live consultations and teleconsultations. In any place, in any way, and at any time that diagnosis of skin tumors or other diseases occurs, dermatoscopy is there.

As doctors, we are privileged to live in an era in which scientific information is accessible and can be acquired through several channels. Therefore, the current book does not contain any information that cannot be found in other sources, and it is not a summary of our previous research efforts.

In this book, we tried to provide essential information on the dermatoscopy of skin tumors and other diseases in a structured way, filtered by our conceptual views that undoubtedly are objective. Therefore, we invite all our readers to read it critically and always keep in mind that any established knowledge might be challenged in the future.

We hope you will enjoy reading.

1

Introduction to Dermatoscopy

Fundamental principle

Dermatoscopy should be considered as an integral part of the clinical dermatologic examination, and the interpretation of the dermatoscopic criteria is meaningful and helpful only within the clinical context of each particular patient. Knowledge of dermatoscopy is by no means a substitute for basic knowledge about pathogenesis, epidemiology, clinical morphology, and histopathologic features of skin tumors and other cutaneous diseases. On the contrary, dermatoscopy enriches and complements the cognitive framework of the physician on skin diseases.

1.1 Device

The dermatoscope is a handheld device with 10-fold magnifying optics, combined with a transilluminating light source. The expanded use of dermatoscopy among clinicians is based on the following important strengths: it is a fast and effective method applied with a small and inexpensive device. Therefore, the dermatoscope should be considered not as an imaging device but as a clinical tool that can be routinely used on all skin lesions by any physician dealing with skin disorders, acquiring a role similar to the stethoscope of physicians.

Digital dermatoscopic devices (videodermatoscopes) that allow much higher magnifications (up to ×200) also exist. Although these devices provide further insights into the morphology of skin lesions, they lack three important properties of the handheld dermatoscope: they require some time, space, and cost. Therefore, these devices are not convenient for use on all skin lesions during the daily routine. Instead, digital dermatoscopy has specific indications that are discussed in some chapters of this book. All the patterns, structures, features, or criteria described in this book can be seen with a handheld dermatoscope, unless otherwise clarified in the text.

1.2 Basic Parameters

The use of the dermatoscope reveals a morphological world of macroscopically invisible structures and criteria. The dermatologic patterns are composed of two basic parameters: colors and morphological structures.

1.2.1 Colors

Considering skin color as "neutral," skin lesions are typically divided into two main categories: pigmented and nonpigmented. Pigmented lesions are characterized by one of the following colors: black, brown, blue, or gray (Figures 1.1 through 1.4). Nonpigmented lesions are characterized by the presence of white, red, and yellow or orange (Figures 1.5 through 1.8). Obviously, a lesion may be partially pigmented and partially not. The general rule is that when pigmented structures

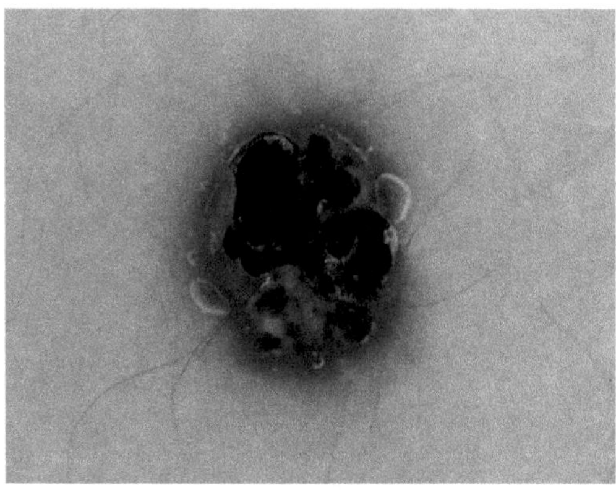

FIGURE 1.1 The black color in dermatoscopy. In this example, it corresponds to coagulated blood (angioma).

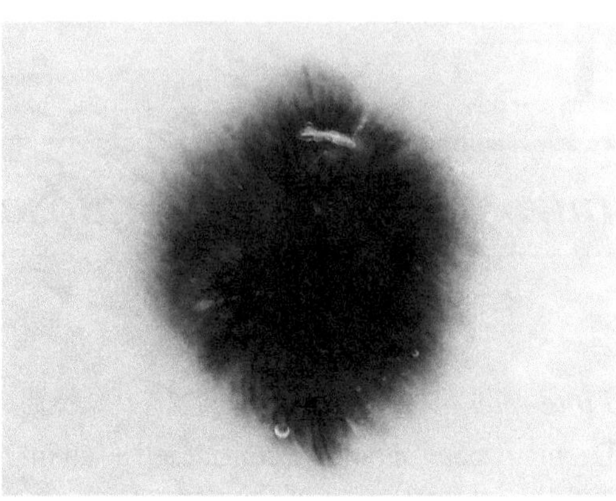

FIGURE 1.2 The brown color in dermatoscopy. In this example, it corresponds to melanin (nevus).

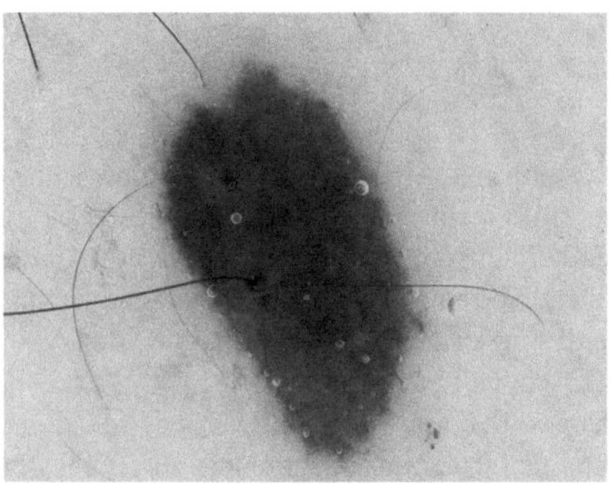

FIGURE 1.3 The blue color in dermatoscopy. In this example, it corresponds to melanin (nevus).

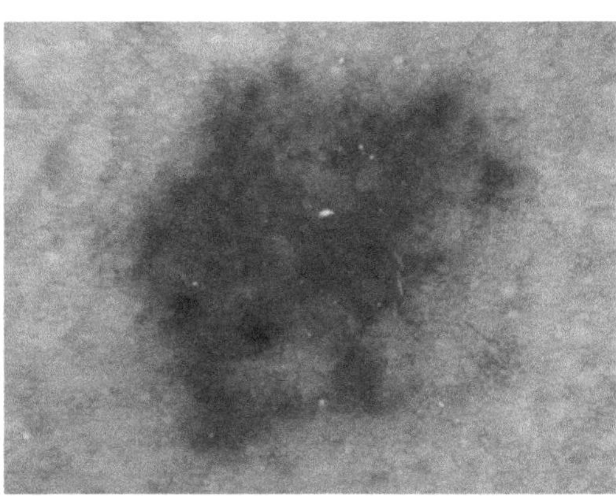

FIGURE 1.4 The gray color in dermatoscopy. In this example, it corresponds to melanin (nevus).

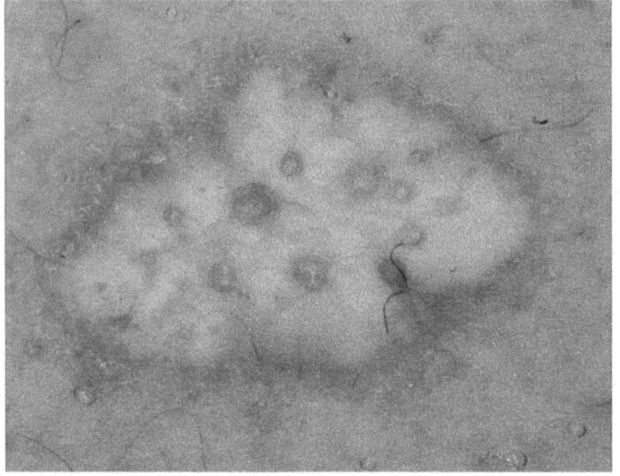

FIGURE 1.5 The white color in dermatoscopy. In this example, it corresponds to fibrosis (lichen sclerosus).

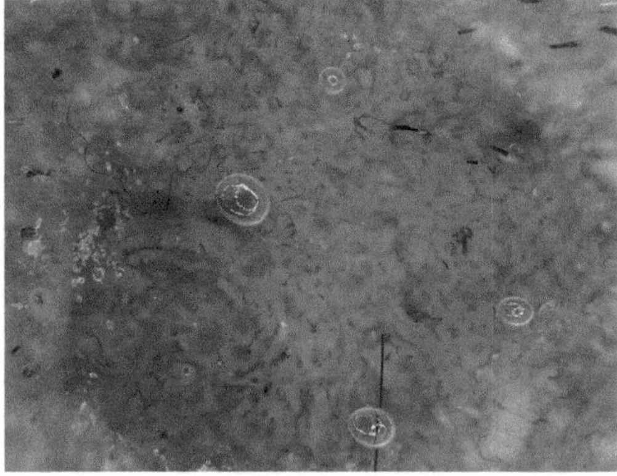

FIGURE 1.6 The red color in dermatoscopy. In this example, it corresponds to vessels (squamous cell carcinoma).

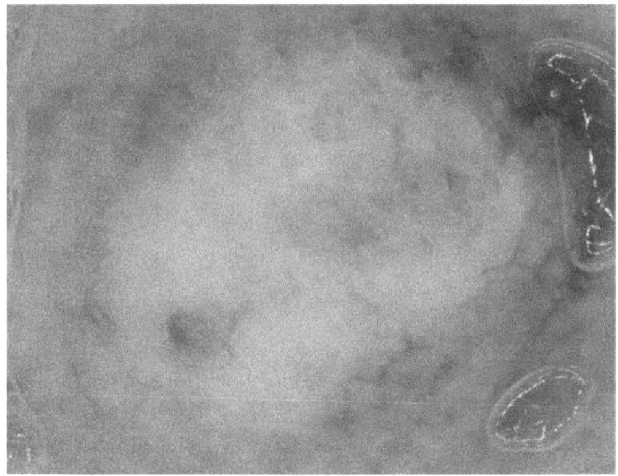

FIGURE 1.7 The yellow color in dermatoscopy. In this example, it results from sebum (sebaceous cyst).

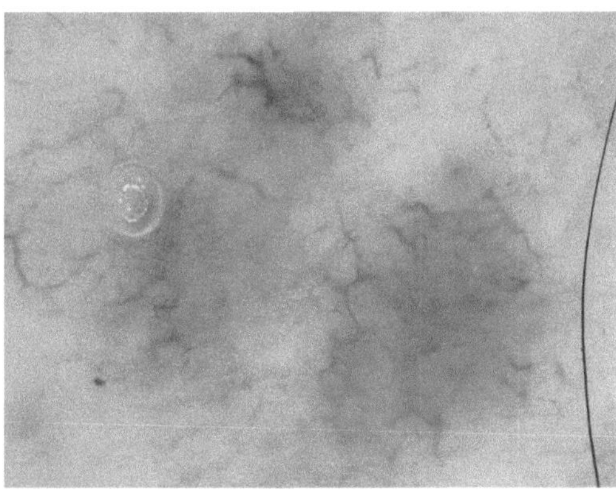

FIGURE 1.8 The yellow-orange color in dermatoscopy. In this example, it corresponds to cutaneous granulomas (sarcoidosis).

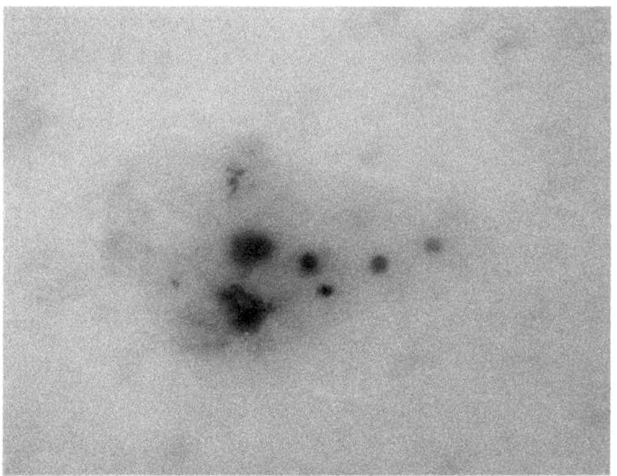

FIGURE 1.9 This lesion is only partially pigmented (blue color). However, the pigmented structures are diagnostically highly valuable (basal cell carcinoma).

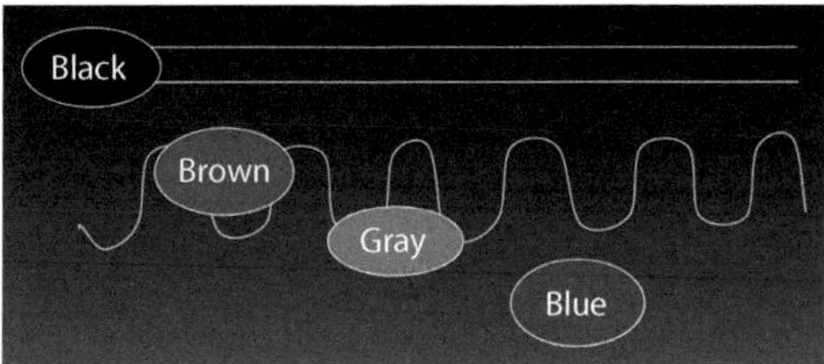

FIGURE 1.10 Melanin, depending on the depth of location, may appear as black, brown, gray, or blue in dermatoscopy.

are present, they are usually diagnostically more important than nonpigmented ones; therefore, they should be evaluated first (Figure 1.9).

The main chromophore component of skin that results in dermatoscopic color is melanin. The dermatoscopic color of melanin might be black, light or dark brown, gray, or blue, depending on its distribution in the epidermis, dermo-epidermal junction, or upper or deeper dermis, respectively (Figure 1.10). The dermatoscopic detection of melanin is not tantamount to the diagnosis of a melanocytic tumor, since it is known that melanin may be found not only in melanocytes but also in keratinocytes, in the neoplastic cells of an epithelial tumor (e.g., pigmented basal cell carcinoma), in macrophages (melanophages), or even free on the epidermis or dermis (pigment incontinence) (Figures 1.11 through 1.15).

The second major chromophore of the skin is hemoglobin, which usually dermatoscopically appears red. However, hemoglobin may also appear blue when it is located deeper in the dermis, or black as a result of thrombosis or oxidation (Figure 1.16). Since hemoglobin is typically found in the vessels, the red color usually corresponds to well-formed vascular structures. However, when blood is extravasated, dermatoscopy will reveal structureless red or black sharply demarcated areas/spots (bleeding) or purpuric dots/globules (purpura) (Figures 1.17 through 1.19).

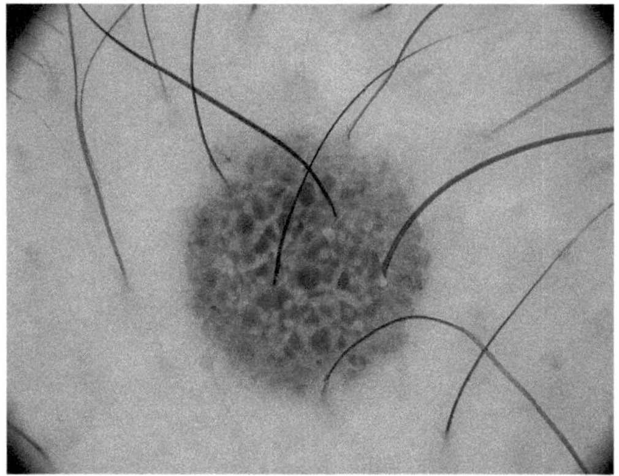

FIGURE 1.11 Melanin in melanocytes (nevus).

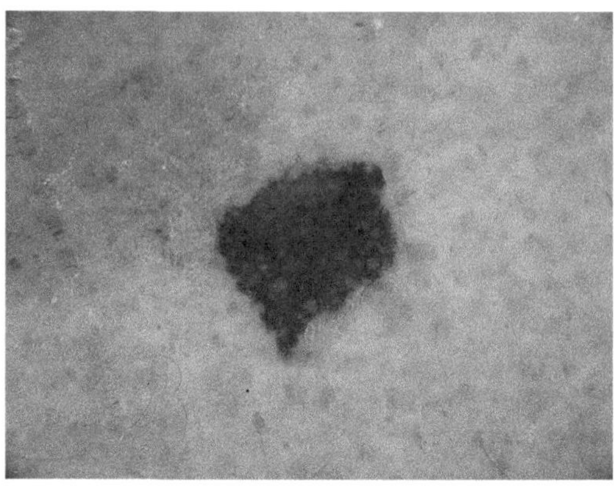

FIGURE 1.12 Melanin in keratinocytes (seborrheic keratosis).

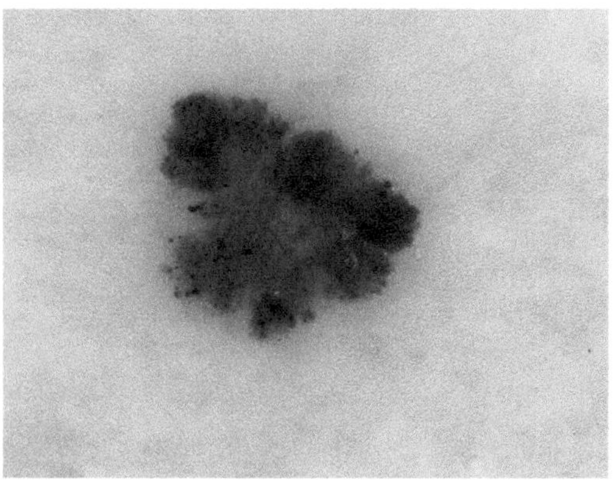

FIGURE 1.13 Melanin in basal neoplastic cells (basal cell carcinoma).

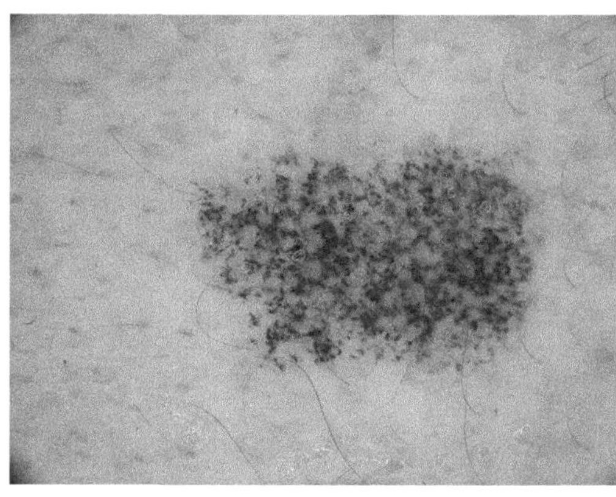

FIGURE 1.14 Melanin in macrophages-melanophages (lichenoid keratosis).

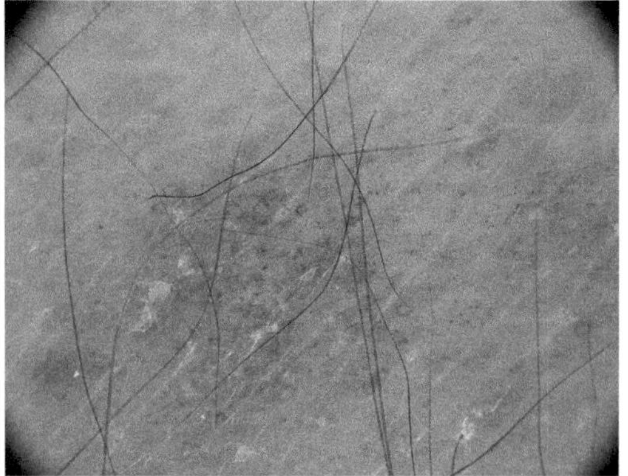

FIGURE 1.15 Melanin free in dermis and in melanophages (ashy dermatosis).

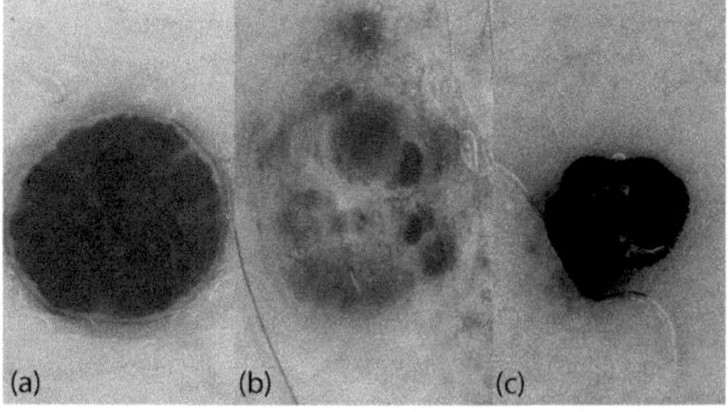

FIGURE 1.16 Depending on the depth of location, the presence of hemoglobin corresponds to a red or blue color in dermatoscopy, which turns into black in the event of thrombosis: (a) angioma; (b) cavernous angioma; (c) thrombosed angioma.

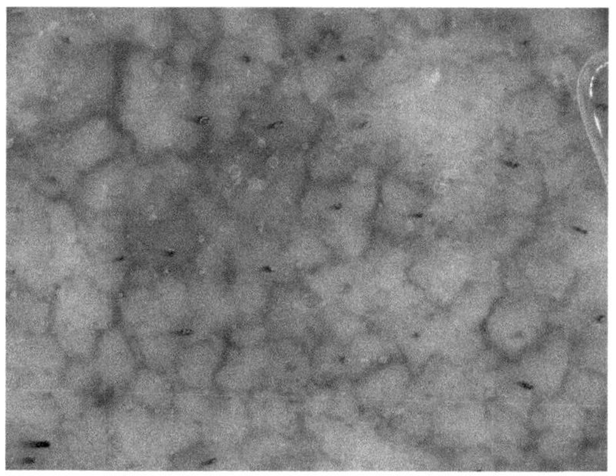

FIGURE 1.17 Hemoglobin in blood vessels (rosacea).

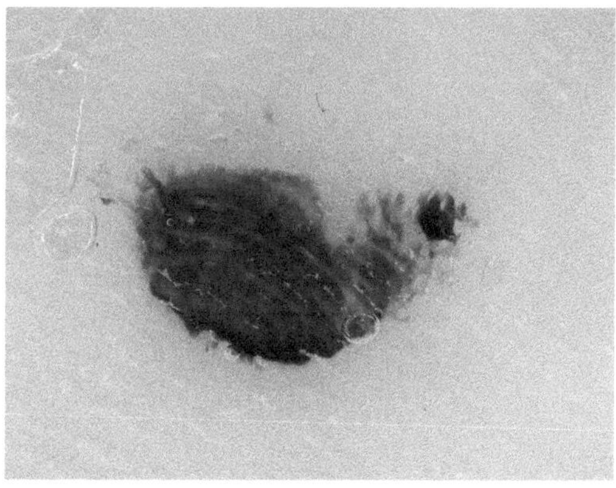

FIGURE 1.18 Extravasated hemoglobin in a hemorrhage (subcorneal hemorrhage).

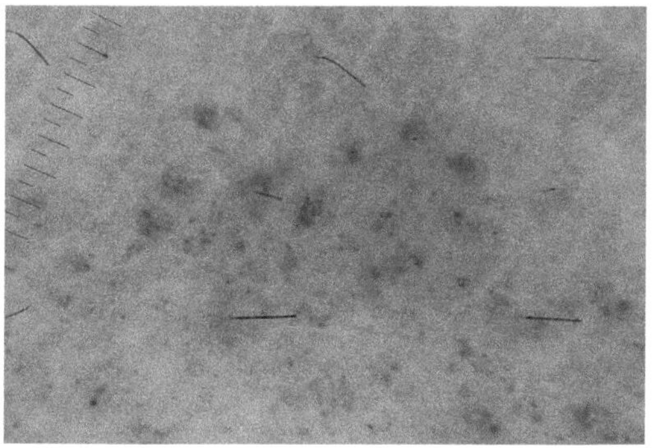

FIGURE 1.19 Extracted hemoglobin in purple (Schamberg disease).

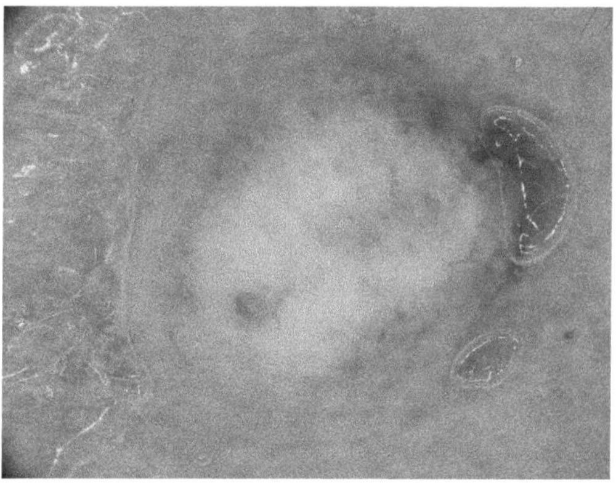

FIGURE 1.20 Yellow color as a result of the presence of sebum (epidermal cyst).

In addition to melanin and hemoglobin, several other skin components might have a chromatic effect on dermatoscopy: sebum, keratin, extravasated plasma serum, cutaneous granulomas, or even the hyperplasia of one or more layers of the epidermis (Figures 1.20 through 1.24).

Figure 1.25 presents a summary of all dermatoscopic colors and the skin chromophores that correspond to each color.

1.2.2 Basic Structures

The aforementioned dermatoscopic colors appear either diffuse or in shaped morphological structures. The morphological structures seen under dermatoscopy can be divided into two main categories: pigmented and nonpigmented structures. In conjunction with the previously mentioned color classification, pigmented structures are black, brown, gray, or blue; nonpigmented structures might be white, yellow, orange, or red.

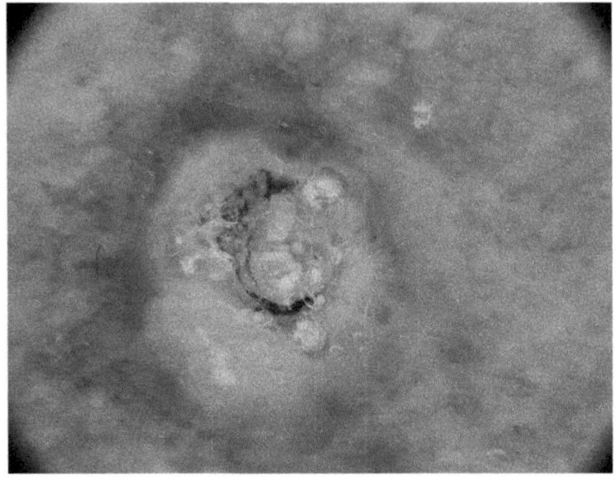

FIGURE 1.21 White color as a result of the presence of keratin (keratoacanthoma).

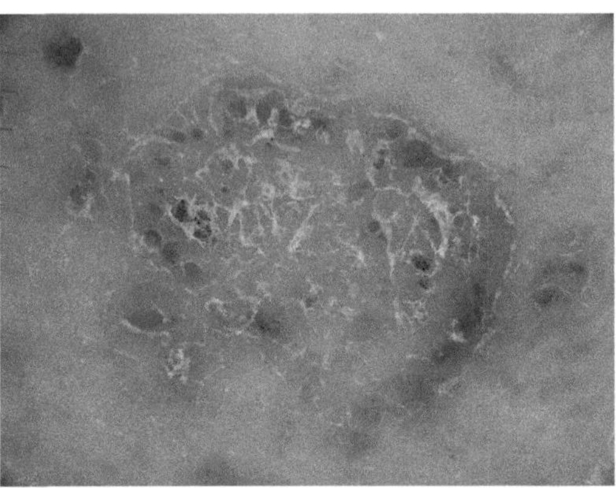

FIGURE 1.22 Yellow color as a result of the presence of extravasated plasma serum (dermatitis).

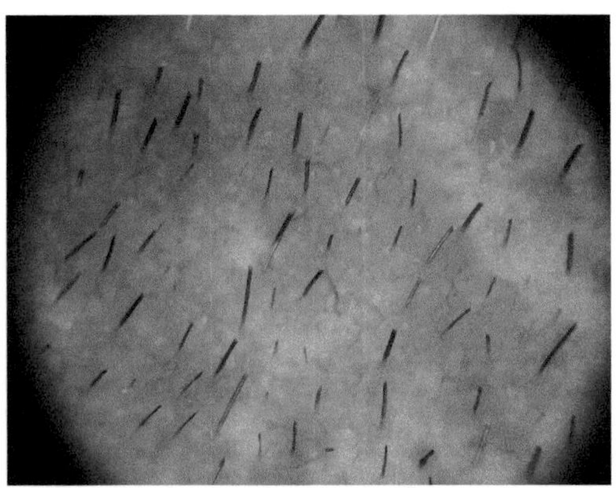

FIGURE 1.23 Yellow-orange color as a result of the presence of cutaneous granulomas (granulomatous drug reaction).

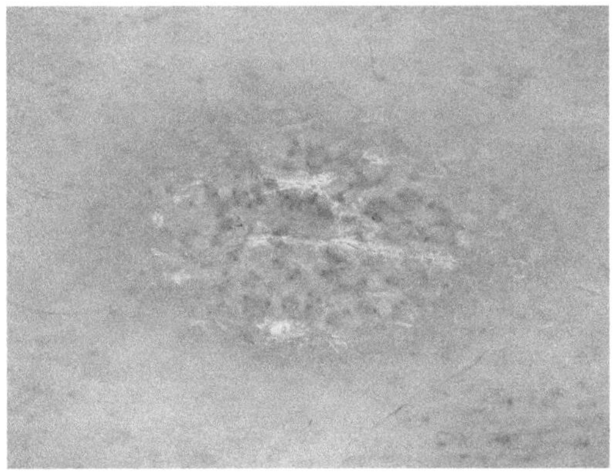

FIGURE 1.24 White color as a result of hypergranulosis (lichen planus).

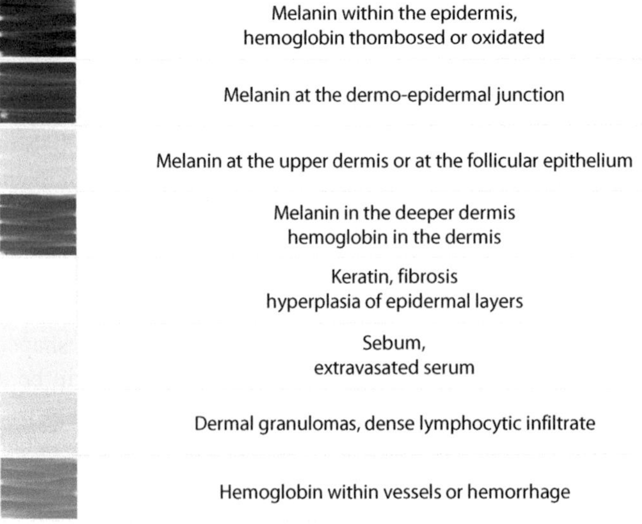

FIGURE 1.25 Colors in dermatoscopy and the chromophores to which they correspond.

Pigmented Structures

- **Structureless (homogeneous) pigmentation:** The presence of a homogeneous region of any color (black, brown, gray, or blue) without the presence of any other identifiable morphological structure.
  - **Most common colors:** Brown, black, and blue (Figure 1.26)
- **Pigment network:** A network of lines intersecting in such a way as to create round or polygonal openings (holes).
  - **Most common colors:** Light and dark brown (Figure 1.27)
- **Globules:** Multiple roundish structures of variable size, usually confluent.
  - **Most common colors:** Light and dark brown (Figure 1.28)
- **Dots:** Roundish structures similar to the globules but smaller in diameter that may appear isolated or in groups. Tiny dots are sometimes called *granules.*
  - **Most common colors:** Dark brown, black, blue, and gray (Figure 1.29)
- **Streaks and pseudopods:** Radial peripheral projections arising from the pigmented center of the lesion. At the peripheral end of the projection there may be a spherical protrusion (pseudopod).
  - **Most common colors:** Dark brown and black (Figure 1.30)
- **Ovoid nests:** Well- or less well-demarcated spherical or oval structures of blue color, larger than globules, that might coalesce to form larger structures.
  - **Most common colors:** Blue and gray (Figure 1.31)
- **Leaf-like areas:** Linear projections originating from a common base, resulting in an appearance reminiscent of the shape of the leaves. These formations are usually distributed to the periphery and, in contrast to streaks, are not associated with pigmented areas in the center of the lesion.
  - **Most common colors:** Light and dark brown (Figure 1.32)
- **Spoke wheel areas:** Radial projections originating from a central darker dot or globule.
  - **Most common colors:** Light and dark brown (Figure 1.33)

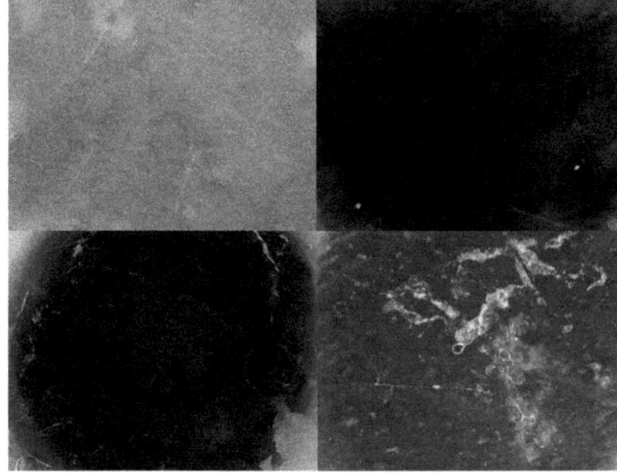

FIGURE 1.26 Homogeneous light brown, dark brown, blue, and gray areas without detectable morphological structures (nevi).

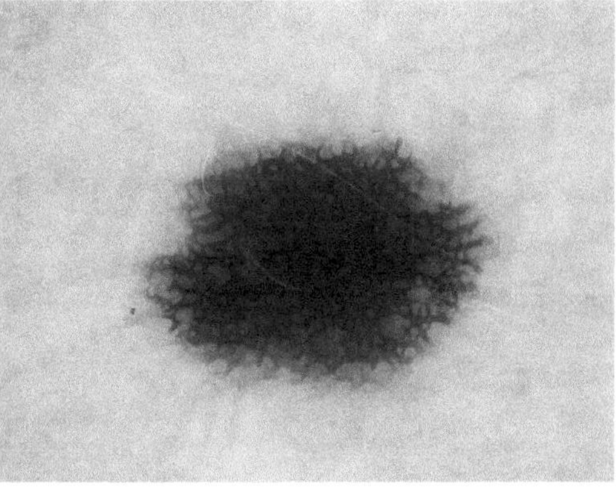

FIGURE 1.27 Pigment network (nevus).

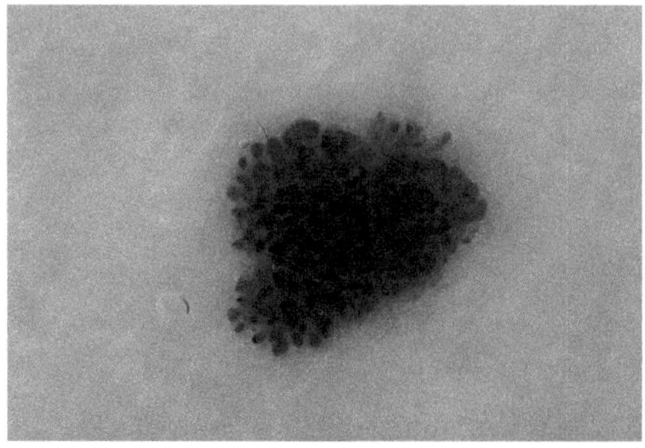

FIGURE 1.28 Multiple aggregated globules (nevus).

FIGURE 1.29 Multiple dots/granules of gray color (lichenoid keratosis).

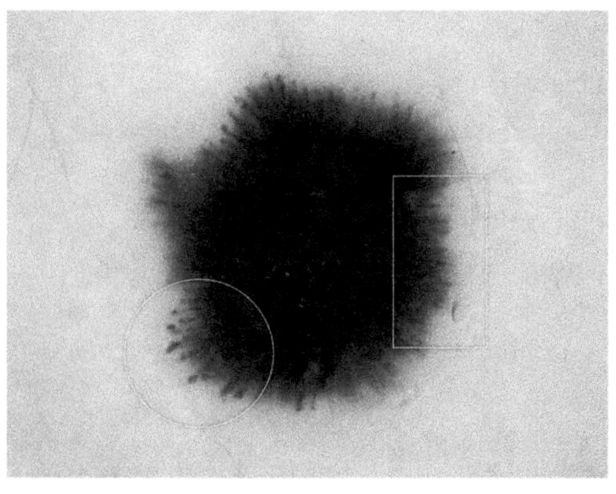

FIGURE 1.30 Multiple peripheral streaks (square) and pseudopods (circle) (spitz nevus).

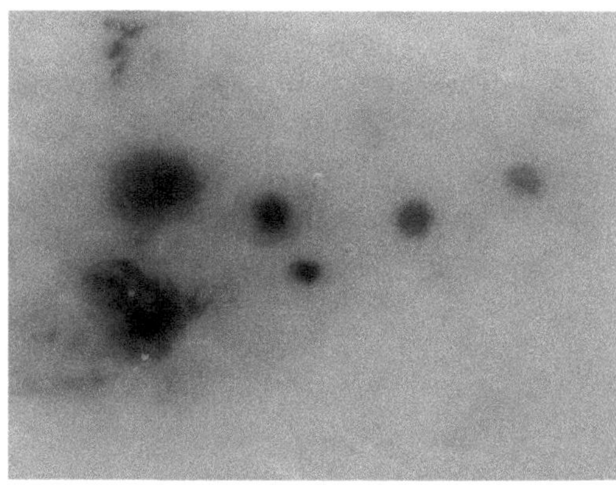

FIGURE 1.31 Multiple round-ish and ovoid blue-gray nests (basal cell carcinoma).

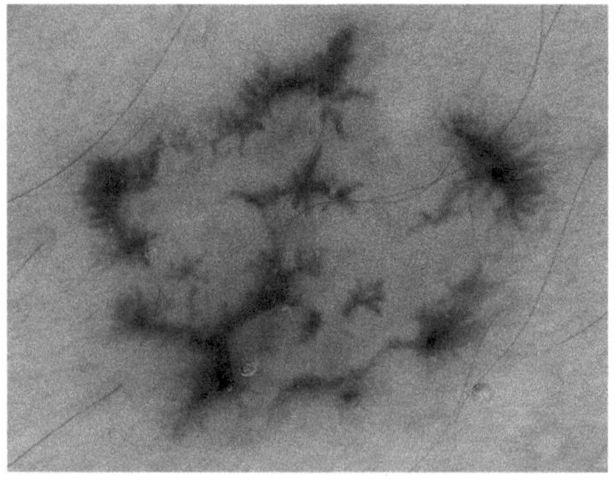

FIGURE 1.32 "Leaf-like areas" (basal cell carcinoma).

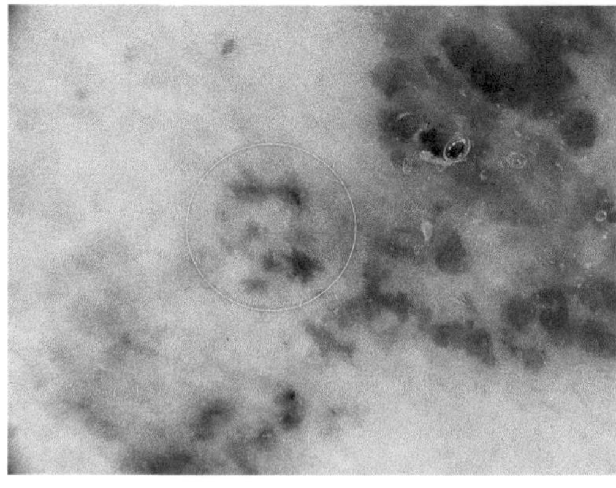

FIGURE 1.33 "Spoke wheel" areas (basal cell carcinoma).

- **Concentric structures:** Roundish pigmented areas with a darker center.
    - **Most common colors:** Light and dark brown (Figure 1.34)
- **Comedo-like openings:** Well-circumscribed roundish, oval, or polygonal structures.
    - **Most common colors:** Brown-yellow and brown-black (Figure 1.35)
- **"Fingerprinting":** Parallel curved pigmented lines, similar to the fingerprints.
    - **Most common colors:** Light brown (Figure 1.36)
- **Cerebriform structures:** Pattern of parallel curved alternating gyri and sulci. The sulci are thinner and usually darker than the ridges.
    - **Most common colors:** Light brown and dark brown (Figure 1.37)

Nonpigmented Structures

- **Uniform structureless area:** Defined as a homogeneous area of any color (white, red, or yellow), without the presence of any other identifiable morphological structure.
    - **Most common colors:** White, red, and yellow (Figure 1.38)
- **Dotted vessels:** Vessels shaped as small rounded structures (dots).
    - **Most common color:** Red (Figure 1.39)

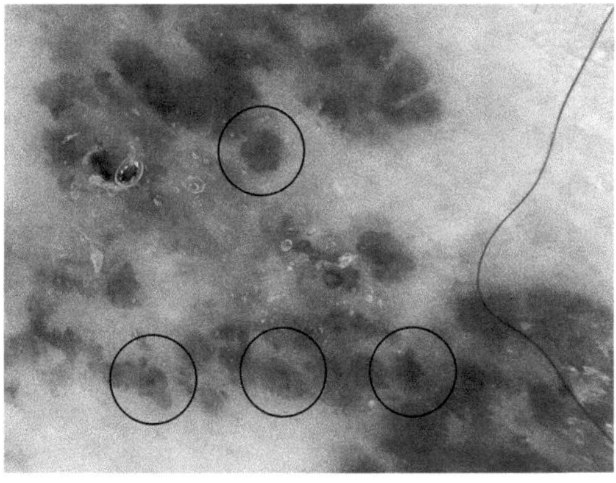

FIGURE 1.34 Concentric structures (basal cell carcinoma).

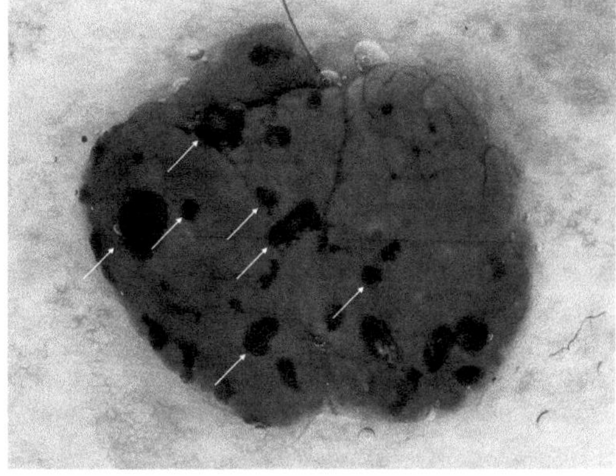

FIGURE 1.35 Multiple round-ish or ovoid comedy-like openings (arrows) (seborrheic keratosis).

FIGURE 1.36 Fingerprinting (seborrheic keratosis).

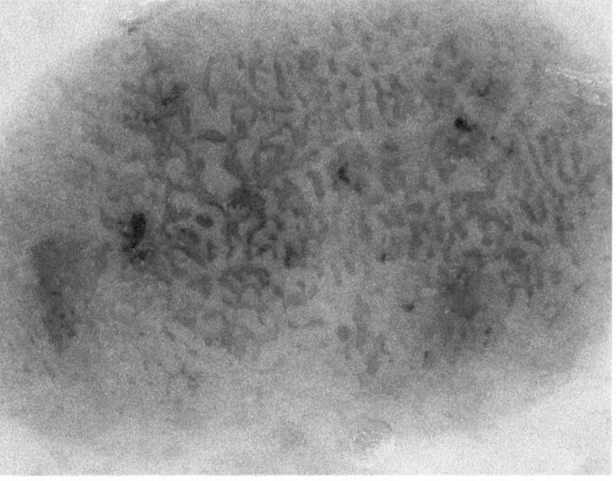

FIGURE 1.37 Cerebriform pattern consisting of gyri and sulci (seborrheic keratosis).

- **Coiled (glomerular) vessels:** Tightly coiled vessels resembling the glomerular apparatus of the kidney. At a small magnification, they often appear as large-sized dotted (globular) vessels.
  - **Most common color:** Red (Figure 1.40)
- **Linear vessels:** Vessels in the form of straight or slightly curved lines.
  - **Most common color:** Red (Figure 1.41)
- **Comma vessels:** Short and usually ticked curved linear vessels.
  - **Most common color:** Red (Figure 1.42)
- **Arborizing (branched) vessels:** Linear vessels of large diameter, ramified into branches of smaller diameter and ultimately capillaries. Branched vessels typically project sharply in-focus and usually cross the center of the lesion.
  - **Most common color:** Red (Figure 1.43)
- **Hairpin vessels:** Linear vessels forming a loop and resembling a hairpin.
  - **Most common color:** Red (Figure 1.44)
- **Linear irregular vessels:** Linear vessels with multiple bends.
  - **Most common color:** Red (Figure 1.45)
- **Vascular lacunes:** Multiple, sharply demarcated, roundish or oval areas of homogeneous color, without vessels inside of them.
  - **Most common colors:** Red, purple, blue, and black (Figure 1.46)
- **Milia-like cysts:** Round, opalescent structures of variable diameter.
  - **Most common colors:** White and yellow (Figure 1.47)
- **White halos:** Cyclic white structures surrounding vessels of any morphological type (Figure 1.48).
- **White circles:** Cyclic white structures surrounding follicular openings (Figure 1.49).
- **Ulceration:** Structureless area of round or irregular shape, often with visible crusts.
  - **Most common colors:** Red and yellow (Figure 1.50)
- **Erosions:** Similar to the erosions but smaller areas, usually roundish and multiple.
  - **Most common colors:** Pale yellow and yellow (Figure 1.51)

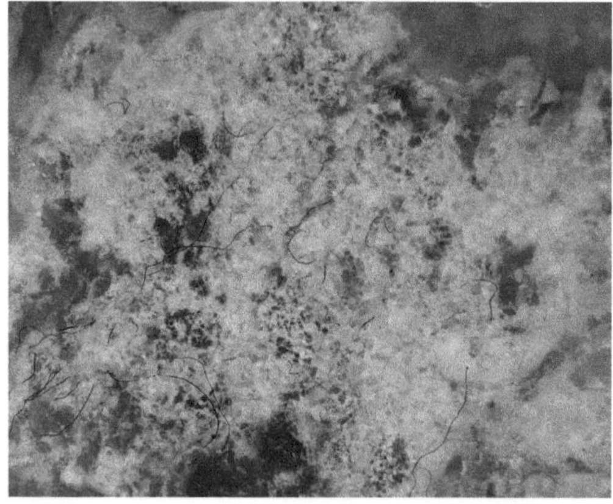

FIGURE 1.38 White area without identifiable morphological structures (squamous cell carcinoma).

FIGURE 1.39 Multiple vessels as dots (psoriasis).

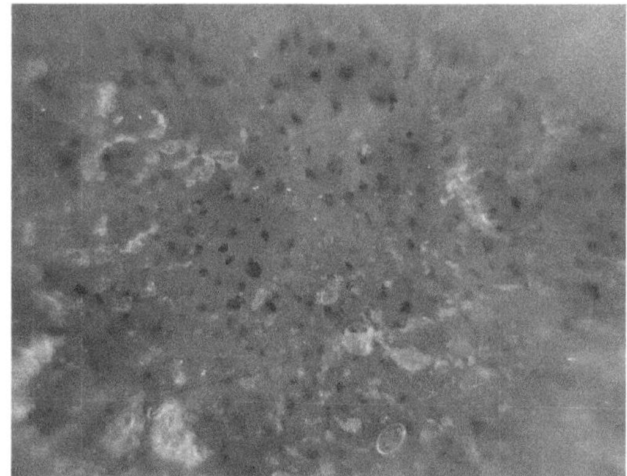

FIGURE 1.40 Multiple glomerular or coiled vessels (Bowen disease).

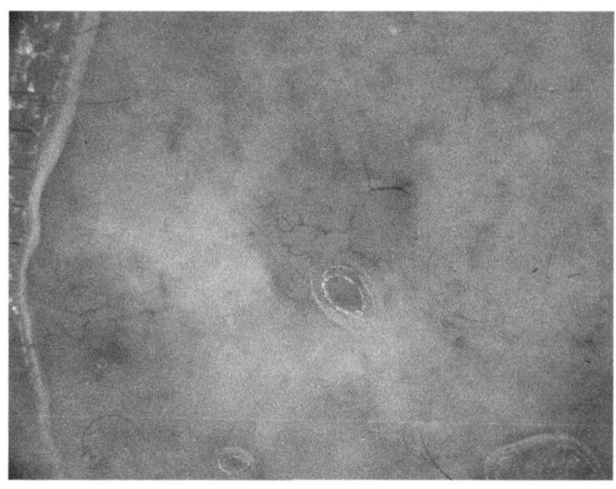

FIGURE 1.41 Linear vessels, some of them curved and with few branches (basal cell carcinoma).

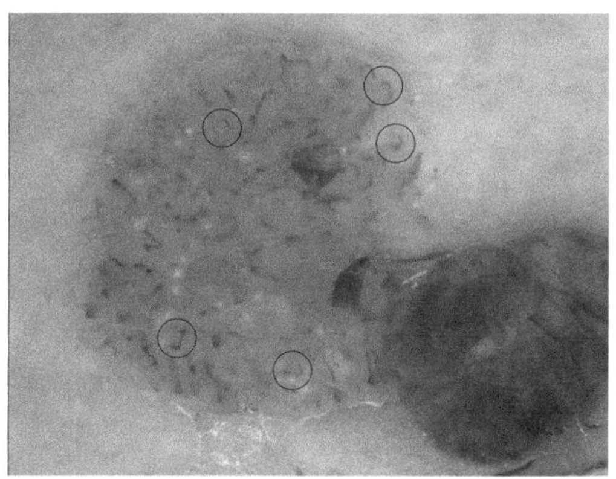

FIGURE 1.42 Comma vessels (circles) (dermal nevus).

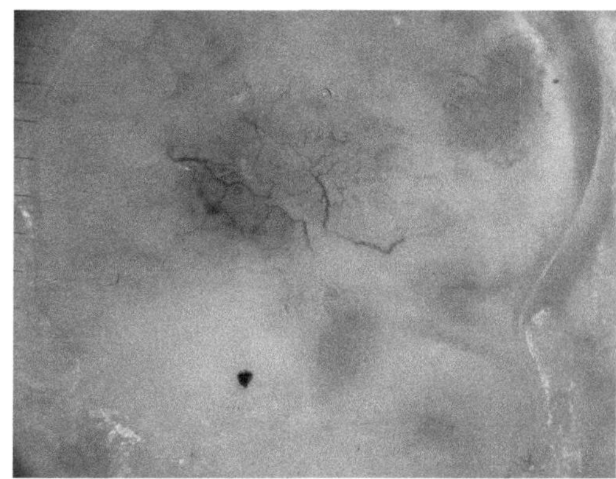

FIGURE 1.43 Branched vessels (basal cell carcinoma).

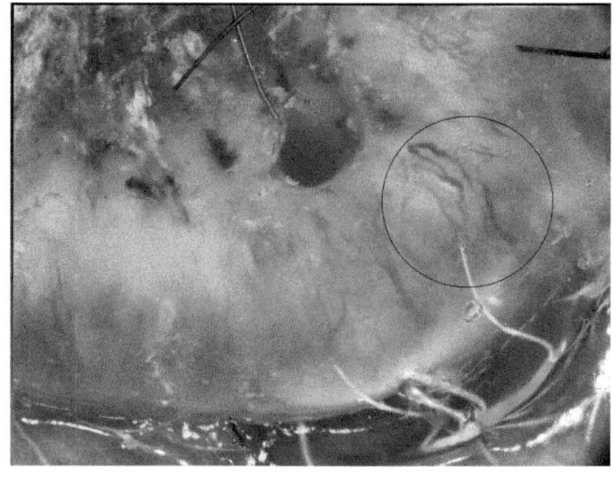

FIGURE 1.44 Hairpin vessels (squamous cell carcinoma).

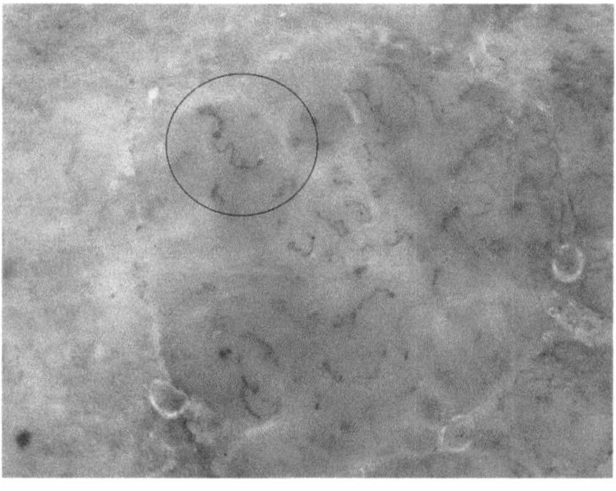

FIGURE 1.45 Linear irregular vessels (melanoma).

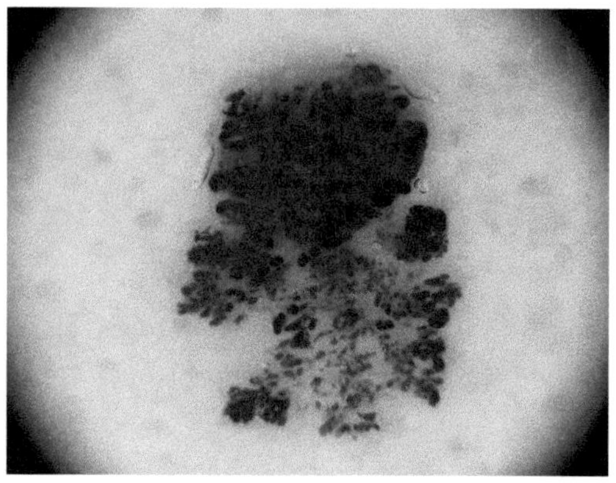

FIGURE 1.46 Multiple sharply demarcated vascular lacunes (angioma).

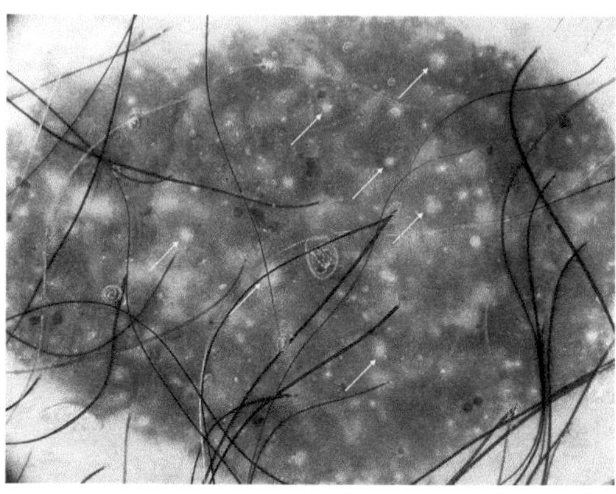

FIGURE 1.47 Multiple shiny milia-like cysts (arrows) (seborrheic keratosis).

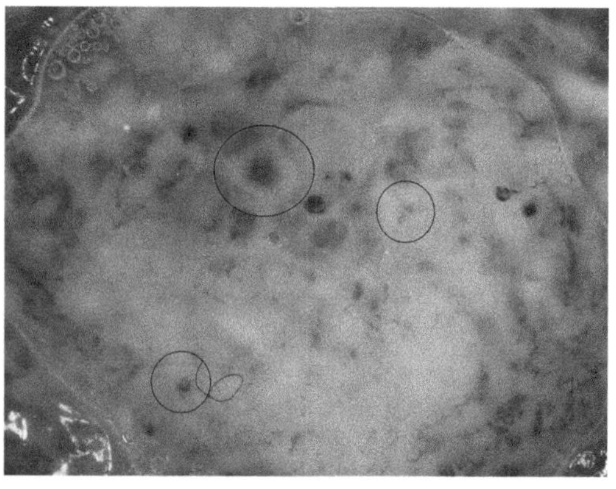

FIGURE 1.48 White halos surrounding vascular structures (squamous cell carcinoma).

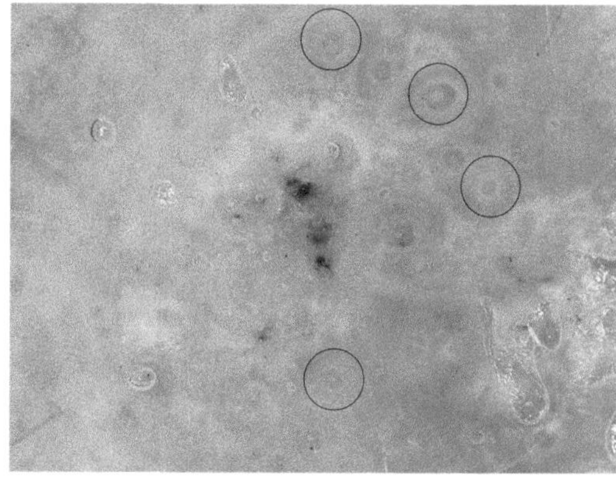

FIGURE 1.49 White circles surrounding follicular openings (squamous cell carcinoma).

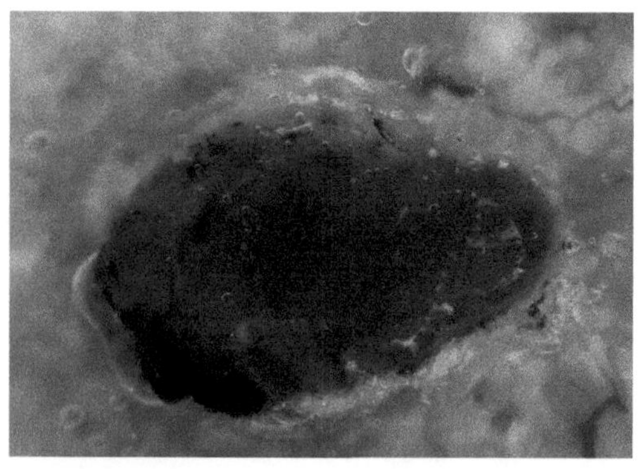

FIGURE 1.50 Large ulceration (basal cell carcinoma).

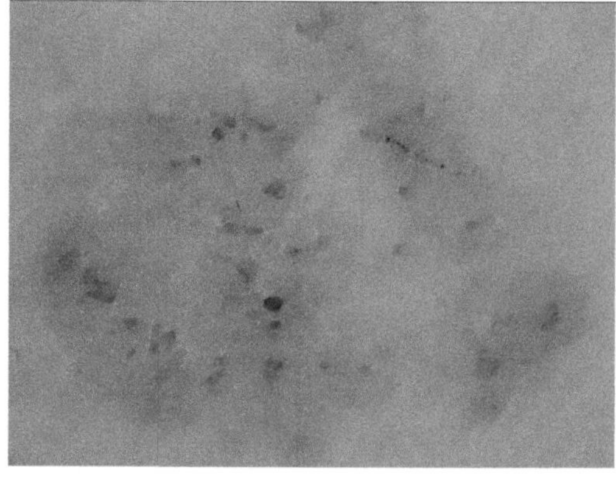

FIGURE 1.51 Multiple superficial small erosions (basal cell carcinoma).

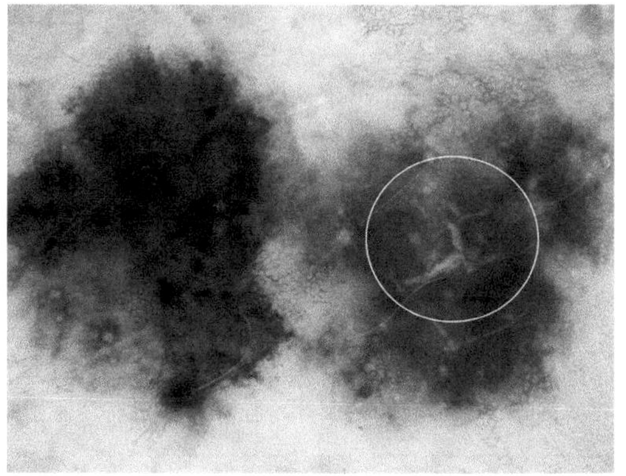

FIGURE 1.52 White shiny streaks (circle) (melanoma).

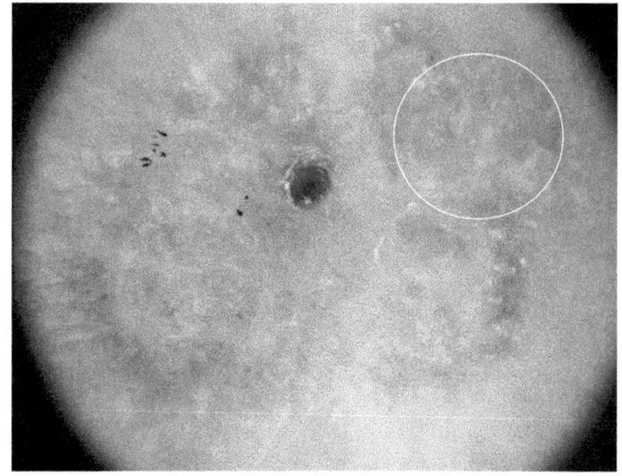

FIGURE 1.53 White shiny blotches/strands (circle) (basal cell carcinoma).

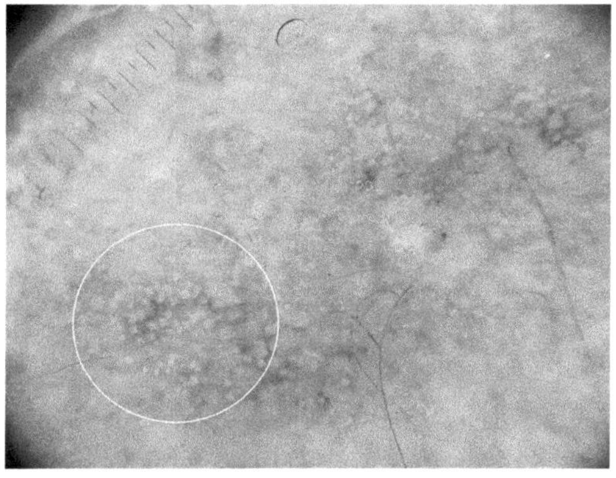

FIGURE 1.54 Rosettes (circle) (actinic keratosis).

- **White shiny streaks:** Short white lines oriented parallel and perpendicular to each other, seen only under polarized dermatoscopy.
  - **Most common color:** White (Figure 1.52)
- **White shiny streaks:** White, roundish, oval or larger areas oriented unspecifically, seen only under polarized dermatoscopy.
  - **Most common color:** White (Figure 1.53)
- **Rosettes:** Four dots arranged as a square within a follicular opening, seen only under polarized dermatoscopy.
  - **Most common color:** White (Figure 1.54)

1.3 Light Modes

Two main light modes in dermatoscopy exist: nonpolarized and polarized. Of note, in several dermatoscopes, both light modes are available. Nonpolarized dermatoscopy requires contact to the skin surface with the use of an immersion fluid or liquid that minimizes the air pockets. Ultrasound gel is considered as the optimal immersion material. Polarized dermatoscopy is based on the use of two polarizing filters positioned perpendicular to each other, does not require immersion fluid, and can be applied with or without contact. From a practical aspect, the possibility of applying it without immersion fluid represents the strongest advantage of polarized dermatoscopy, since it minimizes the required time and allows for fast examination of multiple moles or lesions. In addition to its practical advantage, polarized dermatoscopy also allows for better visualization of deeper skin structures. However, some colors and some structures are better seen with nonpolarized dermatoscopy. Table 1.1 summarizes the features that can be seen

TABLE 1.1

Dermatoscopic Criteria that Differ According to the Light Mode Used

Dermatoscopic Criteria	
Colors	
Brown	Seen with both modes; sharper, darker, and of higher contrast with polarized dermatoscopy
Gray	Better seen with nonpolarized dermatoscopy; under polarization, it appears darker and closer to brown
Blue	Better seen with nonpolarized dermatoscopy; under polarization, it appears darker and closer to brown
Red	More prominent and sharp with polarized dermatoscopy
Structures	
Blue structureless areas	Better seen with nonpolarized dermatoscopy; under polarization, they look darker
Gray dots/granules	Better seen with nonpolarized dermatoscopy; under polarization they might project brown
Blue/gray ovoid nests	Better seen with nonpolarized dermatoscopy; under polarization, they look darker
Comedo-like openings	Much better seen with nonpolarized dermatoscopy
Milia-like cysts	Much better seen with nonpolarized dermatoscopy
All vessels	More prominent and sharp with polarized dermatoscopy
White shiny streaks	Almost exclusively seen with polarized dermatoscopy
White shiny blotches/strands	Almost exclusively seen with polarized dermatoscopy
Rosettes	Almost exclusively seen with polarized dermatoscopy

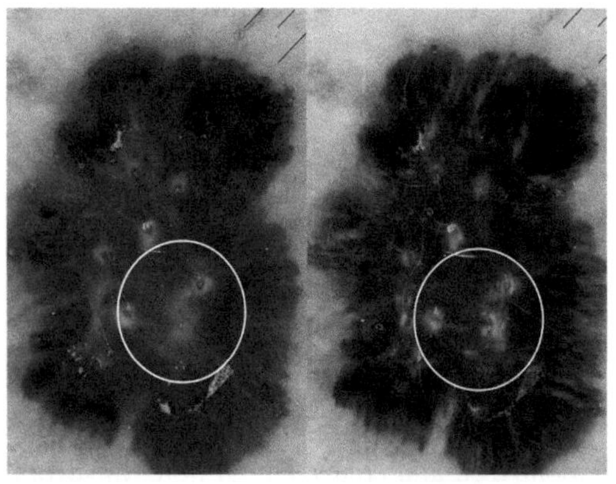

FIGURE 1.55 A melanoma dermatoscopically displaying white shiny streaks (circles), visible only with polarized light (right).

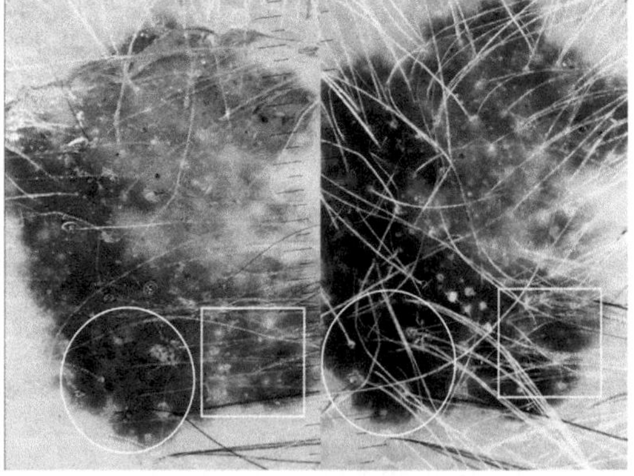

FIGURE 1.56 A seborrheic keratosis dermatoscopically typified by comedo-like openings (circle) and milia-like cysts (square), which can be seen only with nonpolarized dermatoscopy (left).

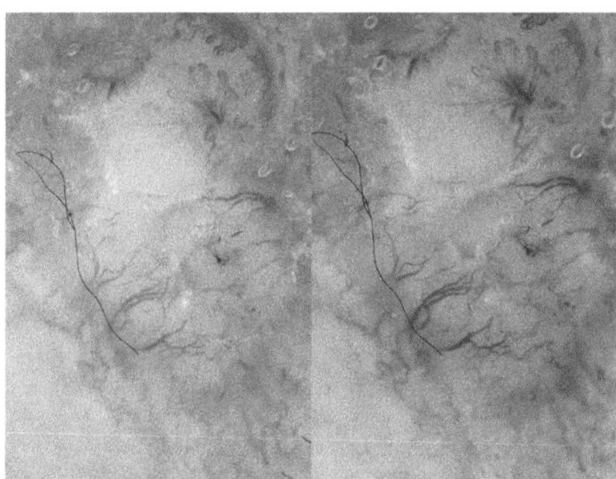

FIGURE 1.57 A basal cell carcinoma with evident vessels, which project more sharp and light red under polarized dermatoscopy (right).

only with one mode and those that their visualization is significantly better with one of the two modes. All features not mentioned in Table 1.1 can be almost equally seen with both modes. In Figures 1.55 through 1.57, some examples of significant differences between the two modes are illustrated. Our recommendation is that the two modes should not be considered as competitive but as complementary to each other. Because of its easier applicability, polarized dermatoscopy should be used for the routine examination of numerous moles/lesions, but the nonpolarized mode will be required quite often.

BIBLIOGRAPHY

Argenziano G, Catricalà C, Ardigo M et al. Seven-point checklist of dermoscopy revisited. *Br J Dermatol.* 2011;164:785–90.

Argenziano G, Soyer HP, Chimenti S et al. Dermoscopy of pigmented skin lesions: Results of a consensus meeting via the Internet. *J Am Acad Dermatol.* 2003;48:679–93.

Balagula Y, Braun RP, Rabinovitz HS et al. The significance of crystalline/chrysalis structures in the diagnosis of melanocytic and nonmelanocytic lesions. *J Am Acad Dermatol.* 2012;67:194.e1–8.

Benvenuto-Andrade C, Dusza SW, Agero ALC, Scope A, Rajadhyaksha M, Halpern AC, Marghoob AA. Differences between polarized light dermoscopy and immersion contact dermoscopy for the evaluation of skin lesions. *Arch Dermatol.* 2007;143:329–38.

Braun RP, Rabinovitz HS, Oliviero M, Kopf AW, Saurat J-H. Dermoscopy of pigmented skin lesions. *J Am Acad Dermatol.* 2005;52:109–21.

Kittler H, Marghoob AA, Argenziano G et al. Standardization of terminology in dermoscopy/dermatoscopy: Results of the third consensus conference of the International Society of Dermoscopy. *J Am Acad Dermatol.* 2016;74:1093–106.

Lake A, Jones B. Dermoscopy: To cross-polarize, or not to cross-polarize, that is the question. *J Vis Commun Med.* 2015;38:36–50.

Lallas A, Apalla Z, Argenziano G et al. The dermatoscopic universe of basal cell carcinoma. *Dermatol Pract Concept.* 2014;4:11–24.

Lallas A, Zalaudek I, Argenziano G et al. Dermoscopy in general dermatology. *Dermatol Clin.* 2013;31:679–94.

Zalaudek I, Kreusch J, Giacomel J, Ferrara G, Catricalà C, Argenziano G. How to diagnose nonpigmented skin tumors: A review of vascular structures seen with dermoscopy: Part I. Melanocytic skin tumors. *J WAm Acad Dermatol.* 2010;63:361–74, quiz 375–6.

2

Nevi

Melanocytic nevi are benign melanocytic tumors characterized by a very high incidence in the population, especially in Caucasians.

Classification of nevi

Several classifications of nevi have been proposed according to the time of appearance (congenital or acquired), the histopathologic distribution (junctional, compound, or dermal), or the origin of the stem melanocyte (epidermal or dermal). This chapter follows a combined classification of nevi that takes into consideration all of the factors mentioned previously plus the dermatoscopic pattern.

a. Common nevi
    i. Nevi of the trunk and the extremities
    ii. Facial nevi
    iii. Acral nevi
    iv. Subungual nevi
    v. Mucosal nevi
b. Spitz and Reed nevi
c. Blue nevi
d. Special nevus types
    i. Traumatized nevus (targetoid hemosiderotic nevus)
    ii. Inflamed nevus (Meyerson nevus)
    iii. Halo nevus (Sutton nevus)
    iv. Balloon cell nevus
    v. Sclerosing nevus (with pseudomelanoma features)
    vi. Recurrent nevus

Total nevus count and time of appearance of nevi

The number, distribution, and morphological type of nevi that each individual will develop are mainly genetically determined, and ultraviolet radiation has a synergistic effect in the appearance of some of them. Most nevi appear within the first three decades of life, and most nevi disappear within the next three decades. Therefore, the nevi count is very low in newborns and elderly individuals. Some nevi are already present at birth (congenital). Most nevi develop in the second, third, and fourth decades of life, whereas the appearance of a new nevus after the age of 50 years is uncommon and after the age of 60 years exceedingly rare. Most common nevi will disappear within the fifth, sixth, or seventh decade of life. As compared to common nevi, Spitz and Reed nevi are more dynamic (grow and involute faster) and blue nevi much more stable, usually remaining unaltered throughout the lifetime.

Dermatoscopic pattern of nevi: General principles

The dermatoscopic pattern of nevi depends on several factors, including the histopathologic type (junctional, compound, or intradermal), the morphological characteristics of the melanocytes (e.g., Spitz/Reed nevi and blue nevi), and the anatomical site. Four predominant dermatoscopic nevus patterns exist: reticular, globular, starburst, and homogeneous or diffuse.

As a general rule, the reticular dermatoscopic pattern (Figure 2.1) typifies junctional nevi and the globular pattern dermal nevi (Figure 2.2), whereas a combined globular-reticular pattern is usually seen in compound nevi (Figure 2.3). The "starburst" pattern (Figure 2.4) typifies pigmented Spitz or Reed nevi, and the homogenous dermatoscopic pattern characterizes blue nevi (Figure 2.5). Congenital nevi might be junctional, compound, or intradermal, displaying a reticular, mixed, or globular pattern, respectively.

The benign nature of nevi is usually reflected also morphologically, meaning that most nevi are clinically and dermatoscopically symmetric (or harmonic). The dermatoscopic colors and structures are combined in an organized way, which results in a morphological order. This is the fundamental morphological difference between nevi and melanoma. However, exceptions to this rule exist, especially in the context of individuals with "atypical mole syndrome."

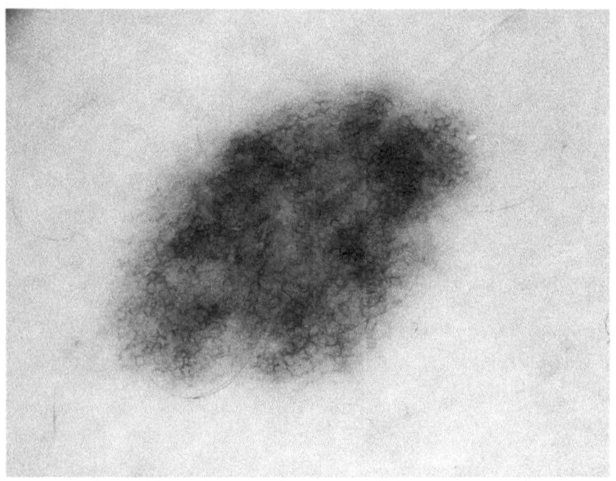

FIGURE 2.1 Reticular pattern.

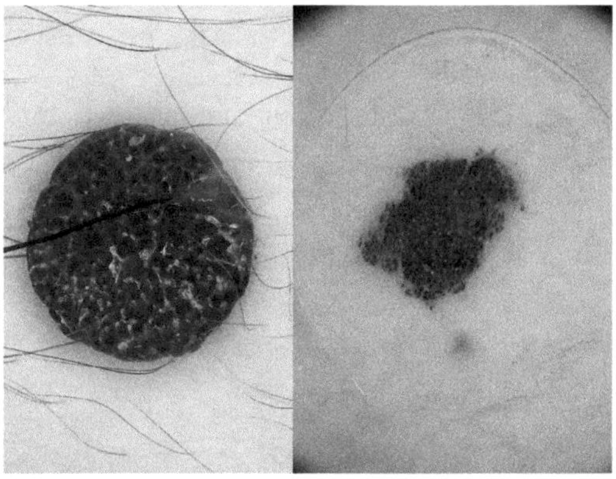

FIGURE 2.2 Globular pattern.

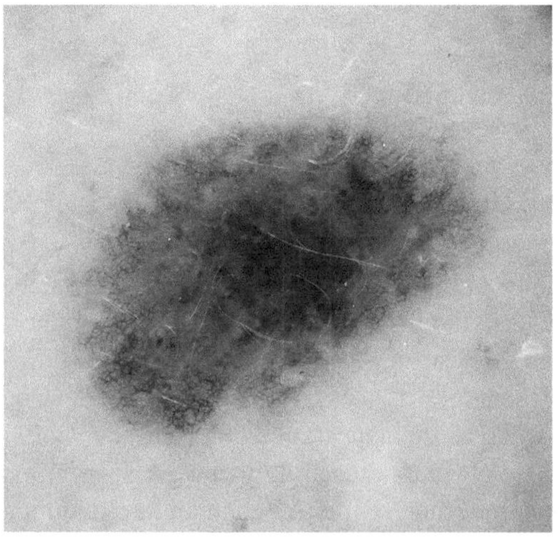

FIGURE 2.3 Nevus with a combination of reticular and globular patterns.

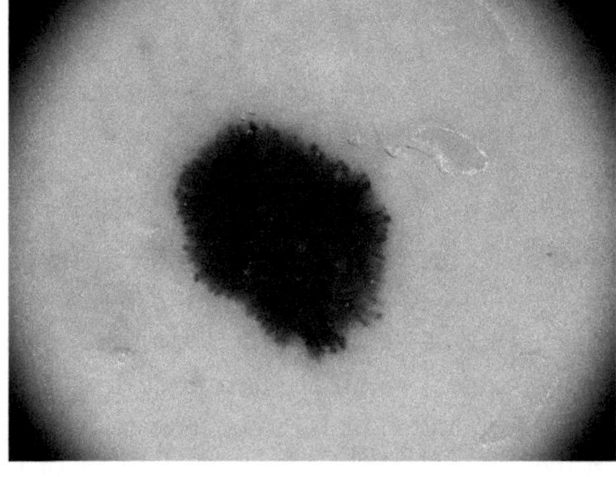

FIGURE 2.4 "Starburst" pattern, characteristic of Spitz nevus.

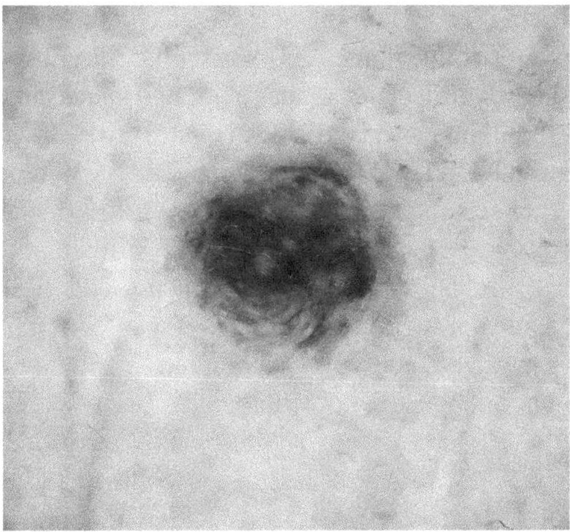

FIGURE 2.5 Homogenous blue pattern of the blue nevus.

2.1 Common Nevi

2.1.1 Nevi of Trunk and Extremities

Common nevi of the trunk and the extremities are dermatoscopically typified by two global patterns that might be combined: reticular and globular.

The reticular pattern consists of intersecting brown lines that form a pigment network (Figure 2.6). Histopathologically, the reticular pattern corresponds to the presence of continuous pigmentation along the dermo-epidermal junction, combined with a normal papillomatosis (alternating rete ridges and dermal papillae). Therefore, the reticular pattern typifies junctional nevi. Ideally, the pigment network of nevi is "uniform" or "symmetric," in the sense that it is characterized by minimal variability in the color and thickness of the lines, as well as the distribution of pigmentation. Typically, the pigment network smoothly fades out at the periphery of the nevus (Figure 2.7).

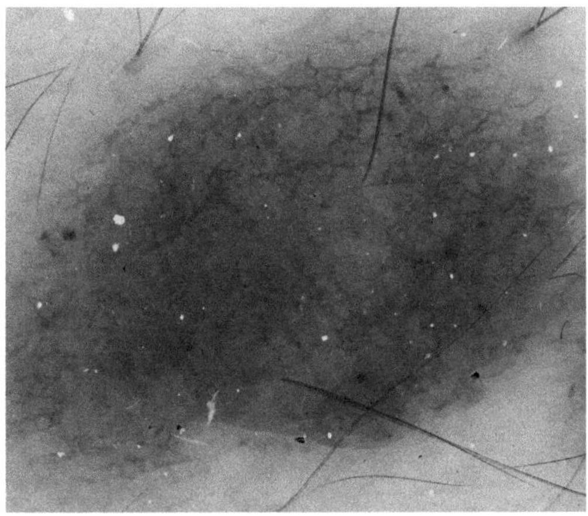

FIGURE 2.6 The reticular pattern is defined by intersecting brown lines that form a network.

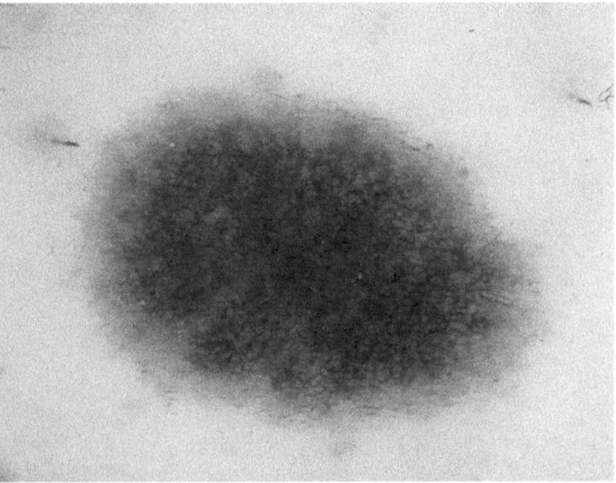

FIGURE 2.7 The pigment network in nevi is relatively uniform in terms of color, thickness of the lines, and distribution of the pigmentation and smoothly fades in the periphery of the nevus.

However, a minority of reticular nevi might lack symmetry. In fact, "atypical" nevi are almost always dermatoscopically reticular. Their dermatoscopic "atypia" results from an uneven distribution of pigmentation over the lesion's surface and/or an increased variability in the thickness of the network lines and the diameter of the holes (Figure 2.8). Obviously, this dermatoscopic "atypia" represents a morphological overlap with melanoma. No single dermatoscopic clue can confidently differentiate between an atypical nevus and an early melanoma. However, atypical nevi usually occur as multiple lesions in the context of individuals with the "atypical mole syndrome." In this context, the dermatoscopic assessment of the lesions should be done in a comparative manner. This peculiar clinical scenario is discussed separately in Chapter 9.

The globular pattern is characterized by well-demarcated, round or oval structures (globules) that are brown in color. The globules histopathologically correspond to nests of melanocytes located at the upper dermis. Therefore, the globular pattern is considered to typify intradermal nevi. The size of the globules may differ, but within a nevus the globules usually remain similar in size, color, and distribution (Figures 2.9 and 2.10). When the globules are very large in size, resembling polygonal structures, the pattern is called "cobblestone" (Figure 2.11). On the contrary, in the case of particularly small globules, the pattern might be referred to as dotted (Figure 2.12).

Globular nevi are the main morphological category of nevi that often display vessels on dermatoscopy. The typical morphological type of vessel has been described as "comma-like." Comma vessels are relatively thick, short, and curved linear vessels (Figure 2.13). They usually project unfocused (blurred) and are typically located within the pigmented globules (Figures 2.14 and 2.15). However, when nevi lose their pigmentation with age or in individuals with fair skin and hypopigmented nevi, the vessels might project more focused and not associated with the globules, since the globules can hardly be seen (Figure 2.16). Finally, in some nevi, the vessels are longer and ramified. In the latter scenarios, the differential diagnosis from basal cell carcinoma, on a dermatoscopic basis, might be very challenging (Figure 2.17).

The reticular and the globular patterns might be combined in a single nevus. This is because in several nevi, a junctional component coexists with a dermal one (compound nevi). However, even when combining two patterns, nevi tend to retain their dermatoscopic symmetry in terms of overall architecture and distribution of structures and colors (Figure 2.18). A peculiar combination frequently seen in growing nevi, especially in children, consists of a reticular, globular, or homogeneous pattern in the center and a rim of globules at the periphery (Figures 2.19 and 2.20). The presence of this rim of peripheral globules is only a sign of radial growth and

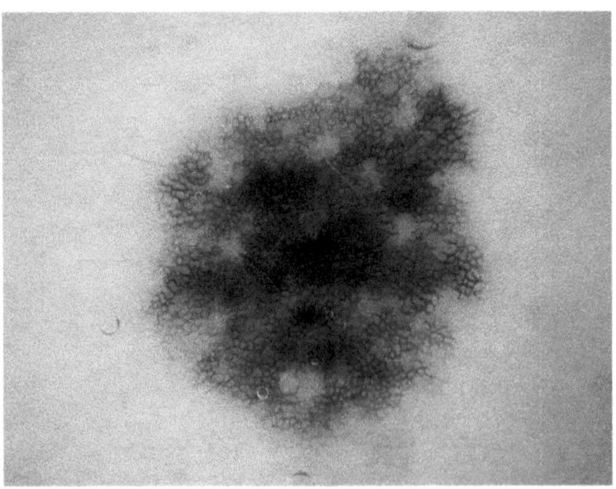

FIGURE 2.8 A reticular nevus that displays areas of darker pigmentation and thickened network lines focally.

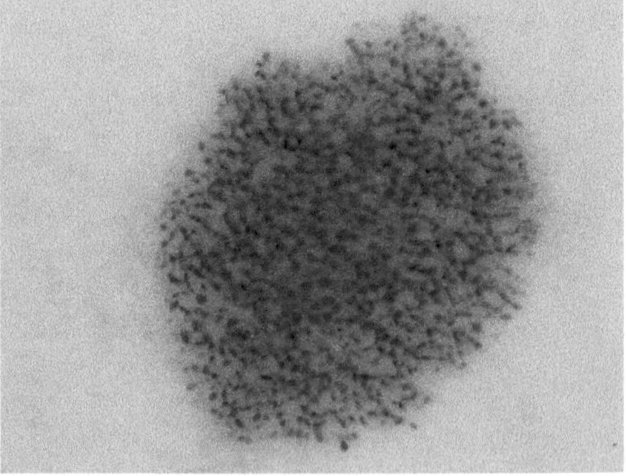

FIGURE 2.9 A globular pattern characterized by clearly demarcated, brown in color, round-ish, or oval structures.

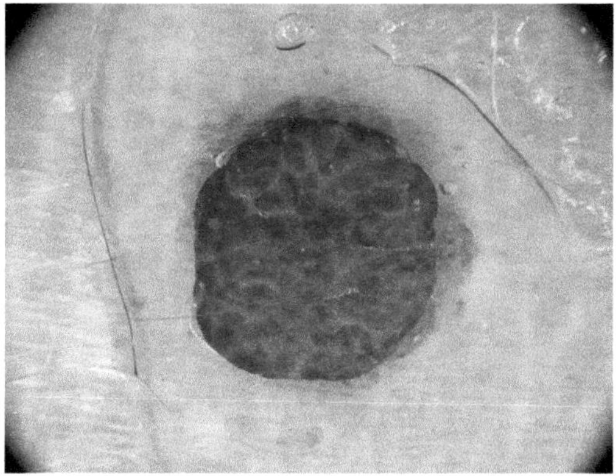

FIGURE 2.10 A classic intradermal nevus with globules that are large but uniform in terms of size, color, and distribution.

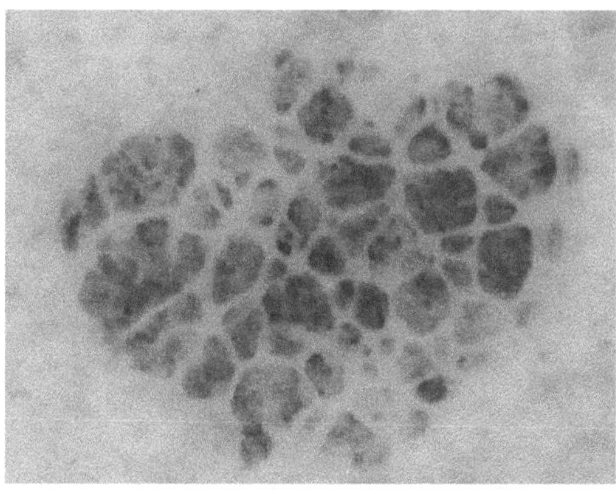

FIGURE 2.11 The "cobblestone" pattern consists of large and somehow polygonal globules.

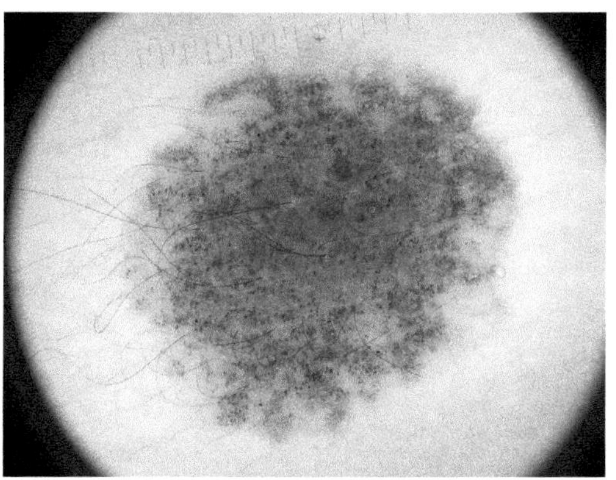

FIGURE 2.12 A nevus displaying multiple small globules that could be characterized as dots.

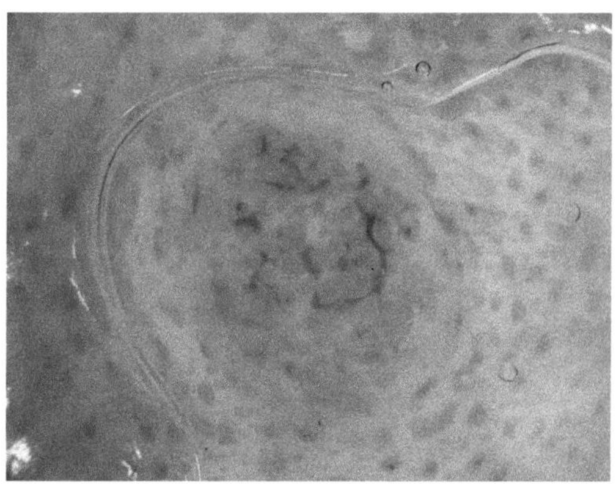

FIGURE 2.13 "Comma" vessels are thick, short, and curved linear vascular structures.

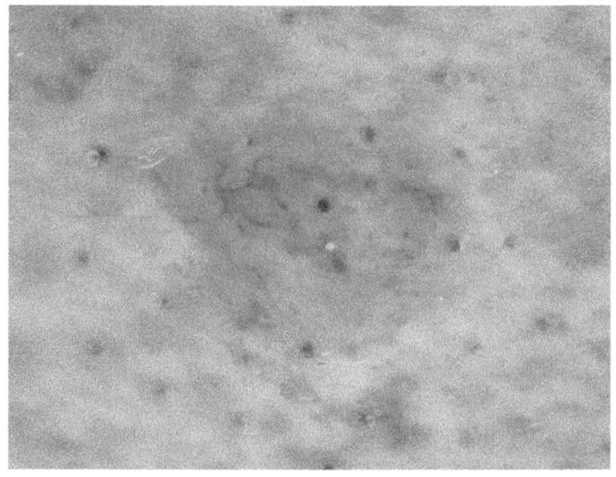

FIGURE 2.14 Comma vessels usually project unfocused or blurred.

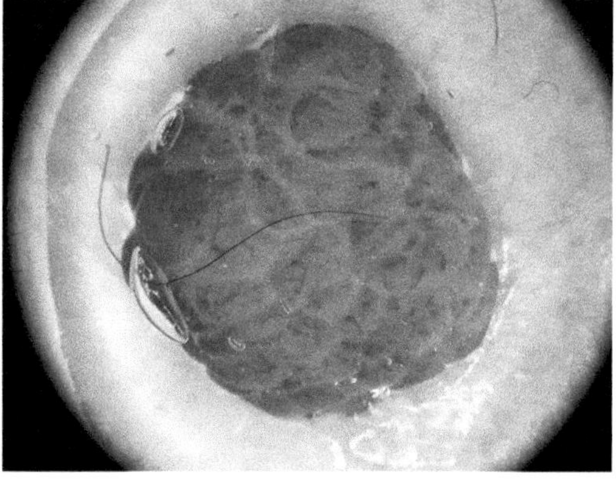

FIGURE 2.15 Typically, comma vessels are located within the pigmented globules.

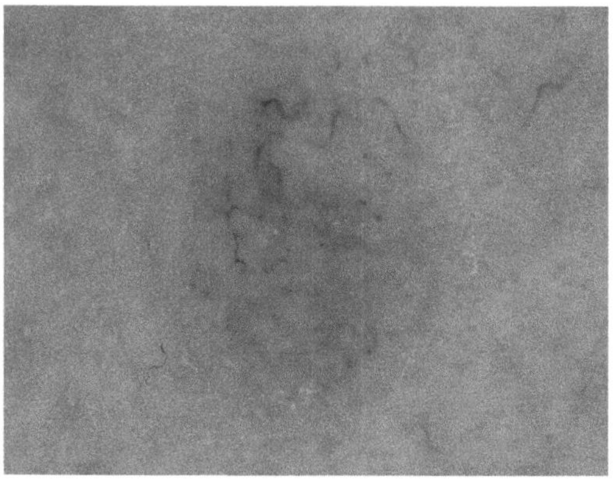

FIGURE 2.16 In a hypopigmented nevus, the comma vessels are not associated with globules, since the globules cannot be seen.

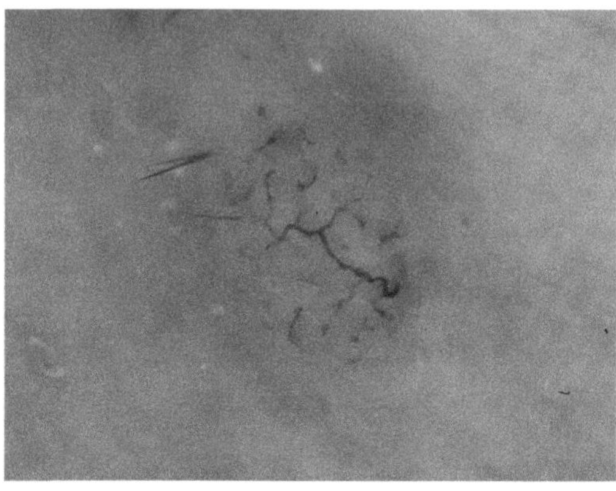

FIGURE 2.17 A nevus dermatoscopically displaying long linear branched vessels that look similar to the vascular structures typically seen in basal cell carcinoma.

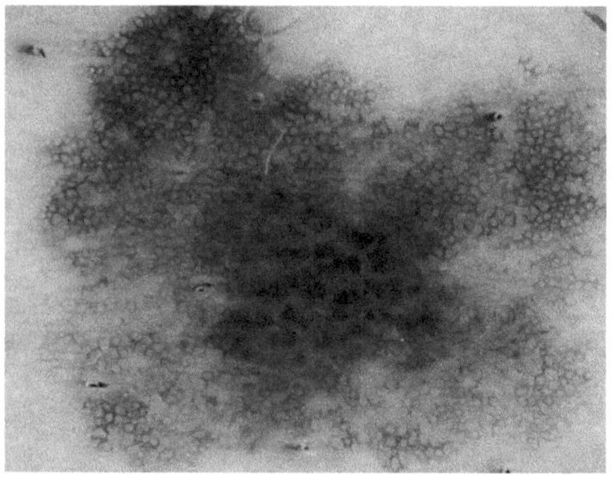

FIGURE 2.18 A nevus with a combined pattern consisting of globules in the center and a network at the periphery.

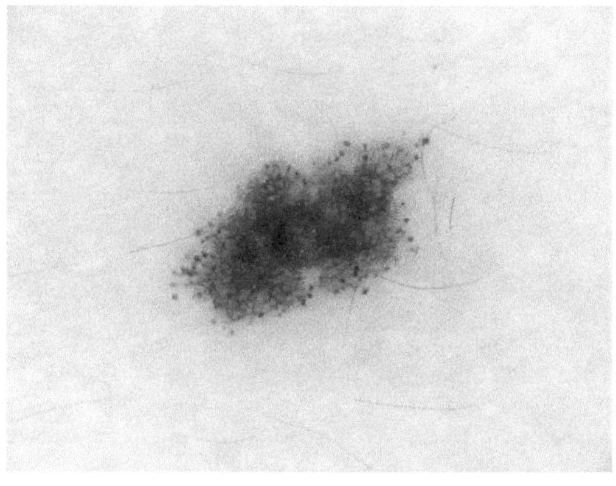

FIGURE 2.19 A nevus characterized by a reticular pattern and a peripheral rim of brown globules.

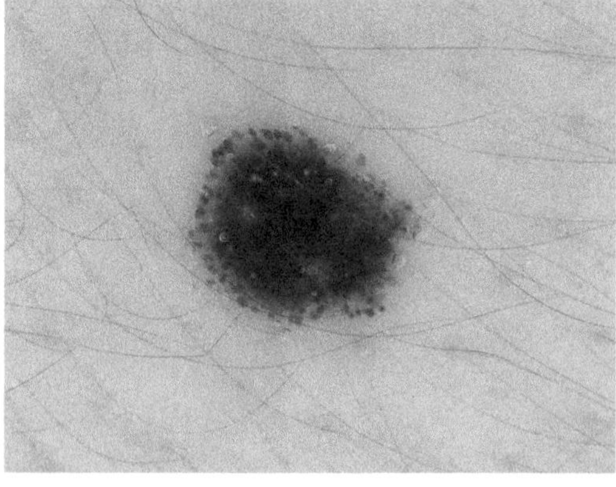

FIGURE 2.20 A nevus characterized by a globular pattern and a peripheral rim of brown globules.

should be considered suspicious only in patients at an age that does not justify growth of nevi. Traditionally, the age threshold for "tolerating" a rim of peripheral globules has been proposed at 45 years. However, our experience suggests that even after this age and until the age of 60 years, a peripheral rim of globules can be seen in some (few) nevi.

Congenital Nevi

Congenital nevi might be junctional, compound, or intradermal and, therefore, display a reticular, mixed, or globular pattern, respectively. This is why they are not described separately in the present chapter. Some additional dermatoscopic features that can be seen almost exclusively in congenital nevi are the following:

Terminal hairs. This is obviously a clinical sign, but sometimes the hairs can be better seen with the dermatoscope (Figure 2.21).

Cobblestone pattern. This was previously mentioned as a variation of the globular pattern, typified by large and polygonal globules (Figure 2.22).

Perifollicular hypopigmentation. This feature refers to the presence of a hypo- or depigmented circle surrounding follicular openings within a congenital nevus (Figure 2.23).

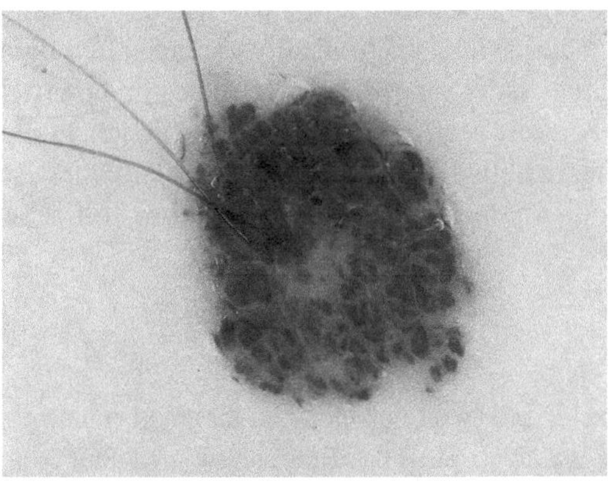

FIGURE 2.21 Terminal hairs are highly suggestive of a congenital nevus.

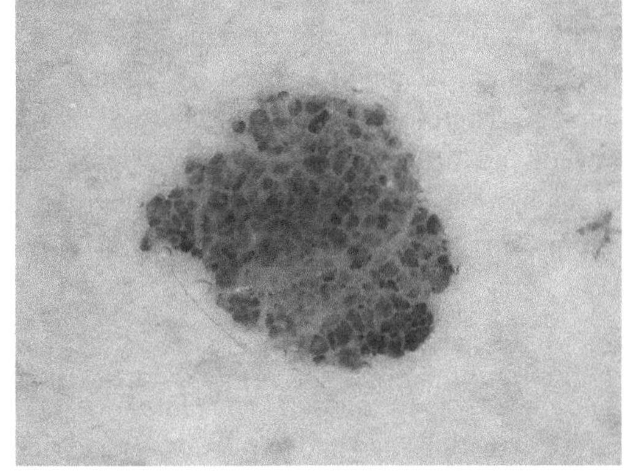

FIGURE 2.22 A congenital nevus typified by a cobblestone pattern (large polygonal globules).

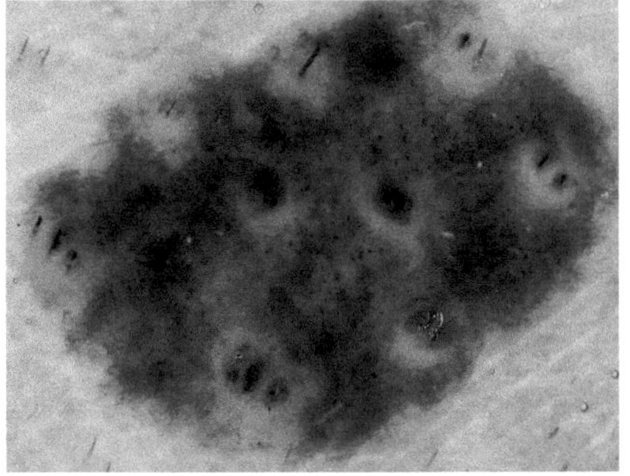

FIGURE 2.23 Perifollicular hypopigmentation is another typical sign of congenital nevi.

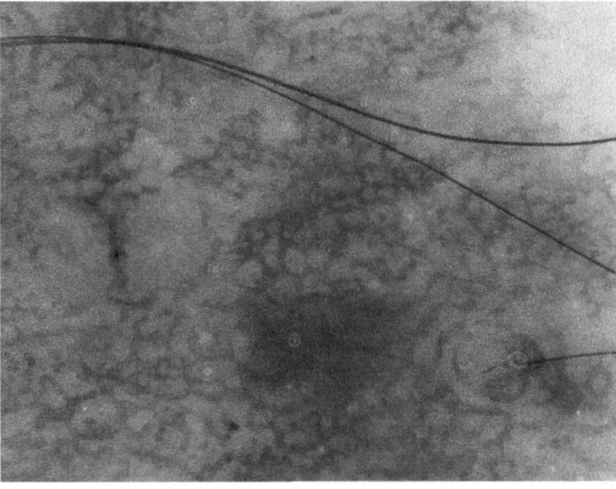

FIGURE 2.24 The "target" network of congenital nevi is typified by the presence of brown dots/globules within the holes of the network.

Target network. This feature results from the presence of a pigmented (brown) dot or small globule inside one or more holes of a network (Figure 2.24).

Target globules. This feature results from the presence of a dark brown dot in the center of a light brown globule (Figure 2.25).

Haloed globules and haloed vessels. These terms refer to the presence of white halo surrounding globules or dotted vessels, respectively (Figure 2.26).

2.1.2 Scalp Nevi

Most nevi on the scalp display a globular pattern (Figure 2.27). Several of them are papillomatous and hypopigmented, dermatoscopically characterized by light brown pigmentation and comma vessels (Figure 2.28). Another peculiar nevus type seen on the scalp is the "eclipse nevus" that dermatoscopically displays central hypopigmentation and peripheral network, globules, or structureless pigmentation (Figures 2.29 and 2.30).

2.1.3 Facial Nevi

The vast majority of nevi on the face are intradermal or compound, whereas purely junctional nevi are rare. Dermatoscopically, intradermal nevi are again typified by a globular pattern (Figure 2.31). In contrast, junctional facial nevi do not follow the dermatoscopic morphology of the trunk and extremities. This is because the facial skin is anatomically characterized by a flattened epidermis that lacks the regular papillomatosis of alternating rete ridges and dermal papillae. Therefore, a pigment network is extremely rarely seen in facial nevi. Instead, junctional nevi on the face dermatoscopically display the "pseudonetwork," which consists of structureless pigmentation interrupted by nonpigmented roundish structures that correspond to follicular openings (Figure 2.32).

2.1.4 Acral Nevi

The anatomy of the palmar and plantar skin is characterized by a thickened and flattened epidermis with alternating sulci and gyri (furrows and ridges). Because of this peculiar anatomy, melanocytic tumors of the acral skin are typified by peculiar dermatoscopic patterns that are completely

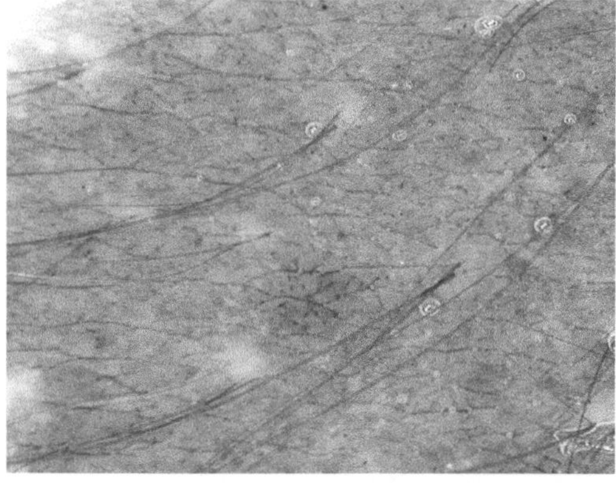

FIGURE 2.25 The "target globules" of congenital nevi are characterized by the presence of a darker dot in the center of the globule.

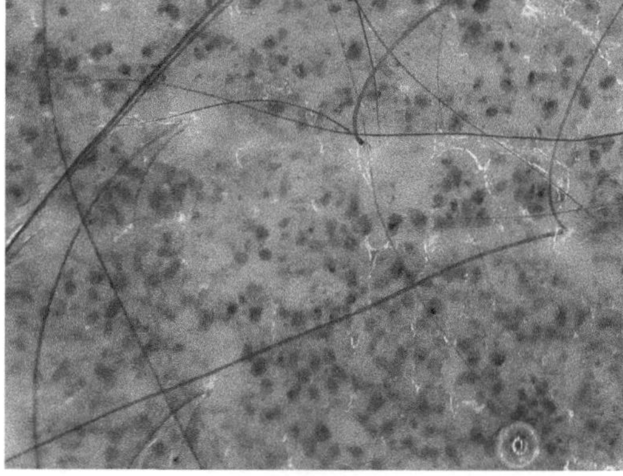

FIGURE 2.26 White halos surrounding globules or dotted vessels represent another common feature of congenital nevi.

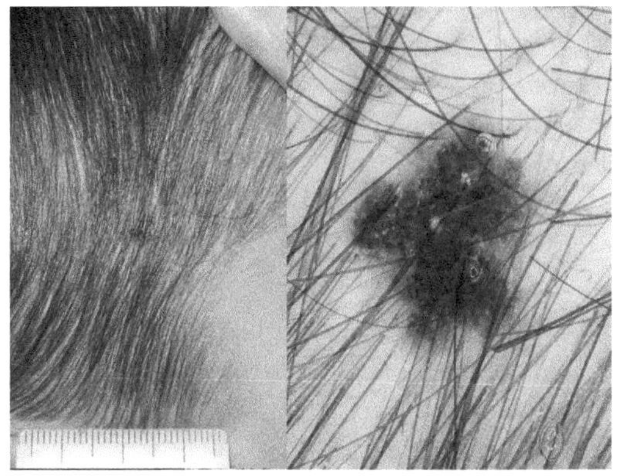

FIGURE 2.27 A scalp nevus dermatoscopically typified by a globular pattern.

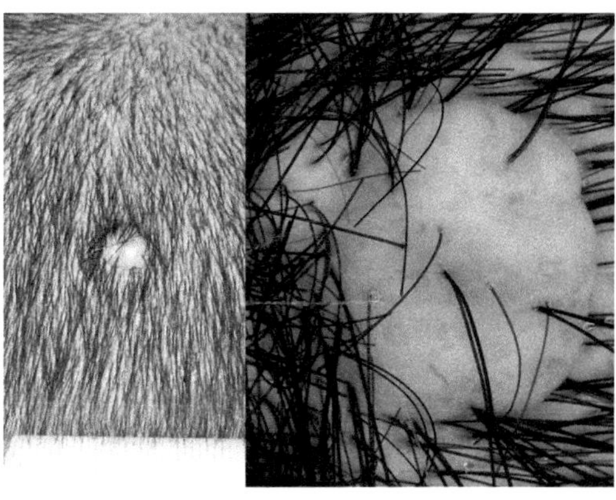

FIGURE 2.28 A papillomatous dermal nevus dermatoscopically displaying hypopigmentation and comma vessels.

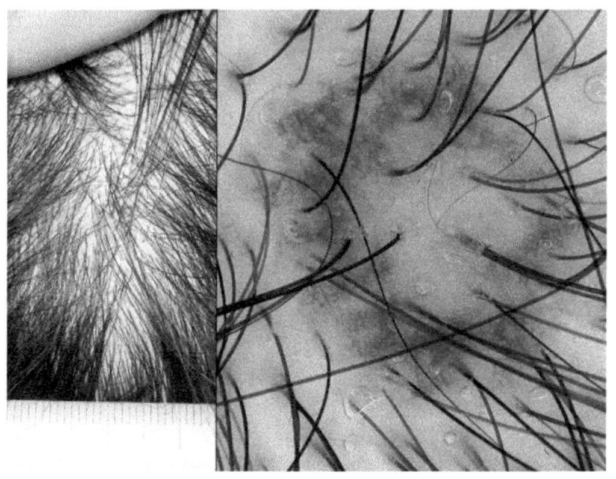

FIGURE 2.29 A typical example of "eclipse" nevus, typified by central hypopigmentation and peripheral network.

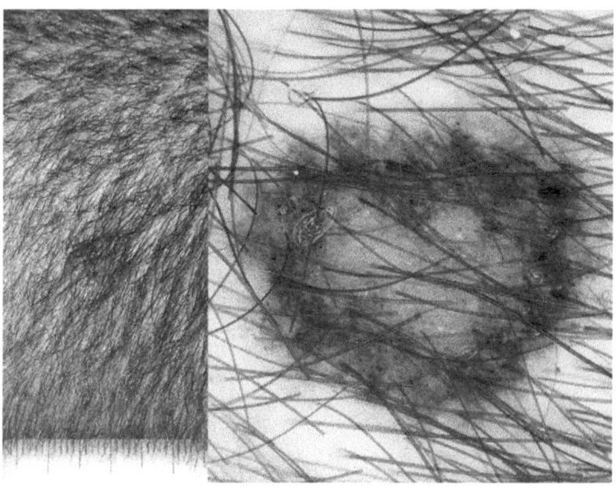

FIGURE 2.30 Another "eclipse" scalp nevus with central hypopigmentation and a globular pattern at the periphery.

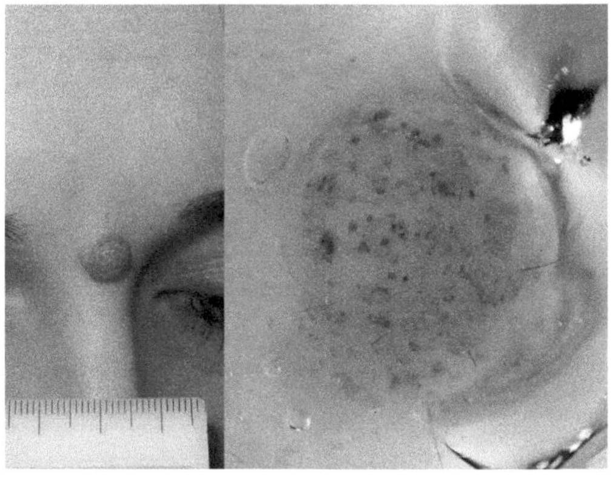

FIGURE 2.31 A dermal nevus on the face, dermatoscopically typified by a globular pattern.

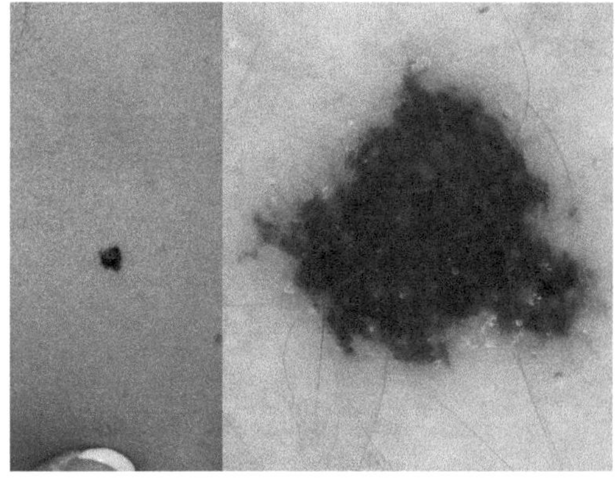

FIGURE 2.32 A hyperpigmented facial nevus dermatoscopically displaying structureless pigmentation interrupted by white follicular openings (pseudonetwork).

different from those seen on nonacral skin. The predominant dermatoscopic patterns of acral nevi are the parallel furrow and the fibrillar pattern, although less frequent patterns also exist.

Discriminating the furrows from the ridges is based on two factors: First, the furrows are much thinner than the ridges. Therefore, in acral nevi, the pigmented lines are much thinner than the nonpigmented ones. Second, the openings of the eccrine sweat glands are usually visible by dermatoscopy, and they are always located on the ridges (Figure 2.33). The dermatoscopic parallel furrow pattern consists of parallel brown lines located on the furrows of the acral skin, whereas the ridges are free of pigmentation (Figure 2.34). If a nevus is hyperpigmented (which is frequent in individuals with dark skin), in the center of the nevus, the pigmentation might cover both the furrows and the ridges. However, at the peripheral part of the nevus, it is usually much more clear that the pigmentation tends to follow the furrows (Figure 2.35). In addition to the classic version of the parallel furrow pattern, the following variations do exist:

Double line pattern. In this pattern, not one but two pigmented lines can be seen on each furrow (Figure 2.36).

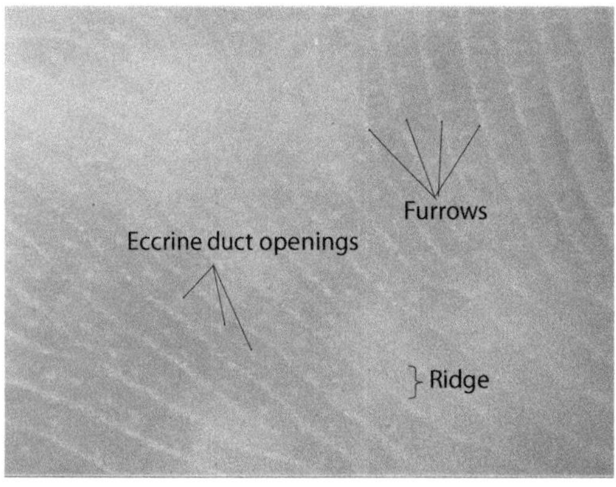

FIGURE 2.33 The acral skin as seen by dermoscopy. Furrows are thinner than the ridges, and the openings of the eccrine sweat glands are located on the ridges.

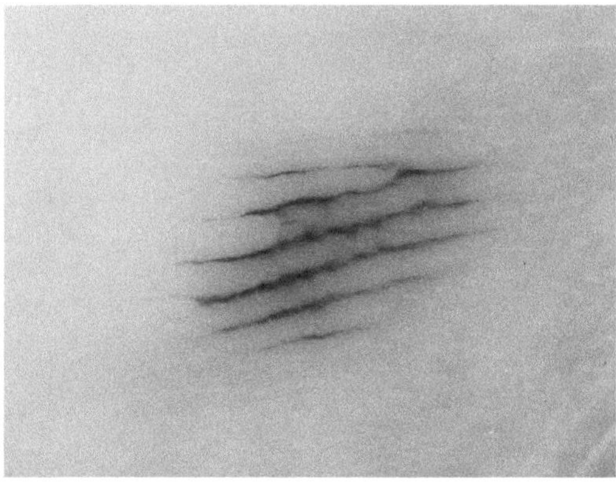

FIGURE 2.34 The parallel furrow pattern is typified by pigmentation on the furrows and not on the ridges.

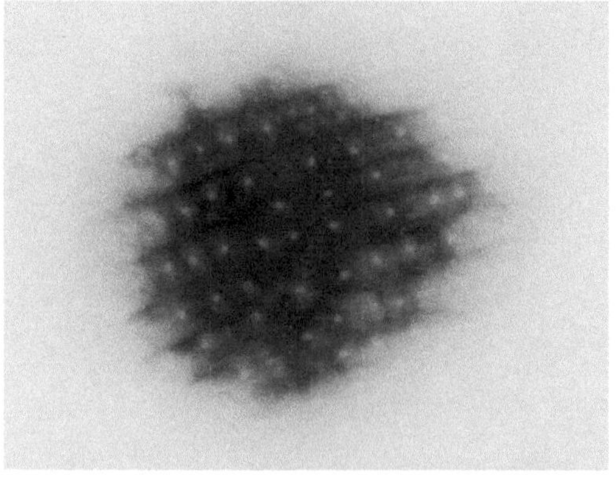

FIGURE 2.35 In hyperpigmented nevi, the central part might be characterized by diffuse pigmentation on the furrows and ridges. At the periphery, it is evident that the pigmentation tends to follow the furrows and spare the ridges.

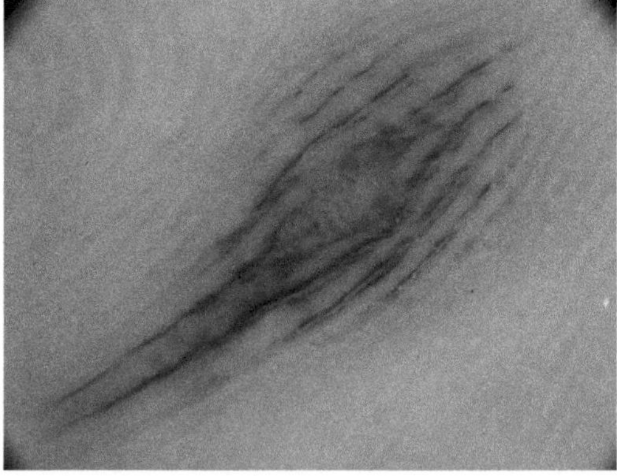

FIGURE 2.36 The double-line parallel furrow pattern consists of two parallel pigmented lines on each furrow.

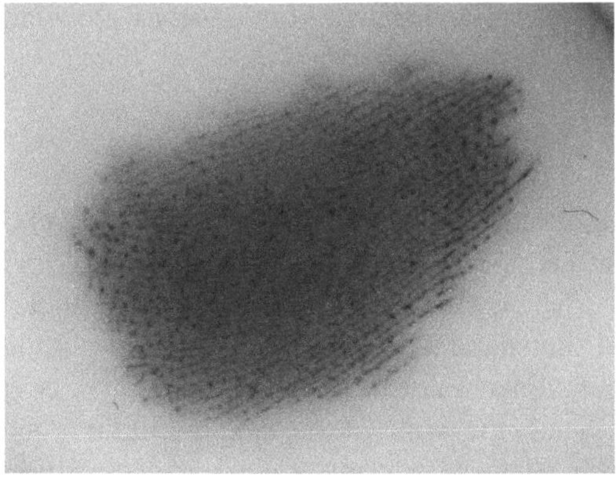

FIGURE 2.37 A congenital acral nevus characterized by the "peas-in-a-pod" pattern, which consists of pigmentation on the furrows and pigmented dots inside the sweat gland openings on the ridges.

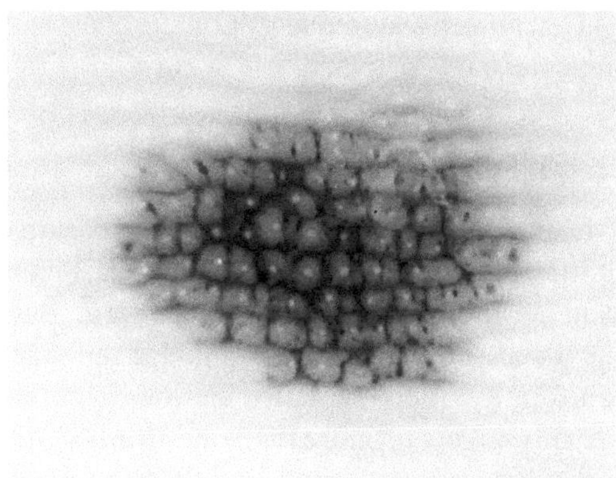

FIGURE 2.38 The lattice-like pattern is in fact a network consisting of parallel furrow lines and vertical pigmented lines crossing the ridges.

Peas-in-a-pod pattern. This variation is mainly seen in congenital acral nevi and consists of parallel furrow lines plus pigmented brown dots precisely inside the openings of the eccrine ducts, which are located on the ridges (Figure 2.37).

Lattice-like pattern. This pattern consists of parallel furrow lines plus perpendicular (vertical) lines on the ridges, resulting in a network-like appearance (Figure 2.38).

The fibrillar is the second main pattern of acral nevi that typifies mainly nevi on weight-bearing areas of the sole. A fibrillar pattern is almost never seen on the palmar nevi, and for this reason, the detection of this pattern in a palmar mole should be considered suspicious. The pattern consists of parallel pigmented lines orientated perpendicular to the direction of the furrows and ridges (Figure 2.39). Ideally, each fibril starts and ends from or at a furrow, and the length and color of fibrils should be uniform within a lesion. Lesions displaying a fibrillar pattern should be managed with caution, especially if they are not symmetric, because fibrillar lines might be seen also in acral melanoma.

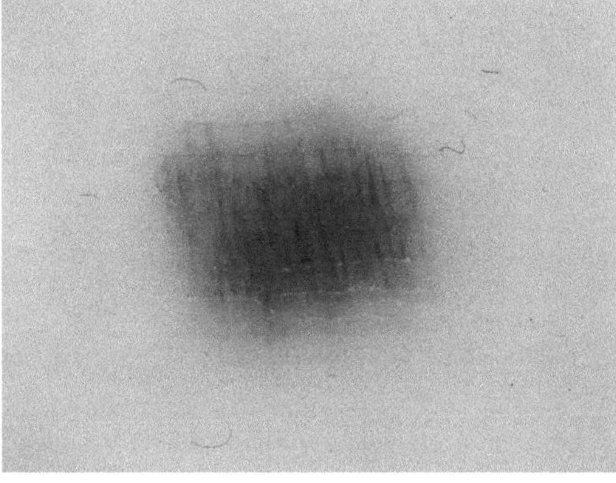

FIGURE 2.39 The fibrillar pattern consists of parallel pigmented lines orientated perpendicularly to the direction of the furrows and ridges.

Other much less frequent dermatoscopic patterns of acral nevi include homogeneous, globular, reticular, and combined.

2.1.5 Subungual Nevi

Melanocytic tumors of the nail apparatus almost always arise on the nail matrix and clinically manifest as a pigmented nail band on the nail plate (melanonychia striata). Nevi and melanoma of the nail bed are extremely rare. The main differences between subungual nevi and subungual melanoma are the size and the shape of the nail band, as well as the uniformity of pigment distribution. In detail, melanonychia resulting from nail matrix nevi usually covers no more than one-third of the nail plate, the width of the band is similar at the proximal and distal edge, and the band is relatively uniform in terms of pigment distribution (Figure 2.40). In contrast, melanoma will gradually grow and cover larger parts of the nail plate (usually more than half). A characteristic clue for melanoma is the increased width of the band at the proximal nail fold, as compared to the distal edge (triangular shape). Finally, the melanonychia resulting from melanoma typically consists of bands of different widths and color shades (Figure 2.41).

2.1.6 Mucosal Nevi

The vast majority of mucosal nevi have been reported to develop within the first three decades of life. The most frequent mucosal surfaces on which nevi might develop are genitalia, followed by oral mucosa. The predominant dermatoscopic patterns of mucosal nevi are globular (including cobblestone) and structureless (Figures 2.42 and 2.43). A reticular pattern is very rare, since the epidermis on mucosa lacks the normal papillomatosis that corresponds to the dermatoscopic pigment network. Most mucosal nevi display light brown, dark brown, or black color, and they are typified by dermatoscopic symmetry of structures. However, a proportion of genital nevi might be quite atypical from a clinical, dermatoscopic, and histopathologic aspects (Figure 2.44).

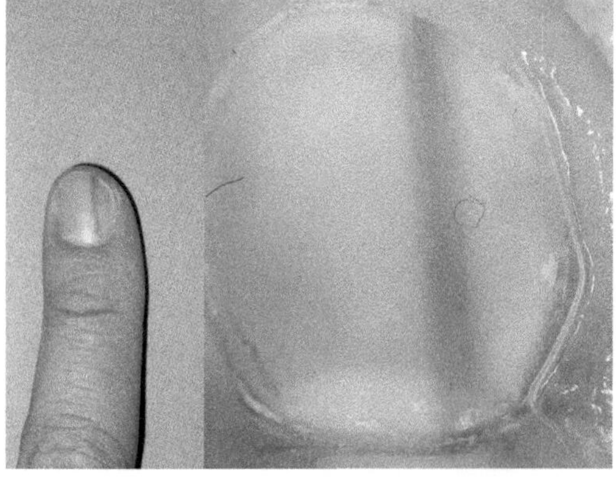

FIGURE 2.40 A subungual nevus projecting as a nail band that covers less than one-third of the nail plate and is relatively uniformly pigmented.

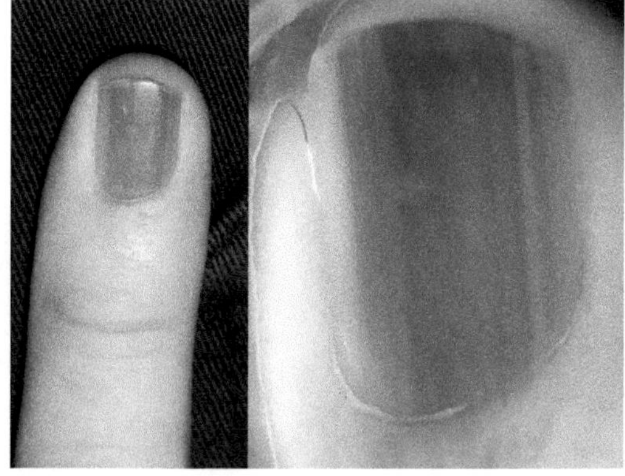

FIGURE 2.41 A subungual melanoma projecting as a nail band that covers more than half of the nail plate and consists of zones of different pigment intensity.

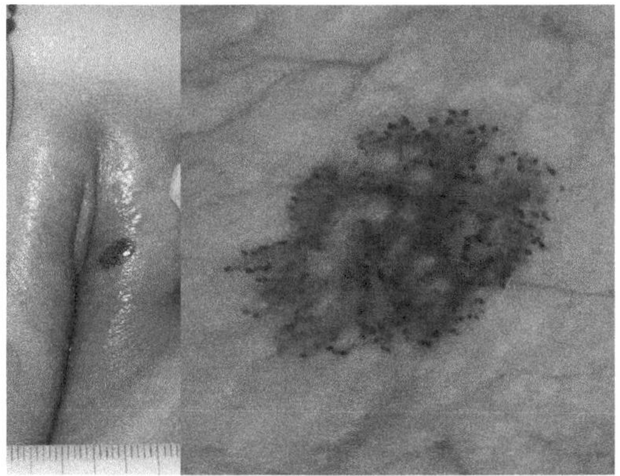

FIGURE 2.42 A vulvar nevus dermatoscopically typified by a globular pattern.

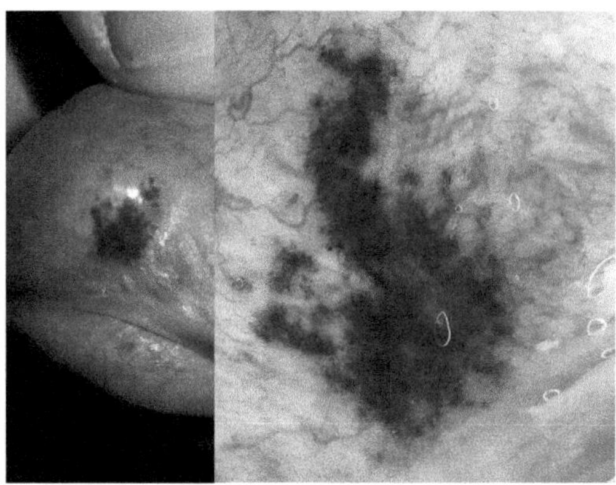

FIGURE 2.43 A nevus on the glans penis dermatoscopically characterized by a brown structureless pattern.

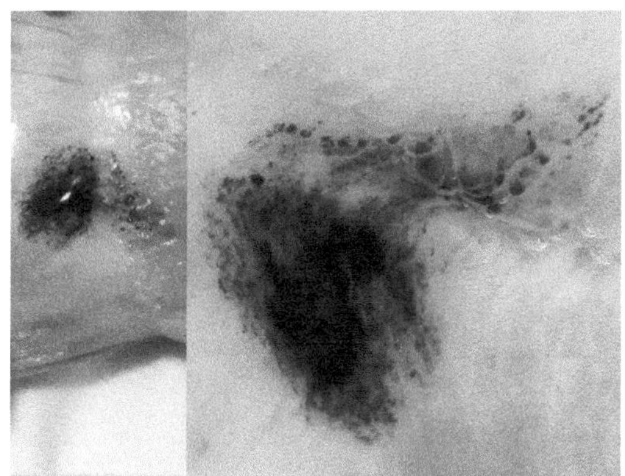

FIGURE 2.44 An "atypical" nevus on the glans penis that is clinically asymmetrical in shape and dermatoscopically characterized by a structureless black area and irregularly distributed brown and black globules.

2.2 Spitz and Reed Nevi

Whether Spitz and Reed nevi represent distinct nevus types or not remains controversial and is rather clinically irrelevant. From a dermatoscopic aspect, three main patterns can be seen in Spitz and Reed nevi, as discussed in the following sections.

2.2.1 Vessels and White Network (Nonpigmented Spitz Nevus)

Dermatoscopy of nonpigmented Spitz nevi typically reveals multiple and relatively regularly distributed dotted vessels (Figure 2.45). In more nodular nevi, the vessels tend to be larger than dots and project as globular, glomerular, and less frequently comma or hairpin vessels (Figures 2.46 and 2.47). A frequent additional finding is the inverse or negative or white network, which corresponds to white crossing lines or areas that surround the vascular structures (Figures 2.45 through 2.47).

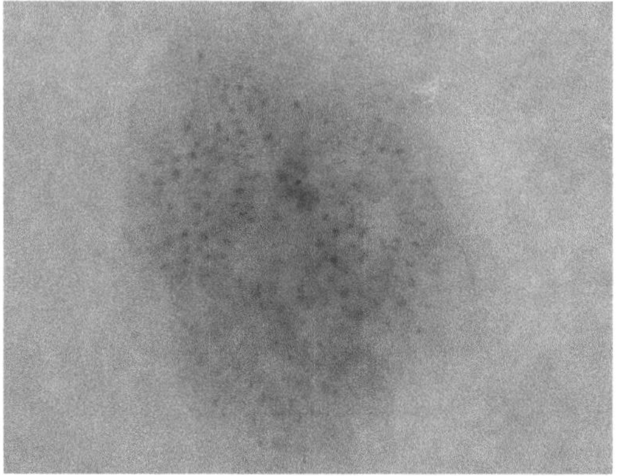

FIGURE 2.45 The typical pattern of nonpigmented Spitz nevi consisting of multiple and relatively regularly distributed dotted vessels surrounded by white color.

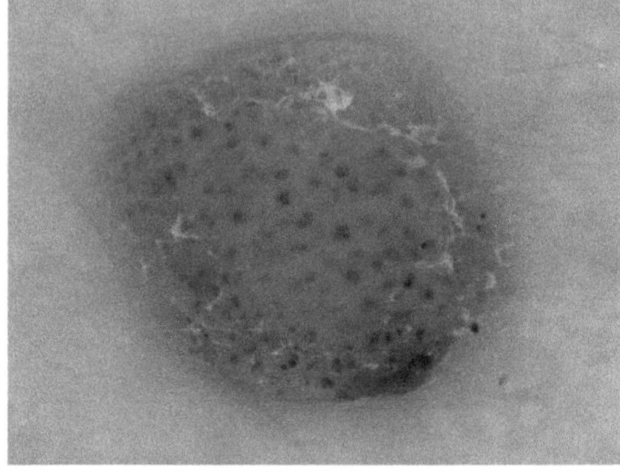

FIGURE 2.46 In this nonpigmented Spitz nevus, the vessels are larger and project as red globules.

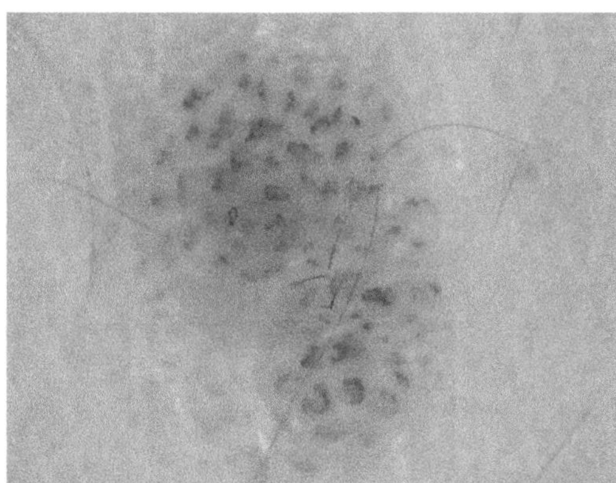

FIGURE 2.47 A nonpigmented Spitz nevus displaying glomerular, hairpin, and highly tortuous vessels.

2.2.2 Globules and White Network (Pigmented Spitz Nevus)

Pigmented Spitz nevi are dermatoscopically typified by variously sized brown and/or black globules, surrounded by white crossing lines or areas (inverse or negative or white network or reticular depigmentation (Figure 2.48). The variability of size and color of the globules as well as the presence of a white network allows for the discrimination of pigmented Spitz nevi from regular dermal nevi (Figure 2.49).

2.2.3 Starburst Pattern (Reed Nevus)

Reed nevus is dermatoscopically typified by the "starburst" pattern. The term derives from the fact that the dermatoscopic structures are arranged in a way that, overall, resembles an exploding star. Typically, it consists of a central area of dark brown/black/blue pigmentation and multiple pigmented streaks and/or pseudopods that arise from the center and radially expand toward the

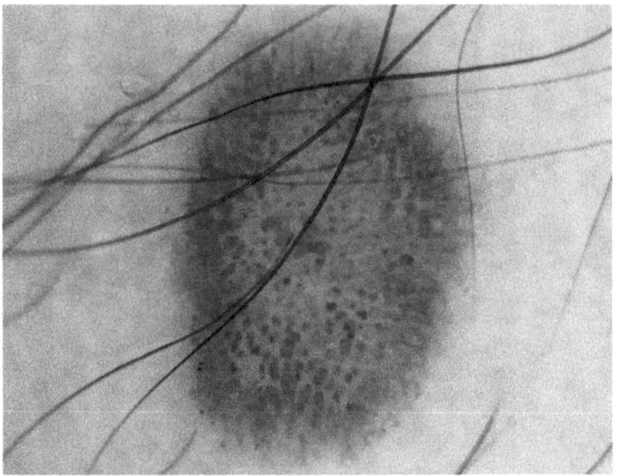

FIGURE 2.48 A pigmented Spitz nevus typified by a globular pattern with a white network (reticular depigmentation) among the globules.

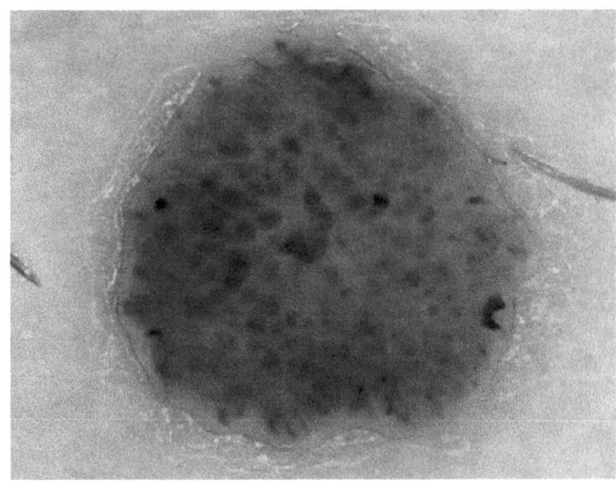

FIGURE 2.49 A nevus displaying globules of variable color and size, and the white network among them is much more likely a Spitz than a common globular nevus.

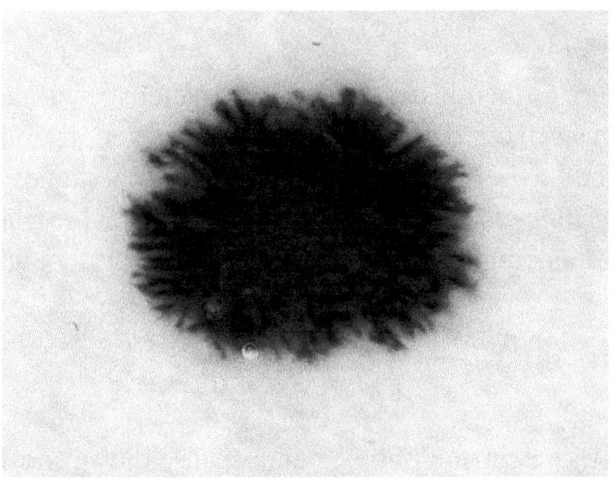

FIGURE 2.50 The typical starburst pattern of Reed nevi consists of a heavily pigmented center and radial peripheral streaks.

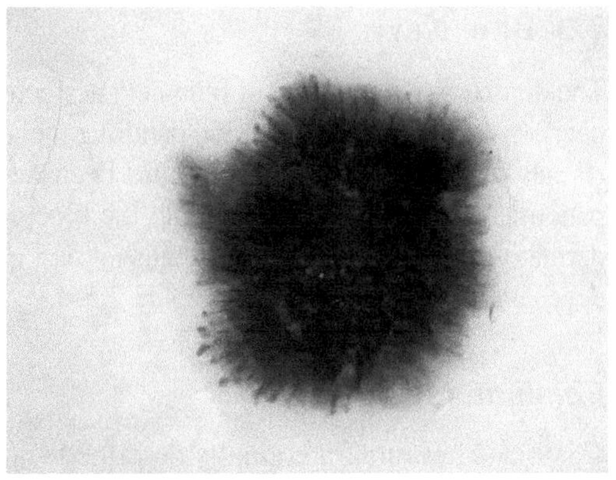

FIGURE 2.51 Radial streaks and pseudopods at the periphery typify Reed nevus.

periphery (Figures 2.50 and 2.51). The starburst pattern is indicative of the radial, rapid growth that biologically characterizes Reed nevi. When the nevus is stabilized, the starburst pattern is replaced by a homogeneous or reticular pattern (Figure 2.52).

Evolution of Spitz Nevi

It has been proposed that very early Spitz and Reed nevi are dermatoscopically typified by a dense globular pattern, which gradually changes into a starburst pattern with peripheral pseudopods and streaks. Subsequently, the starburst pattern is replaced by a homogeneous or reticular pattern, which suggests a termination of growth (Figure 2.53). Eventually, Spitz and Reed nevi will either remain stable or undergo spontaneous involution (partial or complete) over a variable period of months to years.

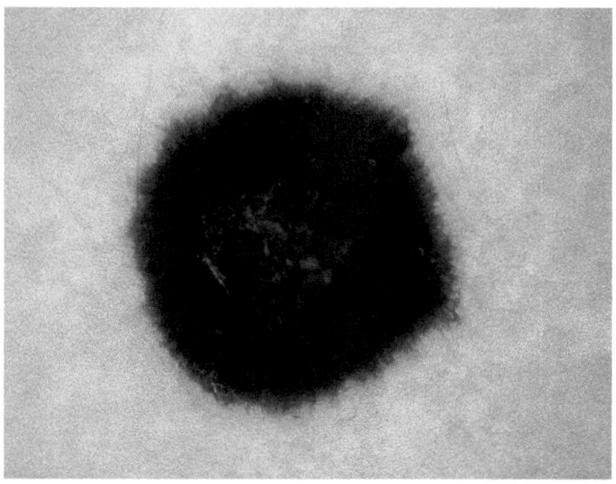

FIGURE 2.52 An "old" Reed nevus dermatoscopically displaying a homogenous black pigmentation.

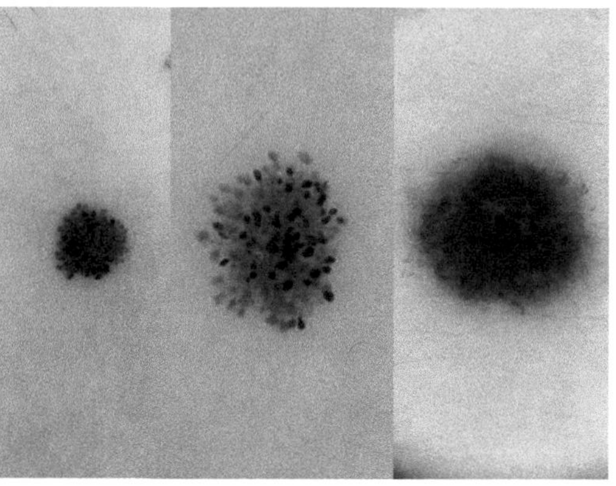

FIGURE 2.53 The proposed evolution of Reed nevi: a globular pattern evolving into a typical starburst pattern and finally central hyperpigmentation and peripheral network.

2.3 Blue Nevi

The dermatoscopic pattern of blue nevi perfectly mirrors their histopathologic characteristics. Blue nevi consist of aggregated dermal dendritic melanocytes; therefore, their dermatoscopic examination reveals diffuse blue color, which has been described as a blue "homogeneous" or structureless pattern (Figure 2.54). In addition to the blue color, long-standing and/or cellular blue nevi might dermatoscopically display also whitish areas, corresponding to dermal fibrosis, or sites of myxoid degeneration within the nevus (Figure 2.55).

Combined Nevi

Combined nevi are traditionally described within the spectrum of blue nevi because they almost always consist of a blue nevus and an overlying common (usually junctional) nevus. Expectedly, dermatoscopy will reveal both components: a blue structureless area and a pigment network, corresponding to the blue and junctional nevus, respectively (Figure 2.56). The blue area might be located in the center of the reticular lesion or eccentrically.

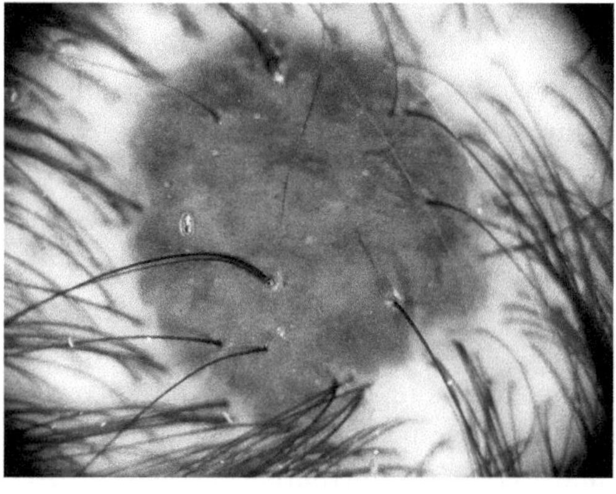

FIGURE 2.54 The typical dermatoscopic pattern of blue nevi consists of homogeneous or structureless blue pigmentation.

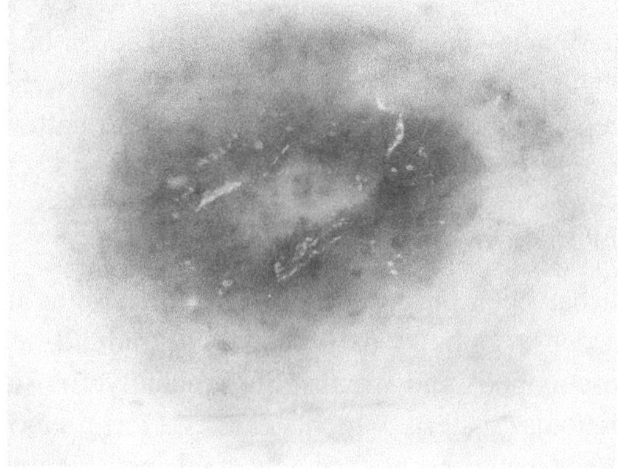

FIGURE 2.55 Quite frequently, blue nevi might dermatoscopically display white areas in conjunction with the predominant blue color.

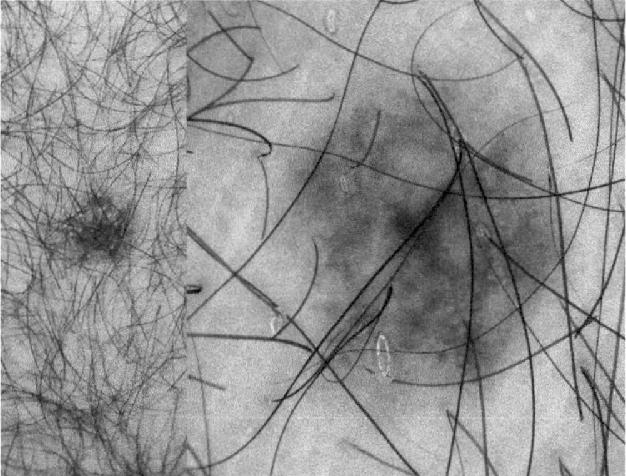

FIGURE 2.56 An example of a combined nevus with a central blue homogeneous area, corresponding to the blue nevus, on a reticular background that corresponds to the junctional nevus.

2.4 Special Nevus Types

2.4.1 Traumatized Nevus (Targetoid Hemosiderotic Nevus)

Random mechanical injury of any nevus might occur, and elevated or nodular nevi are more likely to be traumatized than flat ones. The term "targetoid hemosiderotic nevus" refers to the post-traumatic appearance of an ecchymotic, violaceous halo around a long-lasting centrally elevated nevus (Figure 2.57). Dermatoscopy reveals the typical features of the nevus (usually multiple globules) with vascular-hemorrhagic (red to purple or black) changes superimposed on the nevus or surrounding it (Figure 2.58). In a later stage, the hemorrhagic features disappear, and the nevus acquires its previous morphology. Signs of post-traumatic fibrosis (white scar-like areas) might occasionally remain in case of severe trauma (Figure 2.59).

2.4.2 Eczematous Nevus (Meyerson Nevus)

Meyerson phenomenon is characterized by the development of an eczematous reaction on one or more pigmented nevi. Clinically, it is typified by the appearance of erythematous halo around the nevus, with or without scaling (Figure 2.60). Dermatoscopy reveals the features of the nevus (network or globules) and the characteristic yellow sero-crusts that typify any eczematous reaction (Figure 2.61). Eczematous vesicles and crusts can also be found in the central, darkly pigmented area of Meyerson nevus. The eczematous reaction clears either spontaneously or after topical application of corticosteroids, and the nevus acquires its previous morphology.

2.4.3 Halo Nevus (Sutton Nevus)

The appearance of a white halo surrounding one or more nevi occurs mainly in children and young adults and is considered as an immunologic reaction that might represent a manifestation of vitiligo or other immunologic disorder (Figure 2.62). Dermatoscopy will reveal the global pattern of the nevus, which usually is globular or homogeneous and less frequently reticular

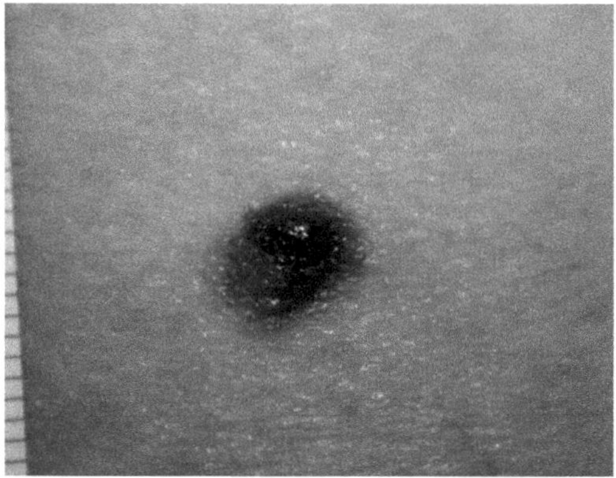

FIGURE 2.57 Targetoid hemosiderotic nevus: an ecchymotic halo appearing at the periphery of a preexisting nevus.

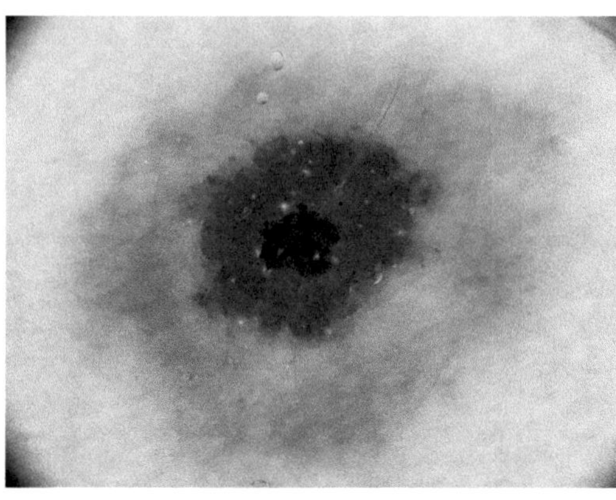

FIGURE 2.58 Dermatoscopy reveals the globules of the nevus in the center and the peripheral post-traumatic erythema.

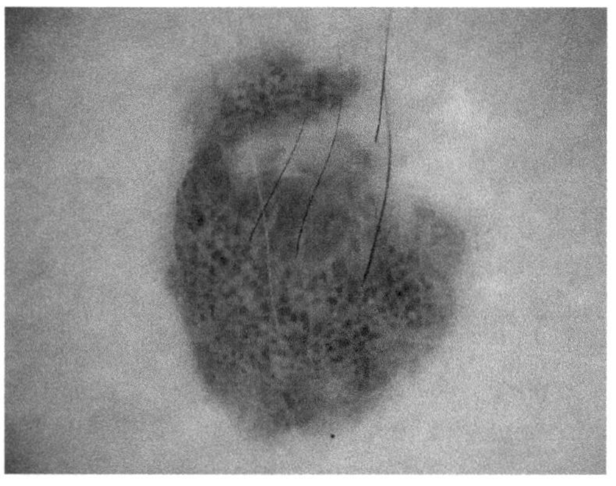

FIGURE 2.59 A scar remaining after healing of a severe trauma in a nevus.

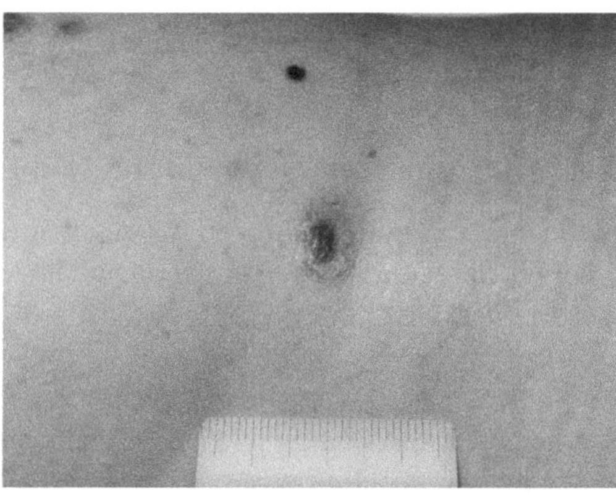

FIGURE 2.60 Meyerson nevus: an erythematous halo with mild scaling appearing at the periphery of a preexisting nevus.

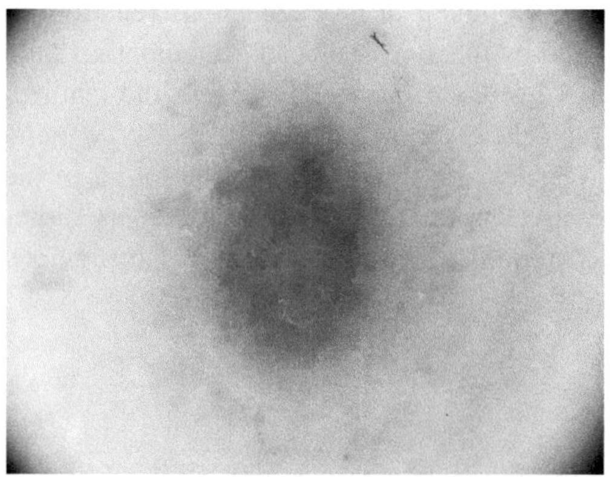

FIGURE 2.61 Dermatoscopy reveals yellow sero-crusts at the periphery, highly suggestive of the eczematous reaction.

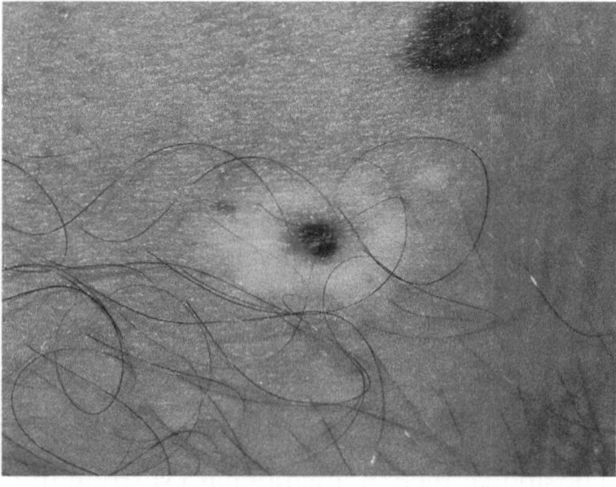

FIGURE 2.62 Sutton nevus: a hypopigmented halo appearing at the periphery of a preexisting nevus.

and the peripheral white halo (Figure 2.63). The halo is typically whiter that the surrounding skin (regression-like or scar-like depigmentation). The most common evolution of halo nevi is the gradual progression of the immunologic process, with the nevus decreasing in size from the periphery to the center. At least half of halo nevi will completely disappear and be replaced by white color (whiter than the surrounding skin). At this stage, dermatoscopy of the central part will reveal red color, possibly with visible vessels from the dermal vascular plexus (Figure 2.64).

2.4.4 Balloon Cell Nevus

This is a peculiar nevus type, histopathologically characterized by large, vesicular, clear cells (balloon cells). Dermatoscopically, the nests of these peculiar cells are seen as aggregated white or yellow globular structures (Figure 2.65).

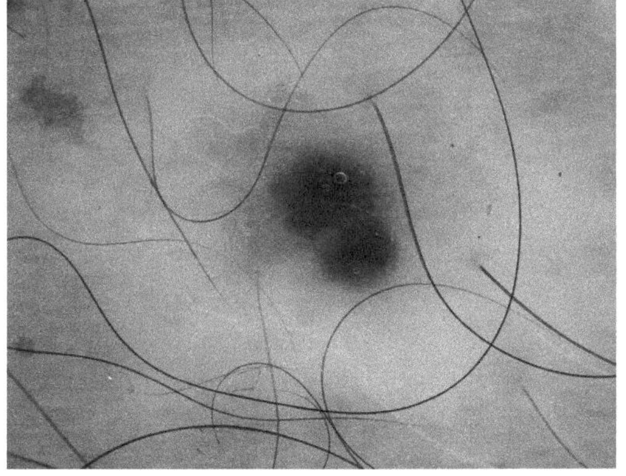

FIGURE 2.63 Dermatoscopy reveals a reticular nevus in the center surrounded by white color, which is clearly whiter than the surrounding skin.

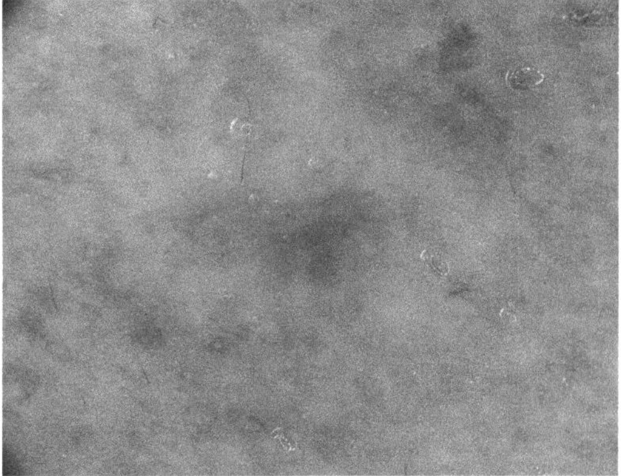

FIGURE 2.64 A Sutton nevus at an end-stage dermatoscopically reveals white color and thin linear vessels corresponding to the underlying dermal vascular plexus.

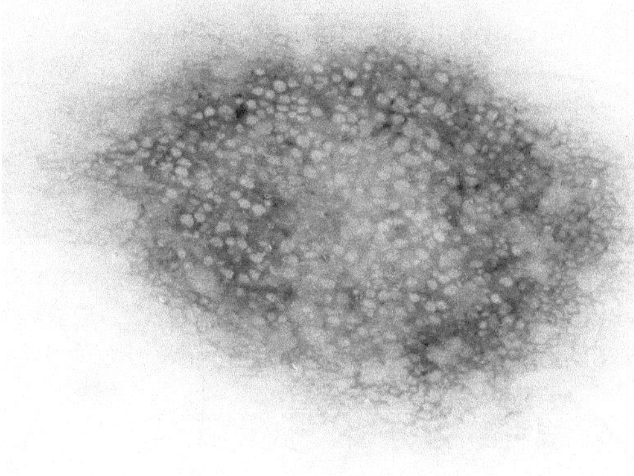

FIGURE 2.65 A balloon cell nevus dermoscopically typified by yellow round-ish structures.

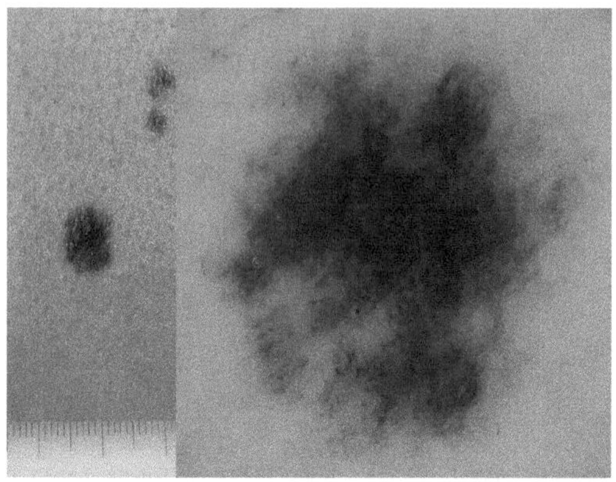

FIGURE 2.66 A sclerosing nevus clinically characterized by an eccentric hyperpigmented area and dermatoscopically displaying blue-gray and white regression structures.

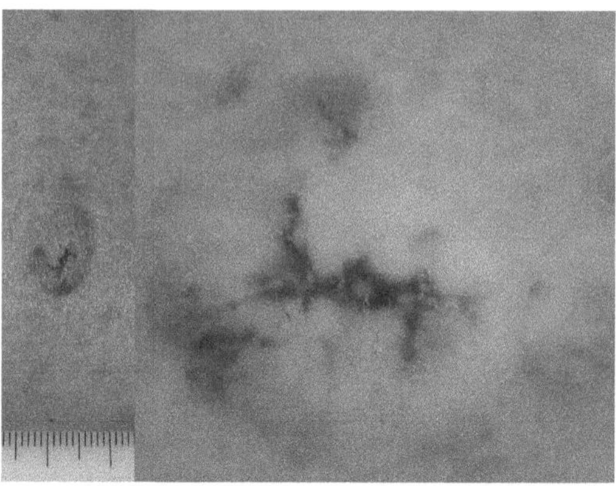

FIGURE 2.67 A nevus recurring after a shave excision: dermatoscopy reveals that the recurrent pigmentation remains restricted within the margins of the scar.

2.4.5 Sclerosing Nevus (with Pseudomelanoma Features)

This nevus type represents a result of minor or unnoticed trauma on a preexisting nevus usually located on the middle upper back of young to middle-aged men. Histopathologically, it is characterized by the presence of dermal sclerosis and architecturally atypical melanocytic nests. Dermatoscopy reveals regression areas covering 10%–50% of the lesion's surface. The regression areas are characteristically "polychromatic," meaning that they consist of blue-gray structures and scar-like or depigmentation (Figure 2.66).

2.4.6 Recurrent Nevus

Nevi excised with regular elliptical or shave excisions might recur. The recurrence is much more likely if a destructive method, such as laser or cryotherapy, had been applied. Most recurrences occur within the first 6 months after excision, in contrast to melanoma that tends to recur later. The recurrent pigmentation of a nevus typically remains restricted within the borders of the scar, whereas recurrent melanoma will grow beyond the scar borders (Figure 2.67). Obviously, in the case of pigmentation appearing on a scar, the availability of histopathologic examination of the previously excised lesion is of paramount importance.

BIBLIOGRAPHY

Aguilera P, Puig S, Guilabert A et al. Prevalence study of nevi in children from Barcelona. Dermoscopy, constitutional and environmental factors. *Dermatology*. 2009;218:203–14.

Argenziano G, Soyer HP, Chimenti S et al. Dermoscopy of pigmented skin lesions: Results of a consensus meeting via the Internet. *J Am Acad Dermatol*. 2003;48:679–93.

Argenziano G, Zalaudek I, Ferrara G et al. Proposal of a new classification system for melanocytic naevi. *Br J Dermatol*. 2007;157:217–27.

Hofmann-Wellenhof R. Special criteria for special locations 2: Scalp, mucosal, and milk line. *Dermatol Clin*. 2013;31:625–36.

Lallas A, Apalla Z, Ioannides D et al. Update on dermoscopy of Spitz/Reed naevi and management guidelines by the International Dermoscopy Society. *Br J Dermatol*. 2017;177:645–55.

Lallas A, Reggiani C, Argenziano G et al. Dermoscopic nevus patterns in skin of colour: A prospective, cross-sectional, morphological study in individuals with skin type V and VI. *J Eur Acad Dermatol Venereol.* 2013;28:1469–74.

Papakonstantinou A, Ioannides D, Vakirlis E et al. Dermoscopic features of melanocytic skin lesions in Greek children and adolescents and their association with environmental factors and skin types. *J Eur Acad Dermatol Venereol.* 2018 April 6. doi: 10.1111/jdv.14996. [Epub ahead of print]

Zalaudek I, Schmid K, Marghoob AA et al. Frequency of dermoscopic nevus subtypes by age and body site: A cross-sectional study. *Arch Dermatol.* 2011;147:663–70.

Zalaudek I, Sgambato A, Ferrara G, Argenziano G. Diagnosis and management of melanocytic skin lesions in the pediatric praxis. A review of the literature. *Minerva Pediatr.* 2008;60:291–312.

Zalaudek I, Grinschgl S, Argenziano G et al. Age-related prevalence of dermoscopy patterns in acquired melanocytic naevi. *Br J Dermatol.* 2006;154:299–304.

Zalaudek I, Schmid K, Niederkorn A, Fink-Puches R, Richtig E, Wolf I, Hofmann-Wellenhof R. Proposal for a clinical-dermoscopic classification of scalp naevi. *Br J Dermatol.* 2014;170:1065–72.

Zalaudek I, Schmid K, Marghoob AA et al. Frequency of dermoscopic nevus subtypes by age and body site: A cross-sectional study. *Arch Dermatol.* 2011;147:663–70.

Zalaudek I, Manzo M, Savarese I, Docimo G, Ferrara G, Argenziano G. The morphologic universe of melanocytic nevi. *Semin Cutan Med Surg.* 2009;28:149–56.

3

Melanoma

Melanoma is a malignant melanocytic tumor that represents the most frequent cause of deaths associated with skin cancer.

Classification

The melanoma family encompasses tumors with different clinical characteristics and biological behavior. Several classifications have been proposed, based on clinical features, histopathologic alterations, and different anatomical locations. Traditionally, four main types of melanoma are described: superficial spreading, nodular, lentigo maligna melanoma, and acral lentiginous melanoma. In this chapter, the selected classification is clinically oriented, aiming to follow the real scenarios that clinicians are faced with in their everyday practice.

It has to be clarified that the biological diversity among various melanoma subtypes (more and less aggressive tumors) refers to the time needed to invade the dermis (and thus, acquire a metastatic potential) and to their vertical growth rate. However, it is well known that the most potent prognostic factor of melanoma is the thickness of the tumor in millimeters (Breslow) at the time of diagnosis. It has been shown that tumors of similar Breslow thickness carry a similar prognosis, irrespective of the time required to acquire this invasion depth. Effectively, although slow-growing melanomas need more time to become invasive, after invading the dermis, they are no longer associated with a better prognosis.

The three main clinical types of melanoma, and their subtypes, include the following:

a. *Conventional melanoma (CM).* Originating from melanocytes at the dermo-epidermal junction, conventional melanoma is initially restricted within the epidermis (melanoma *in situ*) growing mainly peripherally, but after a period that ranges between a few months and many years, it invades the dermis and acquires a significant metastatic potential. The clinical characteristics and the differential diagnoses of CM largely depend on the anatomical site of tumor development and can be subclassified as follows:
   i. Melanoma of the trunk and the extremities. This term corresponds to the superficial spreading melanoma and is the most frequent clinical subtype of the disease, at least in Caucasian populations.
   ii. Facial melanoma, corresponding to lentigo maligna melanoma (LMM).
   iii. Acral melanoma (or acral lentiginous melanoma).
   iv. Subungual melanoma.
   v. Mucosal melanoma.
   vi. Primary extracutaneous melanoma, including ocular, central nervous system (CNS), and soft tissue melanoma. This category will not be analytically described in this book.

b. *Nodular melanoma (NM).* This type of melanoma is less frequent but much more aggressive biologically. Having been proposed to originate from dermal melanocytes, NM immediately grows within the dermis and, from a very early stage, may metastasize through either the lymphatic or the vascular pathway. The clinical characteristics of NM differ significantly from CM, rendering its detection particularly difficult.

c. *Amelanotic melanoma.* This category of tumors is described separately because the lack of pigmentation results in an overall peculiar clinical presentation, significantly increasing the risk of misdiagnosis.

As a general rule, melanoma becomes clinically detectable after a certain point of evolution, as soon as its morphological asymmetry becomes clinically evident. At an earlier stage, melanoma is macroscopically not recognizable because it is small in size and symmetric in terms of shape and color. At this stage, dermatoscopy might uncover the natural asymmetry of the tumor and allow its recognition (Figure 3.1).

3.1 Conventional Melanoma

3.1.1 Melanoma of the Trunk and the Extremities

Clinically, melanoma initially develops as a light to dark brown or black flat macule, gradually enlarging with a rate that varies significantly (Figure 3.2). With time, a palpable elevated or papular component typically develops, multiple colors may appear, while the borders and the overall shape become irregular (Figure 3.3). Several years ago, the clinical criteria of melanoma were summarized in the ABCD clinical rule, which is presented in Table 3.1.

At a later stage, a nodular part might develop, and ulceration or bleeding may occur (Figure 3.4). If left untreated, melanoma invades the deeper and surrounding tissues, resulting in an impressive clinical appearance.

The differential diagnosis of conventional melanoma includes other pigmented skin tumors, mainly nevi, seborrheic keratosis, and pigmented basal cell carcinoma. The clinical discrimination between nevi and melanoma is basically based on the natural symmetry of nevi, in contrast to the irregular morphology that typifies melanoma after a certain progression point (Figure 3.5). Also nevi increase in size, especially in young individuals, but usually they enlarge symmetrically to all directions, remain uniform in color, and retain a regular border. Certainly, morphologically atypical nevi exist, especially in the context of patients with "atypical mole syndrome." In such cases, an accurate diagnosis is impossible without coupling clinical

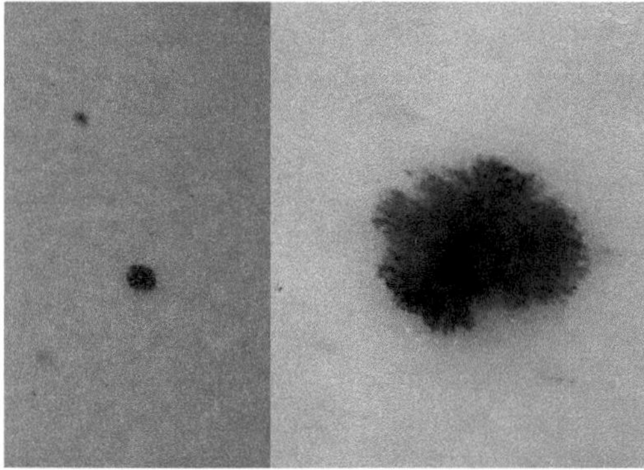

FIGURE 3.1 Dermatoscopy reveals the morphological asymmetry of melanoma before it becomes visible to the naked eye.

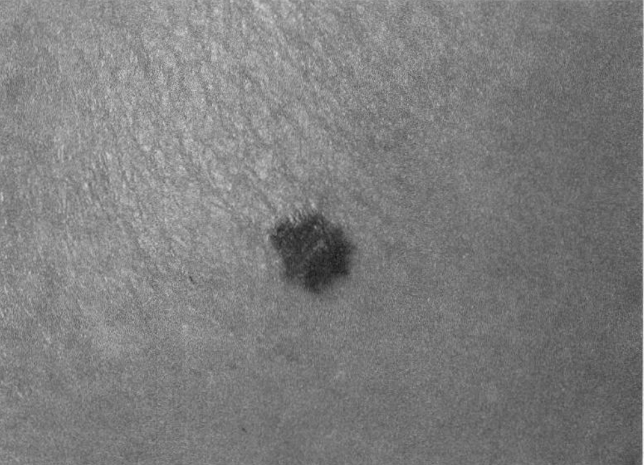

FIGURE 3.2 Early stage melanoma, clinically manifesting as a small, homogenous, light brown macule.

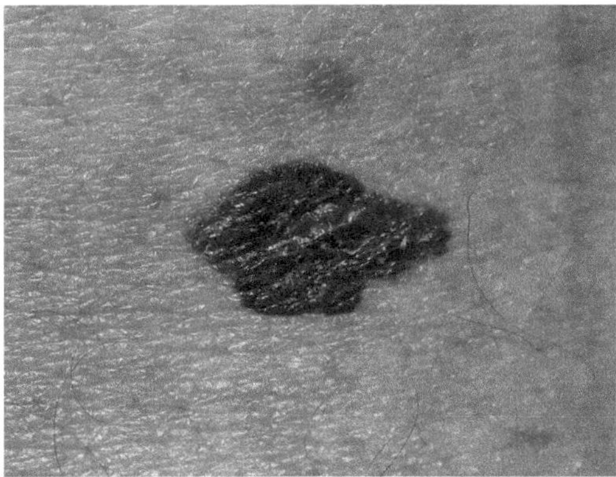

FIGURE 3.3 Melanoma in a later stage characterized by a central darker part and irregular shape.

TABLE 3.1
ABCD Clinical Rule for Detection of Melanoma

A	Asymmetry
B	Border irregularity
C	Color variegation
D	Diameter >6 mm
E	Evolution

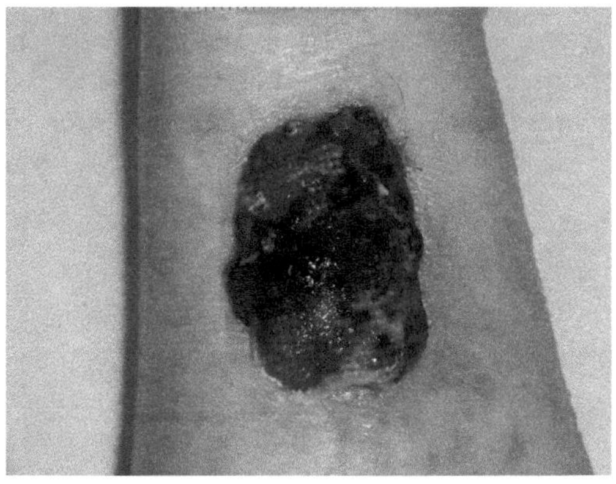

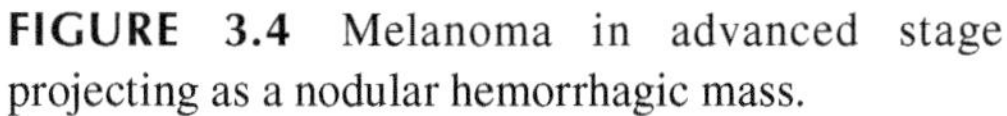

FIGURE 3.4 Melanoma in advanced stage projecting as a nodular hemorrhagic mass.

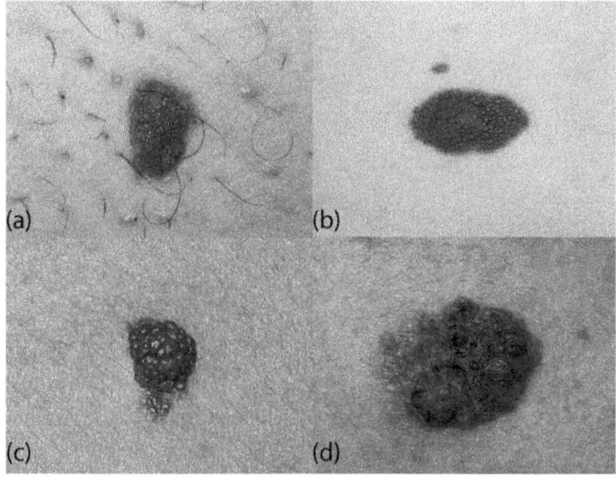

FIGURE 3.5 Nevi are characterized by symmetry of color and shape (a,b,c). In contrast, melanoma is characterized by focal elevated or nodular parts and more than one color (d).

examination with dermoscopy. Seborrheic keratoses are usually easy to diagnose, based on their characteristic "stuck-on" appearance and their sharp demarcation (Figure 3.6). However, sometimes these criteria are not evident enough, while color variegations are not uncommon.

Pigmented basal cell carcinoma might also be very difficult to discriminate from melanoma. An elevated border and a translucent hue are in favor of pigmented basal cell carcinoma, but it is often impossible to differentiate these two tumors on clinical grounds only (Figure 3.7).

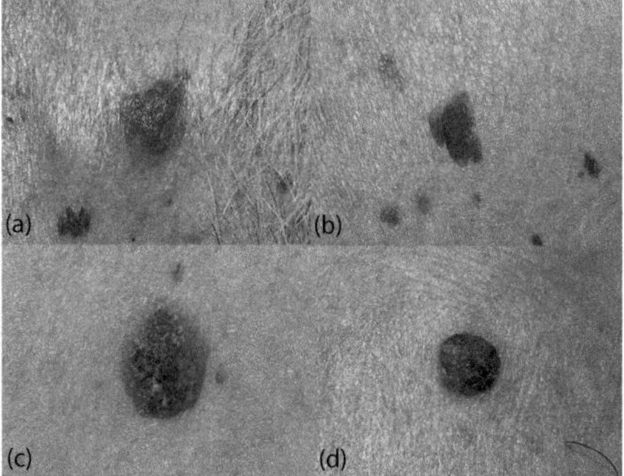

FIGURE 3.6 Seborrheic keratoses are clinically typified by their verrucous surface(a), sharp demarcation (b) and characteristic stuck-on appearance (c,d).

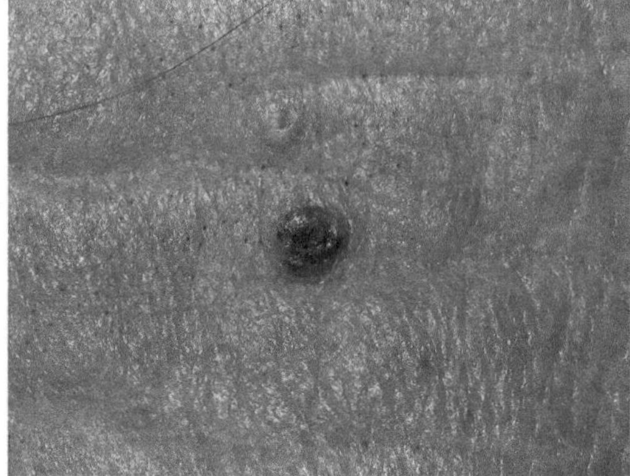

FIGURE 3.7 Pigmented basal cell carcinoma with a slightly elevated and translucent periphery.

Dermatoscopic Features

The natural morphological asymmetry of melanoma is also reflected in its dermatoscopic pattern. As a rule, dermatoscopy of melanoma reveals asymmetry of shape, more than two colors (light brown, dark brown, black, blue, gray, red, white), and asymmetry of structures. Furthermore, local dermatoscopic features associated with melanoma are summarized and analytically described in Table 3.2 (Figures 3.8 through 3.20).

In the real clinical setting, the dermatoscopic diagnosis of melanoma is usually straightforward, based on the immediate recognition of its morphological asymmetry and/or one or more of the structures described in Table 3.2. However, less morphologically evident melanomas do exist, and their recognition requires a more analytic dermatoscopic evaluation of the lesion. Learning the analytic approach is also extremely useful for educative purposes for inexperienced clinicians. The first introduced and more widely adopted method for analyzing the morphology of a pigmented lesion is the two-step algorithm.

Two-Step Algorithm

According to this diagnostic method, the first step when assessing a given lesion is to classify it as melanocytic or not. A lesion is judged as melanocytic when displaying, as a prominent feature, a pigment network or globules or streaks or homogenous pigmentation. Instead, in the presence of criteria specifically associated with basal cell carcinoma, seborrheic keratosis, or angioma, the lesion is classified as nonmelanocytic. Finally, when none of the previously mentioned criteria can be recognized, the lesion is classified as melanocytic. The first step of the algorithm is shown in Table 3.3.

Subsequently, when a lesion is assessed as melanocytic, it enters the second step of the analysis, which aims to differentiate melanoma from nevi. In this step, the morphology of the session is analyzed either by pattern analysis or by using the semiquantitative algorithms that have been suggested.

Pattern Analysis and Semiquantitive Methods

Pattern analysis is a qualitative assessment procedure that evaluates first the global pattern of the lesion and afterward the presence of local features that are associated either to nevus or

TABLE 3.2

Dermatoscopic Criteria for Melanoma

Dermoscopic Criteria	Description
Atypical network	Black, brown, or gray pigment network, irregular holes and irregularly distributed thick lines ending abruptly in the periphery
Irregular blotch	Black or dark brown region without discrete structures non-centrally located in the lesion
Irregular dots/globules	Black or brown round or ovoid structures varying in size, irregularly distributed across the lesion
Irregular streaks/ pseudopods	Radially arranged lines with (pseudopods) or without (streaks) roundish projections in their peripheral part, irregularly distributed in the periphery of the lesion. Varying in color from light brown to dark, starting from the central pigment part of the lesion
Regression structure	Assigning, clinically, in the flat part of the lesion, there are mainly two categories: 1. White, scar-like areas 2. Gray dots
White shiny streaks	Visible only with polarized light, small in length and in vertical, parallel, or angular direction
Blue-white veil	Confluent, irregular, and structureless area of whitish-bluish diffuse depigmentation associated with pigment network, dots, globules, and streaks. Assigning, clinically, the elevated part of the lesion.
Atypical vascular pattern	1. Atypical hairpin vessels 2. Multicomponent vascular pattern consisting of dotted and linear vessels or any other morphological type of vessels
Irregular hyperpigmented areas	Black or dark brown or gray areas with irregular shape or distribution
Prominent skin markings	Hypopigmented skin creases within the lesion
Polygons/angulated lines	Brown or gray angulated lines forming polygons

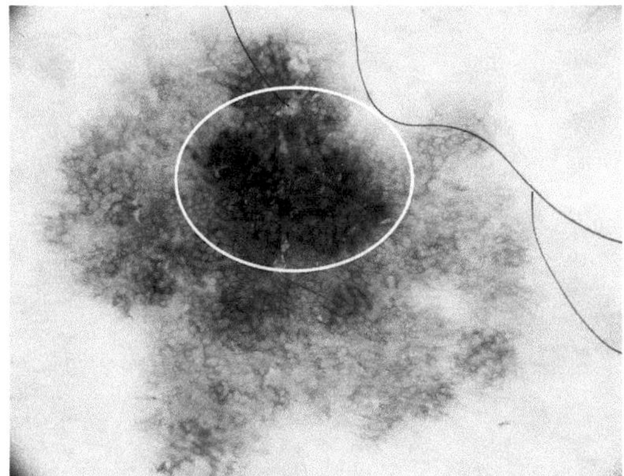

FIGURE 3.8 Atypical pigment network: The area within the circle is characterized by a darker network with thicker lines and smaller holes as compared to the other parts of the lesion.

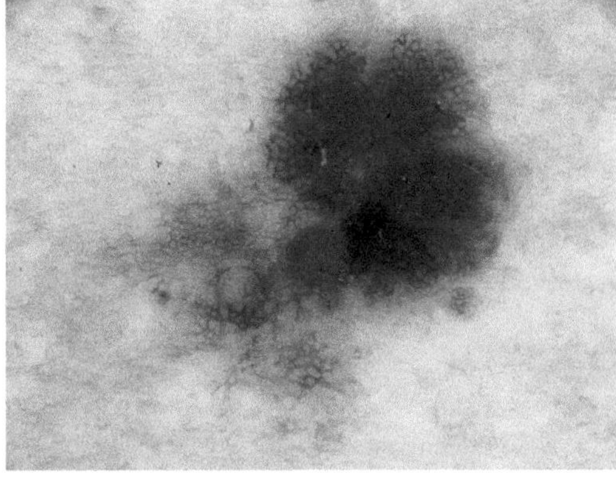

FIGURE 3.9 Atypical pigment network: On the right part, the network is darker, with thicker lines and smaller holes as compared to the left part.

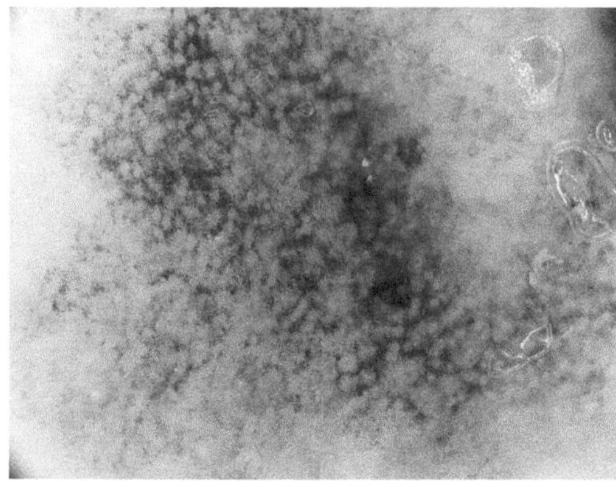

FIGURE 3.10 Regression in early stage melanoma: multiple gray granules, corresponding to diffuse melanophages in the upper dermis.

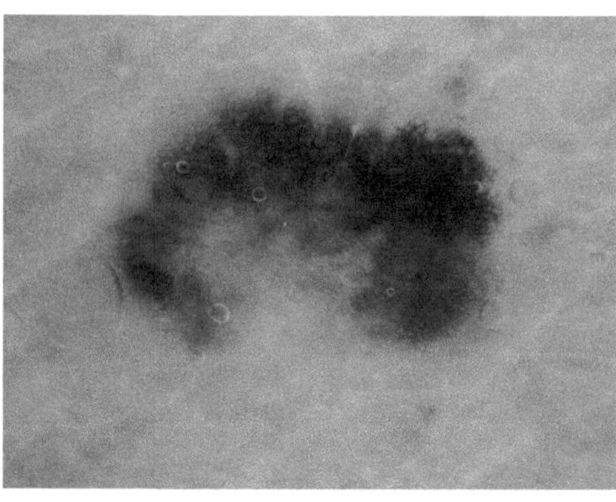

FIGURE 3.11 Regression in advanced melanoma: in the regressed area, the observed color is lighter than the color of the skin surrounding the lesion skin (scar-like depigmentation). Some gray granules can also be found in the regressed area.

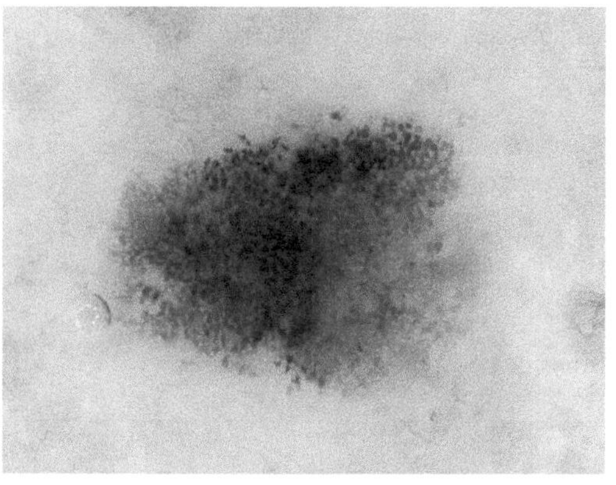

FIGURE 3.12 Irregular globules in terms of size, color, and distribution.

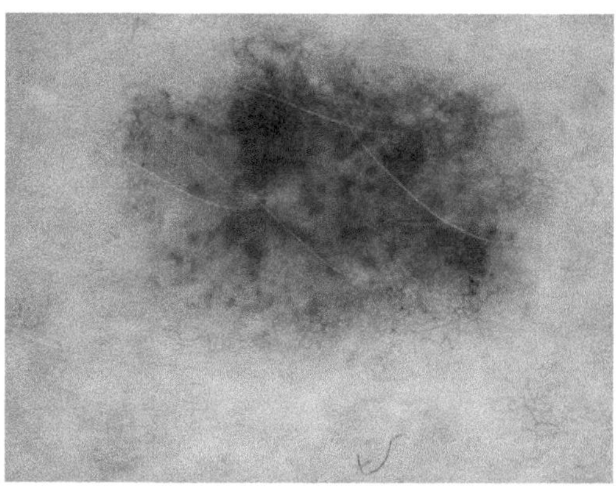

FIGURE 3.13 Irregular gray and brown globules asymmetrically distributed in the lesion.

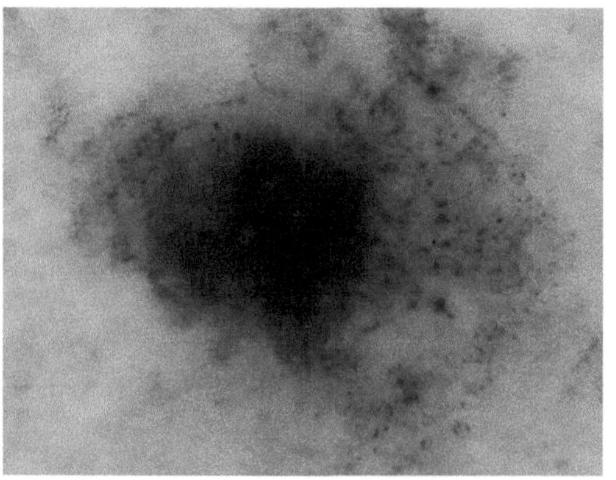

FIGURE 3.14 Eccentrically located blotch.

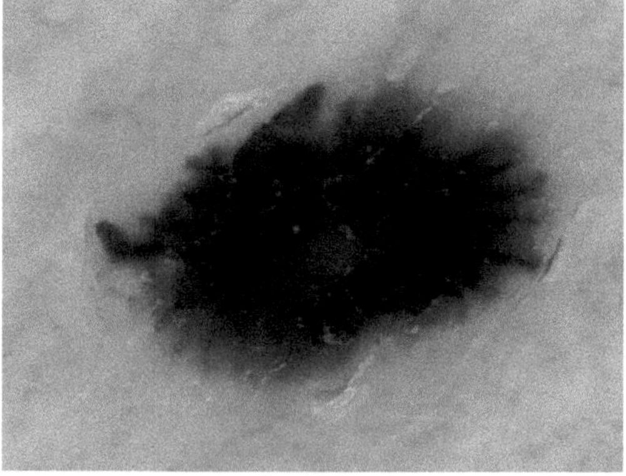

FIGURE 3.15 Peripheral streaks and pseudopods in asymmetrical distribution as they are present in only some parts of the periphery of the lesion.

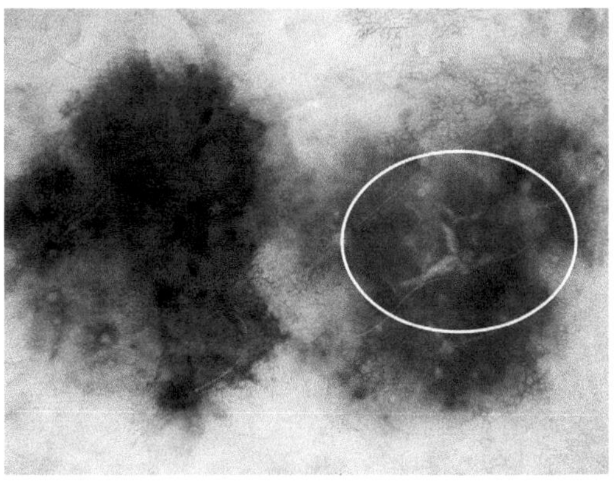

FIGURE 3.16 Irregularly distributed white shiny streaks (circle). This criterion is visible only with polarized light.

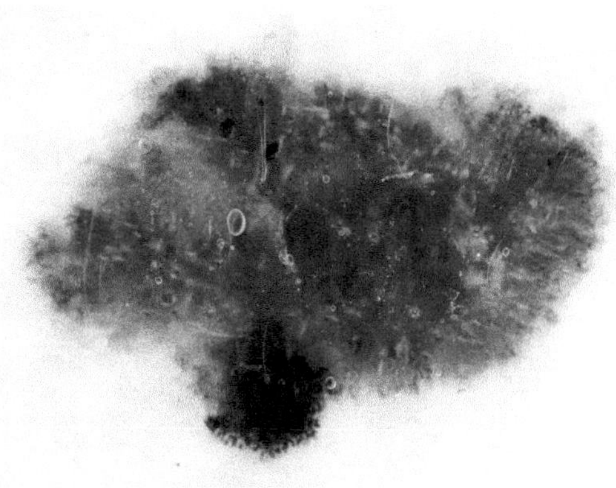

FIGURE 3.17 Multiple white shiny streaks, visible only with polarized light.

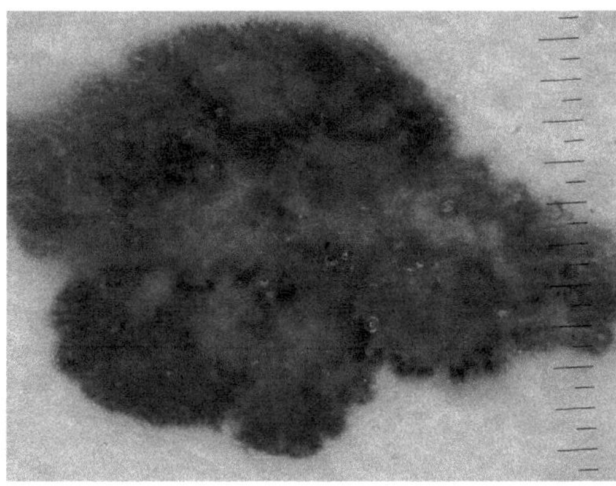

FIGURE 3.18 Blue-white veil in advanced melanoma. Blue color is better seen with nonpolarized light.

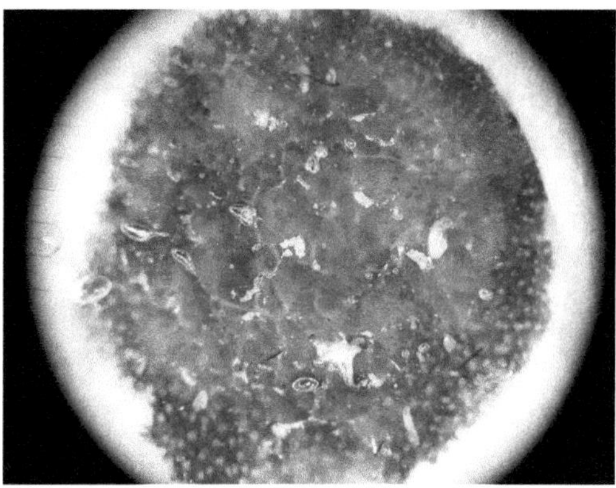

FIGURE 3.19 Blue-white veil in advanced melanoma.

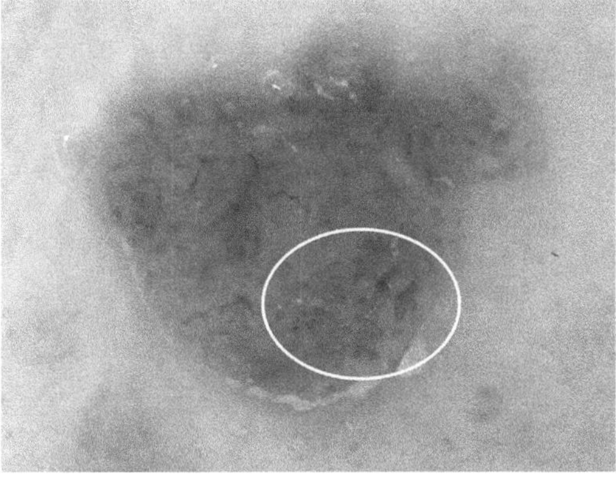

FIGURE 3.20 Polymorphous vascular pattern: multiple highly tortuous vessels (circle), dotted and linear vessels.

TABLE 3.3

First Step of Two-Step Algorithm

Criteria Indicating Melanocytic Lesion	Criteria Indicating Nonmelanocytic Lesion
Pigment network	Milia-like cysts (SebK)
Blotches: dots/globules	Comedo-like openings (SebK)
Streaks/pseudopods	Fingerprint-like structure (SebK)
Homogenous blue pigmentation	Cerebriform pattern (SebK)
	Branching vessels (BCC)
	Blue-gray ovoid nests (BCC)
	Blue-gray globules (BCC)
	Leaf-like structures (BCC)
	Spoke-wheel structures (BCC)
	Red/blue/black lacunes (hemangioma)

Abbreviations: BCC, basal cell carcinoma; SebK, seborrheic keratosis.

to melanoma (Table 3.4). With pattern analysis, the evaluator has to reach a conclusion taking into account all the observed features (global and local) but without using any scoring system. Pattern analysis has the advantage of taking into consideration all the available morphological information but is highly objective, not well-reproducible, and dependent on the experience of each clinician.

To overcome this problem, several semiquantitative methods have been suggested, including the ABCD rule (Table 3.5), Menzies' method (Table 3.6), and the seven-point checklist (Table 3.7). These algorithms are simpler, easier to be used by nonexperts, and have been shown to achieve similar results of diagnostic accuracy.

TABLE 3.4

Second Step in the Two-Step Algorithm in Pattern Analysis

Criteria Indicative for Nevi	Criteria Indicative for Melanoma
Symmetry of structures and colors	Asymmetry of structure and colors
General pattern	General pattern
Reticular	Complexity
Globular	Other criteria
Homogenous	Anything from Table 3.2
Starburst	
Other criteria	
Typical pigment network (homogenous for color, thick lines, and diameters of the holes)	
Black or brown globules similar sized, homogenously distributed in the center of the lesion (e.g., in the center or in the periphery or all over the lesion)	
Streaks or pseudopods in the periphery of the lesion	
Central hyperpigmented region	
Typical vascular pattern (dotted vessels regularly distributed or comma vessels)	

TABLE 3.5

Dermatoscopic ABCD Rule

	Score
Asymmetry in zero to two axons, concerning the contour, colors, structures	0–2
Border: abrupt ending at the periphery in zero to eight segments	0–8
Color: presence of up to six colors (white, red, light brown , dark brown, blue, black)	0–6
Dermatoscopic structures: presence of pigment network, dots, globules, peripheral branched streaks, homogenous blue areas	1–5
Total dermatoscopic score (TDS) = (A score × 1.3) + (B score × 0.1) + (C score × 0.5) + (D score × 0.5)	
TDS: <4.75 = nevus, 4.75–5.45: suspicious lesion, >5.45 melanoma	

TABLE 3.6

Menzies' Method

Negative Criteria	Positive Criteria
Symmetry of pattern	Blue-white veil
Presence of a single color	Multiple brown dots
	Pseudopods
	Radial streaking
	Scar-like depigmentation
	Peripheral dots/globules
	Multiple (five or six) colors
	Multiple blue-gray dots
	Wide network

Note: The diagnosis of melanoma requires the absence of both the negative criteria or the presence of one or more positive criteria.

TABLE 3.7

Seven-Point Checklist

Dermoscopic Criteria	Score
Major criteria	
1. Atypical pigment network	2
2. Blue-white veil	2
3. Atypical vascular pattern	2
Minor criteria	
4. Irregular streaks or pseudopods	1
5. Irregular dots/globules	1
6. Eccentric hyperpigmented region	1
7. Regression structures	1

Note: Total Score: ≥ 3 = melanoma, total score <3 = nevi.

In Situ and Early Invasive Melanoma

All the aforementioned algorithms were introduced several years ago and were constructed by studies including morphologically obvious—and, thus, relatively advanced—melanomas. Therefore, they might fail to detect early melanomas that have not developed, yet have dermatoscopic characteristics evident enough to reach the threshold of each algorithm. This does not meet the modern clinical needs, since our goal today is to recognize melanoma, if possible, before it invades the dermis (melanoma *in situ*). This trend toward earlier diagnosis led to a tapering of the threshold for excision, as highlighted by the recently revised seven-point checklist. According to the "updated" version of the algorithm, the presence of only one of the seven melanoma criteria should be considered enough to warrant excision, provided that the feature is clearly present in a considerable proportion of the lesion. The latter is in line with recent observations suggesting that melanoma *in situ* usually displays subtle dermoscopic characteristics, such as atypical network alone or combined with areas of regression (Figure 3.21). More recently, three new dermatoscopic criteria have been introduced as potent predictors of melanoma *in situ* versus atypical nevi and flat seborrheic and lichenoid keratoses: irregular hyperpigmented areas, prominent skin markings, and angulated lines/polygons (Figures 3.22 through 3.24).

3.1.2 Facial Melanoma

The long-standing controversy whether lentigo maligna represents already a melanoma or a precursor lesion has been resolved. Today, the terms *melanoma*, *lentigo maligna* (LM), and *lentigo maligna melanoma* (LMM) should be considered synonyms, while some authors use the term LM for melanoma *in situ* and LMM for invasive tumors. This subtype of melanoma is characterized by a slow lentiginous growth pattern and represents the less aggressive melanoma subtype. As explained earlier, this does not mean that invasive LM carries a better prognosis but that it takes much more time to become invasive, remaining for years or decades *in situ*.

The association with chronic sun exposure is stronger for LM than any other subtype of melanoma. LM typically develops on the heavily sun-damaged skin of elderly individuals,

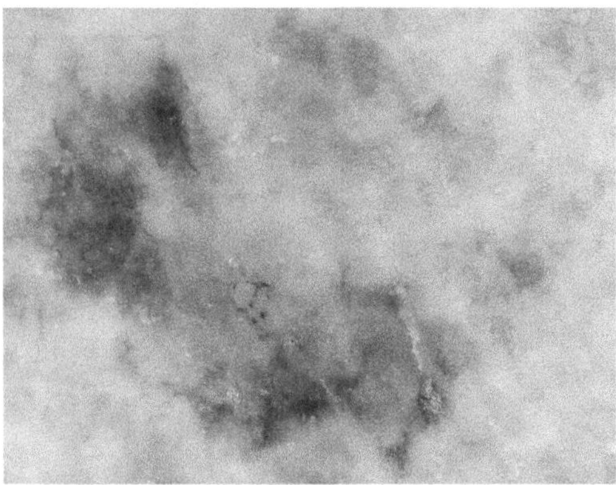

FIGURE 3.21 A melanoma *in situ* characterized by regression in an intermittent stage: a large part of the lesion has regressed but without the development of fibrosis. (There is depigmentation, but the color is not whiter than the surrounding skin.) Gray granules are also present.

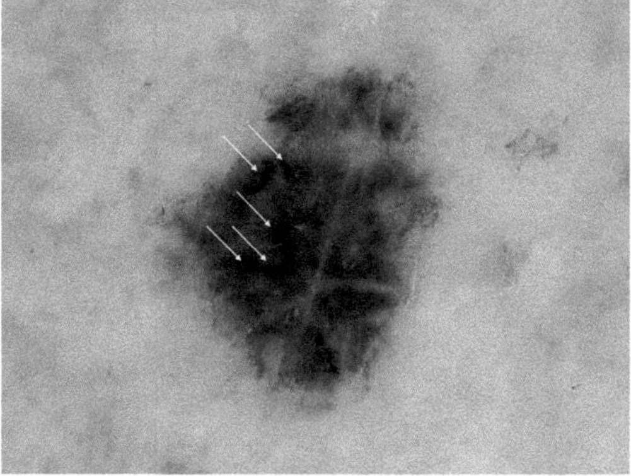

FIGURE 3.22 Small, irregular, hyperpigmented areas (arrows) in a melanoma *in situ*.

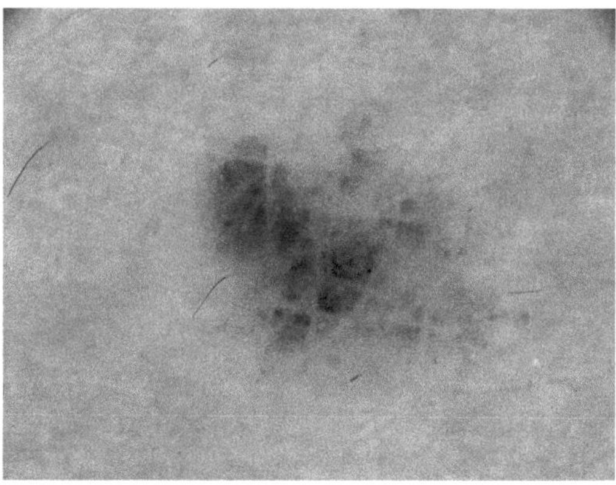

FIGURE 3.23 Melanoma *in situ* with prominent skin markings: skin creases within the lesion are hypopigmented.

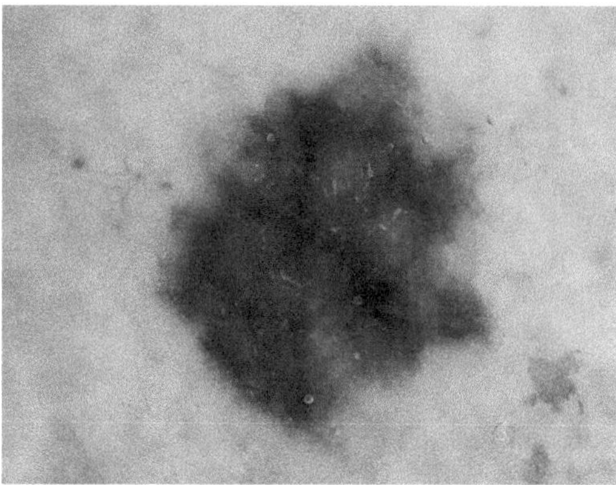

FIGURE 3.24 Angulated lines (polygons) of dark gray/black color in a melanoma *in situ*.

mainly on the face but also on the extremities. Clinically, LM usually is a long-standing tan macule that slowly expands peripherally and with time becomes uneven in color, showing light brown, dark brown, and black areas (Figure 3.25). Regression, seen as whitish areas within the lesion, might also occur. When LM becomes invasive, it may acquire all the characteristics of invasive melanoma (asymmetry, irregularity of shape and border, development of papular/nodular part, ulceration, bleeding) (Figure 3.26).

As opposed to melanoma of the trunk that has to be differentiated mainly from nevi, the differential diagnosis of facial melanoma includes nonmelanocytic tumors, namely, pigmented actinic keratosis (PAK) and solar lentigo/seborrheic keratosis (SL/SK). This is because, as highlighted by recent data, nevi on the face of elderly individuals are mainly dermal and elevated, not being included, thus, in the differential diagnosis of flat pigmented facial lesions of elderly patients (Figure 3.27). The discrimination among LM, PAK, and SL/SK represents one of the most challenging clinical scenarios, even after dermatoscopic examination (Figure 3.28).

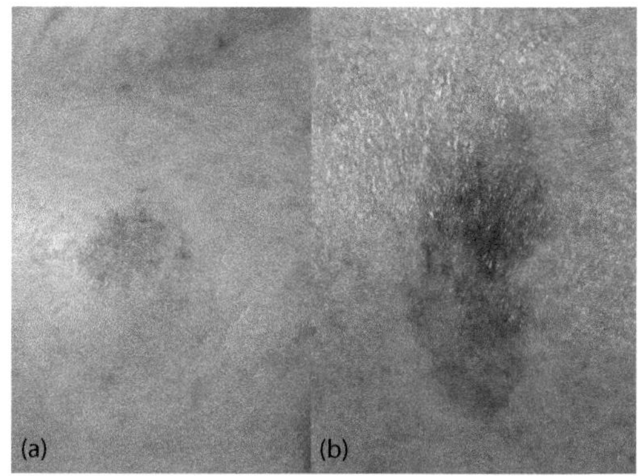

FIGURE 3.25 Lentigo maligna at an early stage, manifesting as a small, homogenous, light brown macule (a). As melanoma expands peripherally, more shades of brown become evident, and the order demarcation is lost (b).

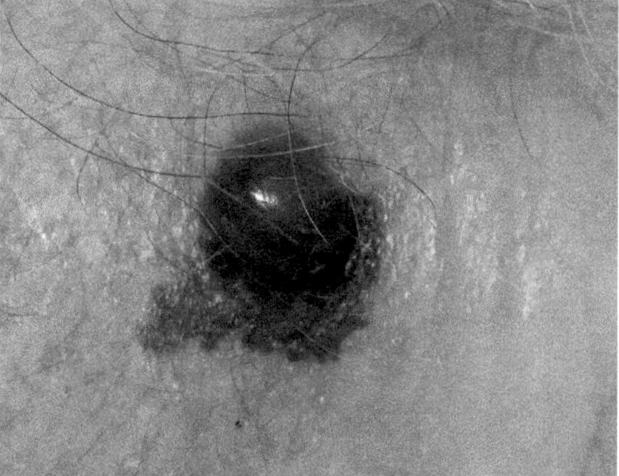

FIGURE 3.26 Lentigo maligna at an advanced stage will develop an elevated or nodular component, similar to other melanoma subtypes.

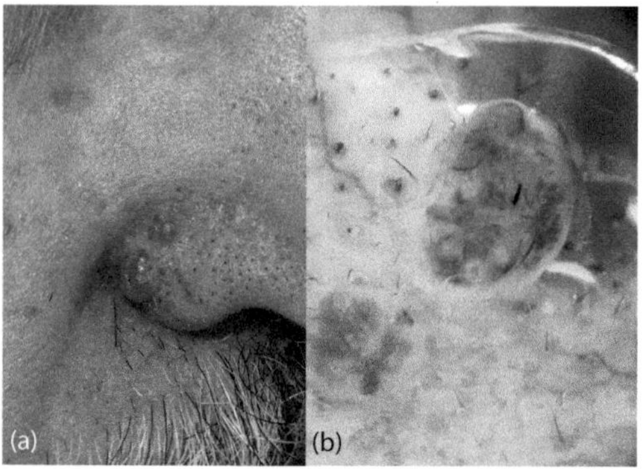

FIGURE 3.27 Nevi on the face of elderly individuals are mainly dermal and elevated (a). Dermatoscopically, they display remnants of pigmented globules and comma vessels (b).

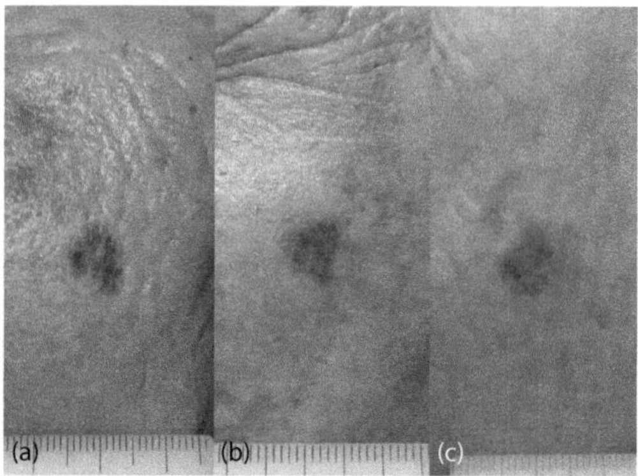

FIGURE 3.28 The differential diagnosis of a flat pigmented facial macule includes lentigo maligna (a), pigmented actinic keratosis (b), and solar lentigo/seborrheic keratosis (c).

Dermatoscopic Features

Facial melanoma is almost always of LM subtype and displays different dermatoscopic characteristics, as compared to the conventional melanoma of the trunk. The most substantial morphological difference is that melanocytic proliferations on the face (both benign and malignant) do not result in a dermatoscopic pigment network because of the relatively flattened dermo-epidermal junction of the facial skin. Instead, junctional melanocytic proliferations on the face are dermatoscopically seen as structureless diffuse brown pigmentation, interrupted by numerous, variably broad hypopigmented holes, which correspond to hair follicles and sweat gland openings. The latter dermatoscopic pattern, which is known by the term *pseudonetwork*, is highly unspecific, since it can be seen in nevi, melanoma, and nonmelanocytic tumors (Figure 3.29).

Several dermatoscopic criteria have been suggested to characterize LM. A dermatoscopic progression model was described several years ago, introducing four main criteria of LM that appear sequentially as the tumor progresses: gray dots, gray globules, asymmetric follicular openings, and rhomboidal structures (Figure 3.30). At a later stage, the pigmentation obliterates

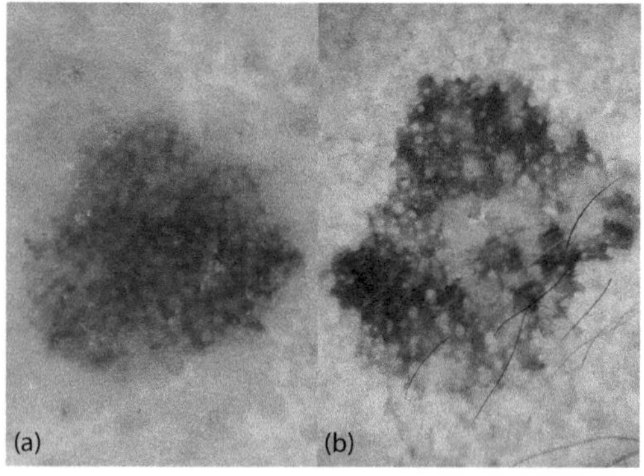

FIGURE 3.29 Pseudonetwork: brown homogenous pigmentation interrupted by nonpigmented follicular openings. It is found in melanocytic lesions as lentigo maligna (a), as well as in nonmelanocytic-like seborrheic keratosis (b).

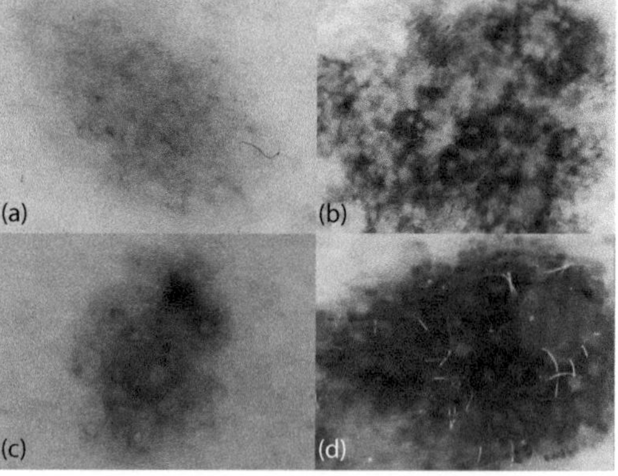

FIGURE 3.30 The four main criteria of LM that appear sequentially as the tumor progresses: gray dots (a), gray globules (b), asymmetric follicular openings (c), and rhomboidal structures (d).

the follicular openings, while blue color and atypical vessels can be seen in advanced tumors (Figure 3.31). More recently, the detection of gray circles surrounding the follicular openings has been suggested as a specific clue of LM, while the presence of gray color (irrespective of the corresponding structure) has been assessed as the most frequent dermatoscopic criterion of LM (Figures 3.32 and 3.33). Vascular criteria have also been described. Table 3.8 summarizes

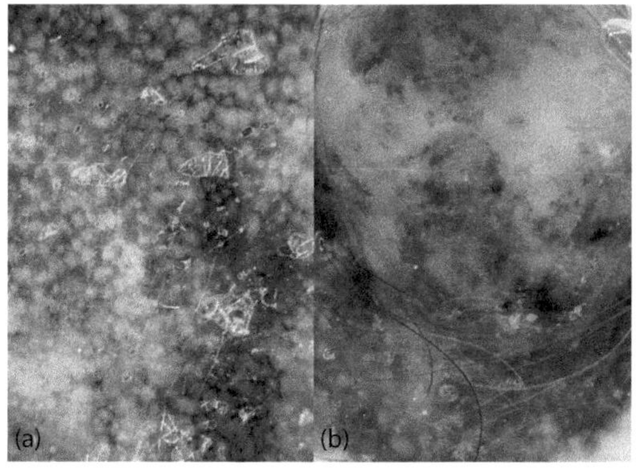

FIGURE 3.31 Advanced lentigo maligna: multiple rhomboid structures obliterating follicular openings (a) and blue color and atypical vessels in the nodular part of the lesion (b).

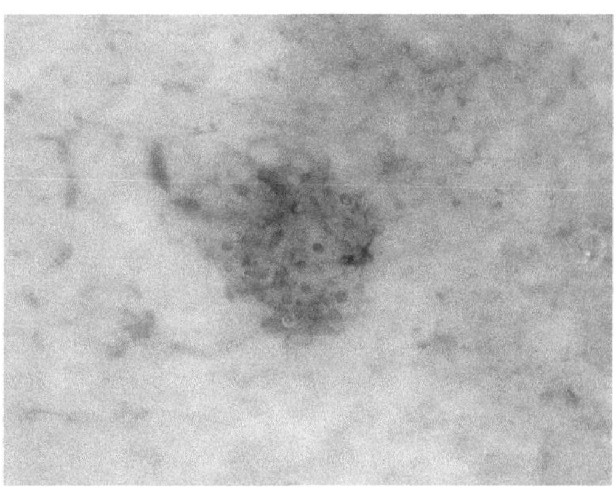

FIGURE 3.32 Gray follicular circles represent the most specific dermatoscopic sign of lentigo maligna.

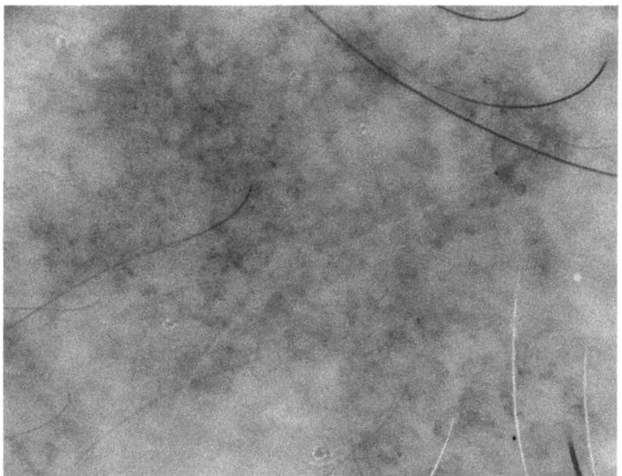

FIGURE 3.33 Gray color, in the form of dots, globules, circles, streaks, or polygons, represents the most frequent dermatoscopic sign of lentigo maligna.

TABLE 3.8

Dermoscopic Criteria for Lentigo Maligna Melanoma

Pseudonetwork	Scar-Like Hypopigmentation
Asymmetrically pigmented follicles	Whitish structures
Gray dots	Increased density of vascular network
Gray globules	Red rhomboid structures
Rhomboid structures	Target-like structures
Granular pattern	Circle into circle
Black/blue homogenous areas	Gray circles

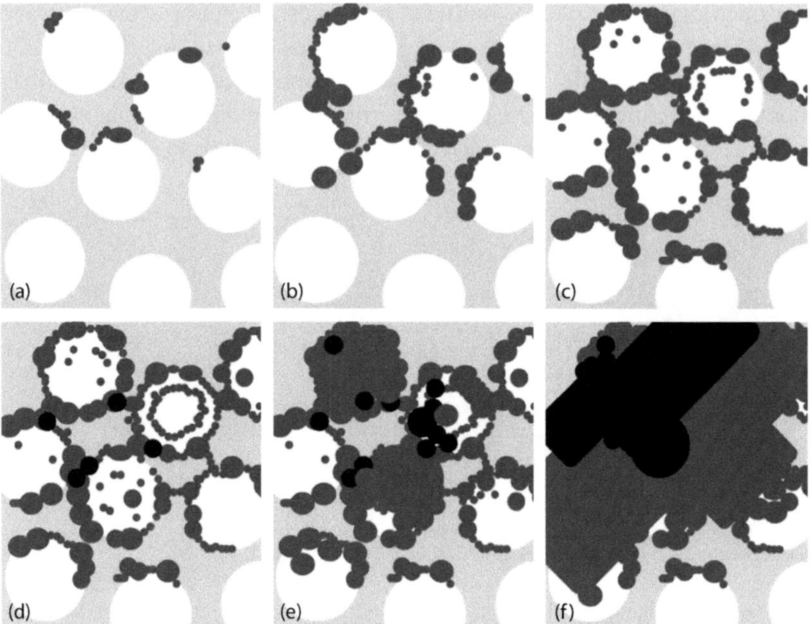

FIGURE 3.34 The dermatoscopic progression model of lentigo maligna: (a) gray dots and globules surrounding follicular openings, (b) semicircles in the outlines of follicular openings, (c) gray follicular circles and rhomboidal structures, (d) "circle within a circle," (e) obliteration of follicular openings, (f) diffuse gray and black pigmentation.

the numerous features that have been reported to characterize LM, and Figure 3.34 shows how these criteria sequentially appear with the tumor progression.

As mentioned, facial melanoma has to be differentiated mainly from nonmelanocytic lesions rather than nevi. This represents one of the most challenging differential diagnoses in clinical practice and includes melanoma, PAK, and SL/SK. With the addition of dermatoscopy, the discrimination between LM and SL/SK is usually feasible, mainly based on the characteristic features of the latter (Figure 3.35). In contrast, PAK may display virtually all the criteria of LM, rendering the differential diagnosis between the two entities highly problematic (Figure 3.36). The differential diagnostic approach for pigmented facial macules is separately discussed in the last chapter of the book.

3.1.3 Acral Melanoma

Acral melanoma (AM) is the most common subtype of melanoma in dark-skin and Asian populations. This, however, is related to the fact that other melanoma subtypes are not so frequent in these populations, while the absolute incidence of AM is similar among all races. AM has long been associated with a worse prognosis compared to other melanoma subtypes, but recent data highlighted that this is rather a result of delayed diagnosis than indicative of more aggressive biological behavior. AM develops much more frequently on the soles, as compared to the palms.

Early AM clinically develops as a pigmented flat lesion with variable shades of brown or black color. Initially, thc lesion might be uniform in color and regularly shaped, but as gradually enlarging at a diameter more than 6–7 mm, acquires an irregular shape and multiple colors

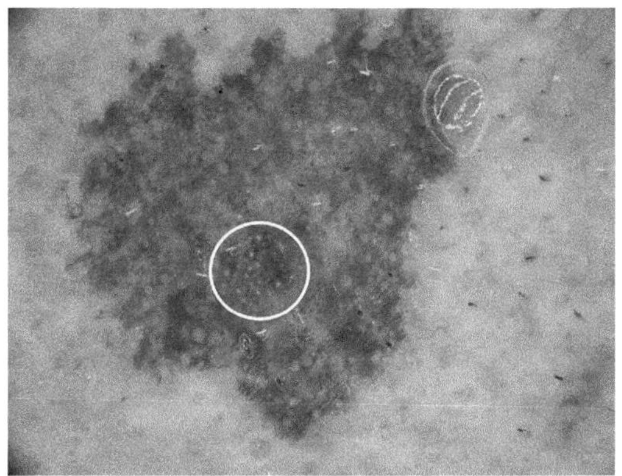

FIGURE 3.35 A seborrheic keratosis dermatoscopically displaying milia-like cysts (circle) and fingerprint-like structures at the periphery.

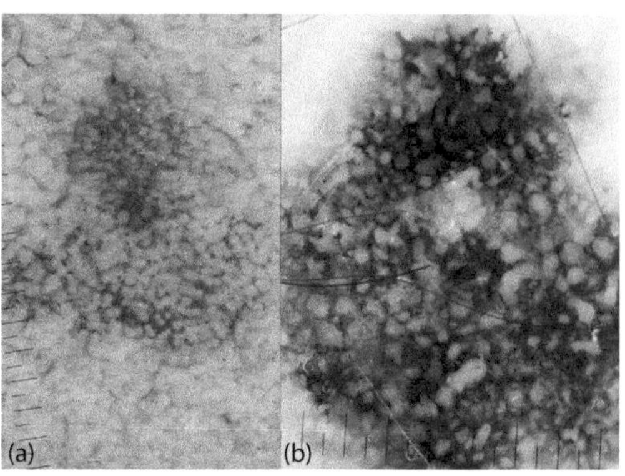

FIGURE 3.36 Pigmented actinic keratoses share similar dermatoscopic findings with lentigo maligna, such as gray dots on the follicular outline (a) and asymmetrically pigmented follicles and rhomboidal structures (b).

(Figure 3.37). At the time of diagnosis, the diameter of AM is usually 9 mm or more. More advanced tumors might develop a papular or nodular component, ulcerate, or bleed (Figure 3.38).

The main differential diagnosis of AM is acral nevi, which also develop as pigmented macules. However, nevi typically remain smaller, with a diameter not exceeding 7 mm, and are characterized by a uniform light brown, dark brown, or black color and a regular shape (Figure 3.39). Subungual hemorrhage is also included in the differential diagnosis of AM but usually can be recognized based on its sharp demarcation and by scratching the epidermal surface (Figure 3.40). Finally, several misdiagnosed advanced AM have long been treated as viral warts or diabetic ulcers (Figure 3.41).

Dermatoscopic Features

From a dermatoscopic aspect, AM deviates the criteria of melanoma of the trunk, and this is explained by the characteristic anatomy of the acral skin, which is characterized by

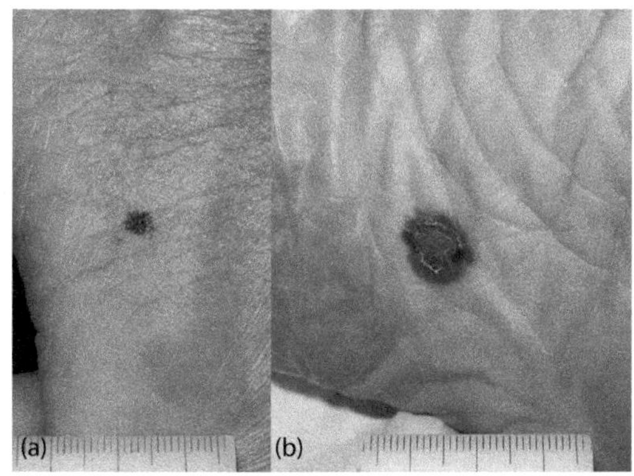

FIGURE 3.37 An early plantar melanoma manifesting as a small homogenous brown macule (a) and a more advanced palmar melanoma displaying an irregular border and multiple colors (b).

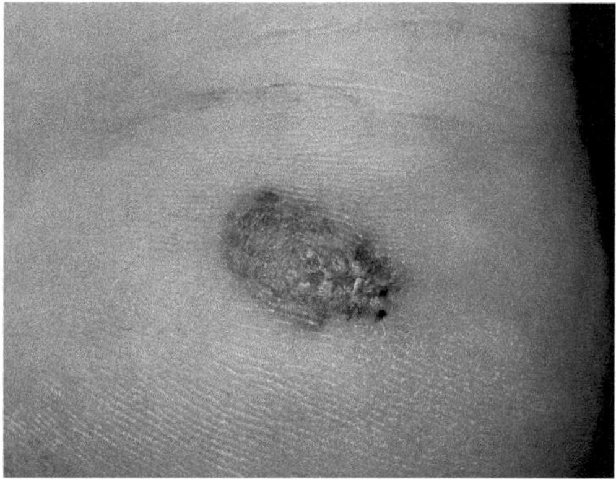

FIGURE 3.38 An advanced palmar melanoma characterized by the development of a nodular part, ulceration, and hemorrhage.

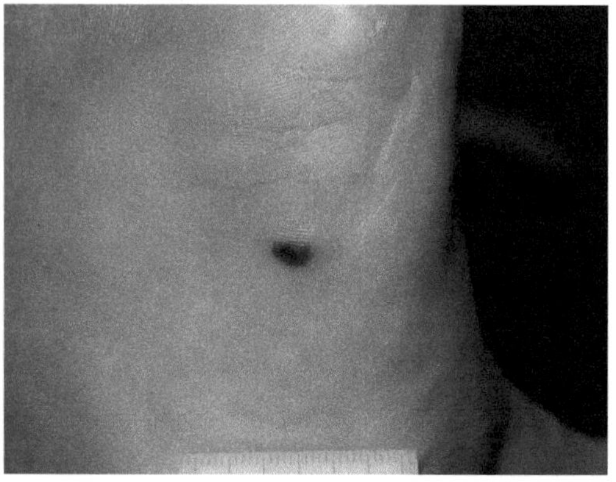

FIGURE 3.39 A palmar nevus with a maximum diameter of 5 mm and morphological symmetry.

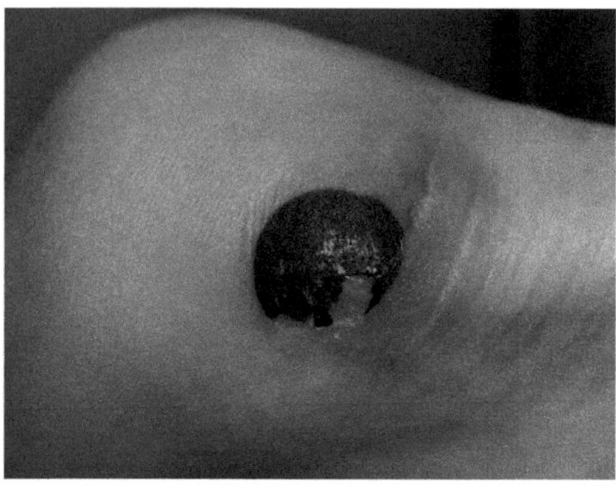

FIGURE 3.40 The most specific sign of subungual hemorrhage is the sharp demarcation at the periphery. Mechanical removal of the stratum corneum often enhances the diagnosis.

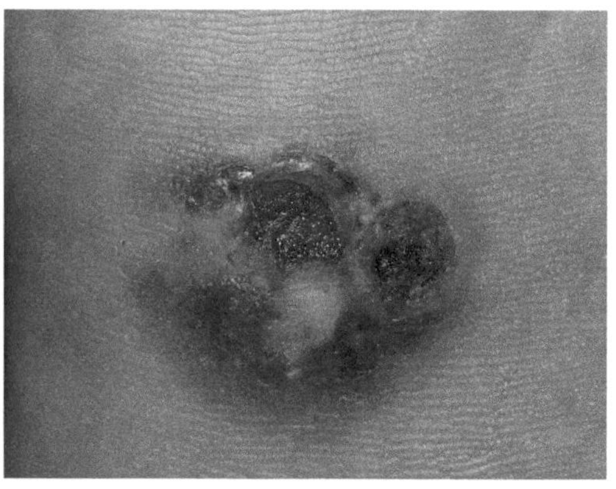

FIGURE 3.41 Advanced plantar melanoma that had been treated as a plantar wart.

FIGURE 3.42 The normal skin of palms and soles as seen under the dermatoscope, with the typical alternating parallel ridges and furrows. The sweat gland openings on the ridges can also be seen.

marked orthokeratosis and the presence of skin markings, namely, parallel furrows and ridges (Figure 3.42). Accordingly, melanocytic proliferations on the acral skin do not dermatoscopically display a pigment network but an accentuation of the pigmentation along these parallel skin markings (pattern of parallel lines).

Dermatoscopy might be very useful for the discrimination between AM and acral nevi, since in AM the pigmentation is distributed on the dermal ridges (parallel ridge pattern [PRP]), whereas in nevi it is accentuated along the epidermal furrows (parallel furrow pattern [PFP]) (Figure 3.43). As analytically described in Chapter 2, plantar nevi may exhibit several variations of the PFP (fibrillar pattern, lattice-like pattern, double-line pattern), depending on the precise localization of the nevus on the sole (Figures 3.44 through 3.47). The discrimination between ridges and furrows is usually feasible since ridges are much broader than furrows and by the visualization of the openings of the sweat glands on the ridges. In heavily pigmented tumors, it might be difficult to assess whether the pigmentation follows the ridges or the furrows, but this is often clarified by focusing on the peripheral parts of the lesion (Figure 3.48).

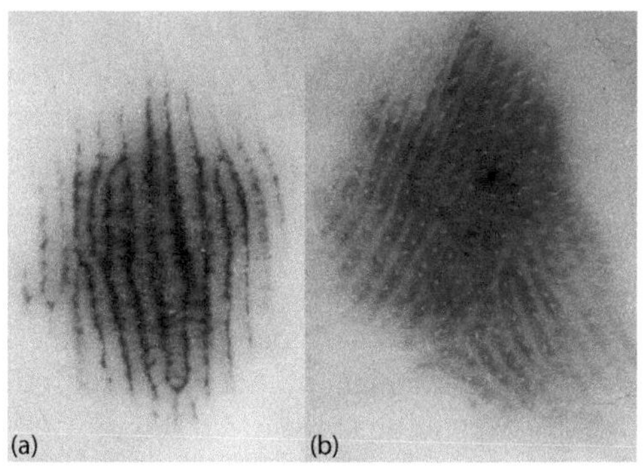

FIGURE 3.43 The parallel furrow pattern of an acral nevus (a), and the parallel ridge pattern of acral melanoma (b).

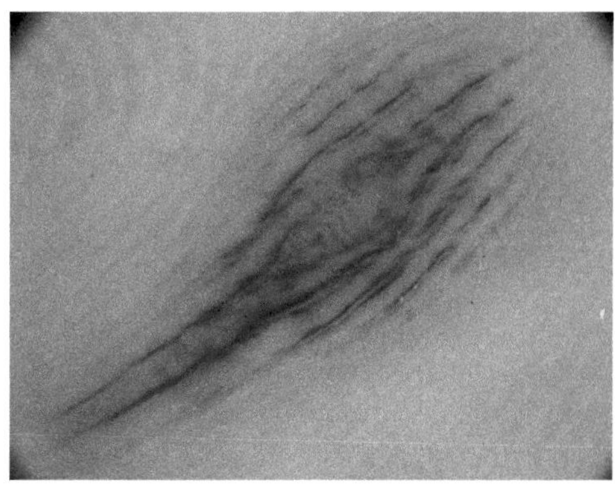

FIGURE 3.44 Acral nevus. The "double-line pattern" is a common variant of the parallel furrow pattern, and it is characterized by the presence of two parallel pigment lines in each furrow.

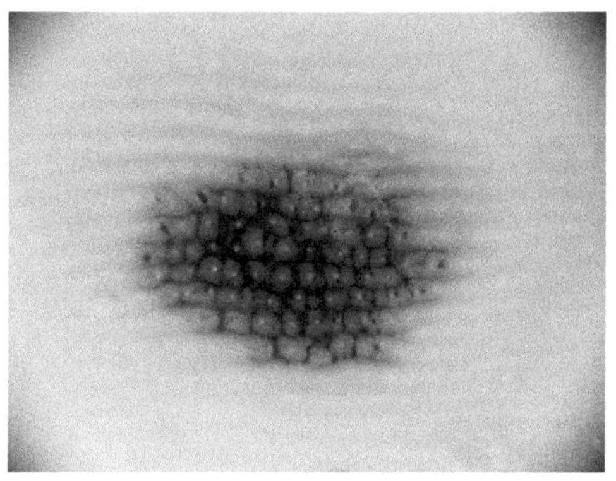

FIGURE 3.45 Acral nevus. The "lattice-like pattern" is characterized by the combination of parallel pigment lines across the furrows and, additionally, vertical pigment lines on the ridges.

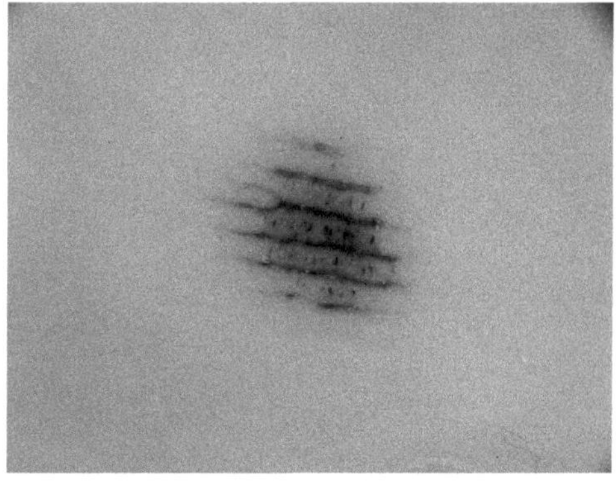

FIGURE 3.46 Acral nevus. The "peas-in-a-pod pattern" combines parallel pigment lines across the furrows with brown globules inside the sweat glands openings on the ridges. This pattern is highly suggestive of congenital nevi.

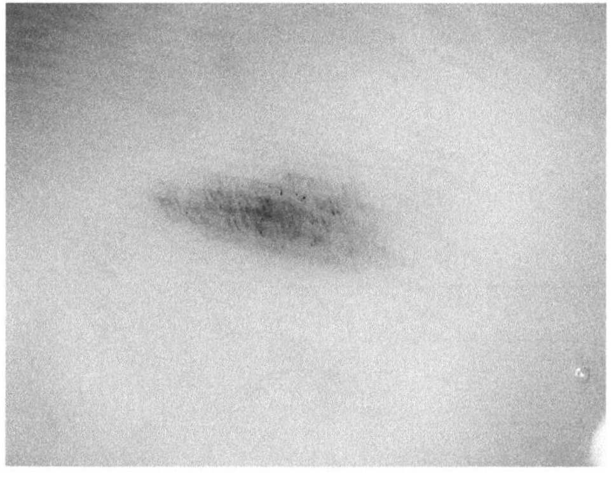

FIGURE 3.47 Acral nevus. The "fibrillar pattern" consists of parallel pigment lines oriented perpendicularly to the furrows and the ridges. This pattern is seen in weight-bearing areas of the sole.

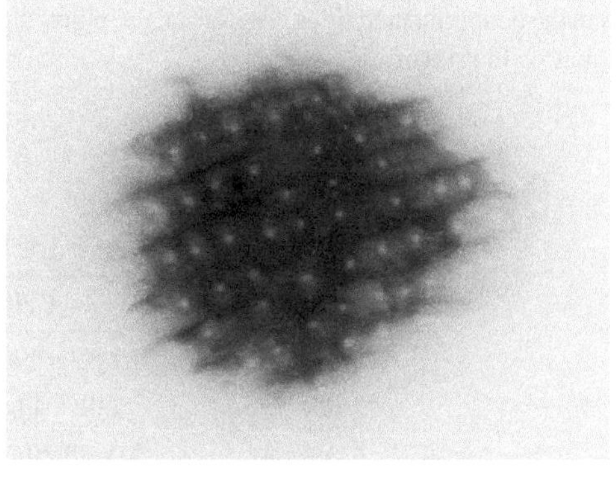

FIGURE 3.48 Acral nevus. In heavily pigmented nevi, the evaluation of the peripheral part will possibly reveal the tendency of the pigmentation to follow the furrows.

Although PRP represents a highly specific melanoma pattern, several AMs lack this criterion (Figures 3.49 and 3.50). In order not to miss these melanomas, a more global morphological assessment should be applied, considering several additional criteria that have been summarized in a recently introduced algorithm (BRAAFF checklist, Table 3.9) (Figures 3.51 through 3.55).

3.1.4 Subungual Melanoma

Nail or subungual melanoma originates from melanocytes of the nail matrix and clinically develops as a pigmented nail band (longitudinal melanonychia or melanonychia striata), initially appearing at the proximal nail fold and gradually linearly expanding to the distal (Figure 3.56). At an early stage, a thin linear band of light brown, dark brown, or black color develops. With progression, the band increases in thickness and loses the uniform hue, developing sequential bands of different shades of brown or black color. A useful clinical characteristic is the triangular shape that the band gradually acquires, with its basis (thicker part) on the proximal fold and its top (thinner part) on the distal, reflecting the rapid growth of the melanoma of the nail matrix. As the tumor grows, it may cover all the surface of the nail bed and might also affect the nail plate, causing onychodystrophy, while advanced tumors may also ulcerate or bleed

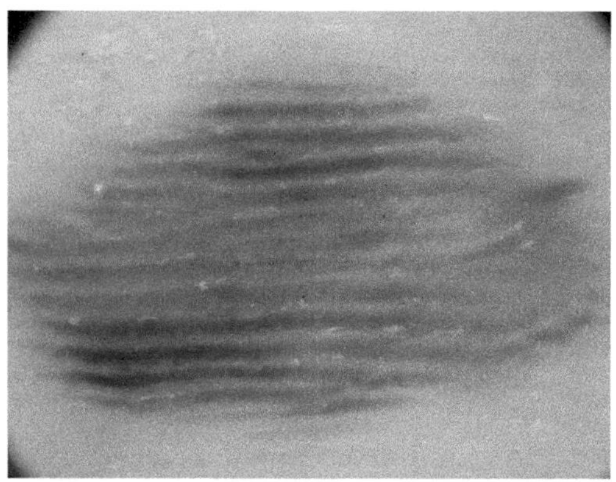

FIGURE 3.49 Parallel ridge pattern in acral melanoma. The brown-colored pigment lines are thicker than the nonpigmented lines. Therefore, the pigmentation is on the ridges.

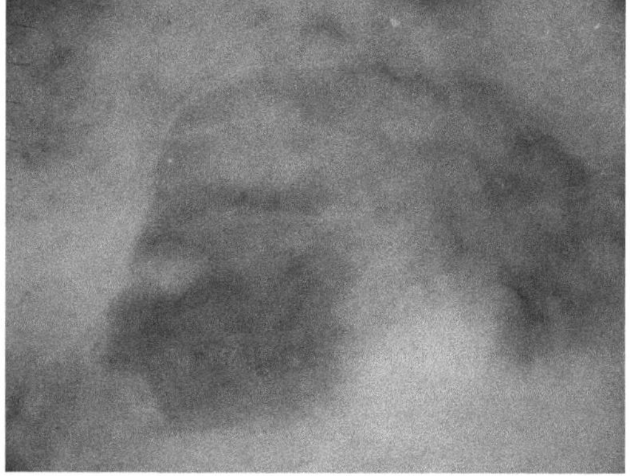

FIGURE 3.50 Melanoma of the soles lacking a parallel ridge pattern. Dotted vessels and brown pigmentation with an unspecific distribution are seen.

TABLE 3.9

Algorithm BRAAFF for Diagnosis of Acral Melanoma

	Criterion	Points
B	Irregular blotch	+1
R	Parallel ridge pattern	+3
A	Asymmetry of structures	+1
A	Asymmetry of colors	+1
F	Parallel furrow pattern	−1
F	Fibrillar pattern	−1

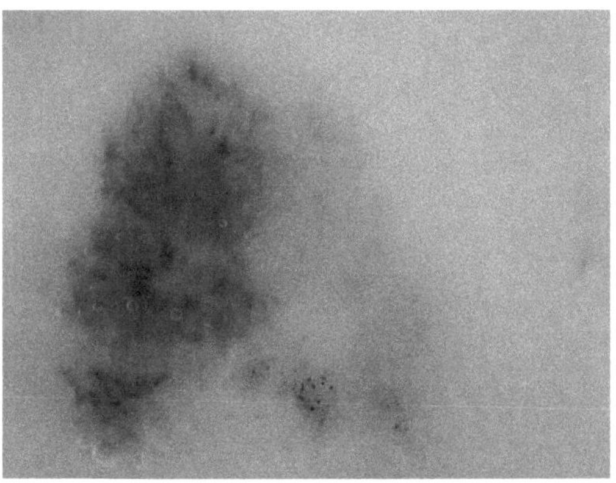

FIGURE 3.51 A melanoma that does not display a parallel ridge pattern but can be detected using the BRAAFF algorithm, due to the asymmetry of colors and structures.

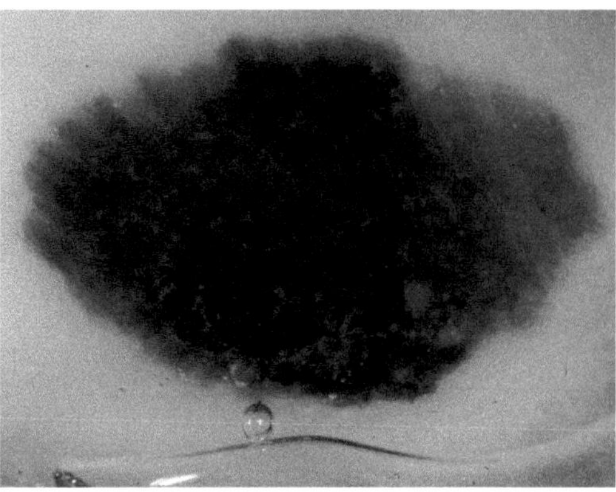

FIGURE 3.52 A melanoma that lacks a parallel ridge pattern but can be detected by the BRAAFF algorithm, due to the presence of an eccentric hyperpigmented blotch.

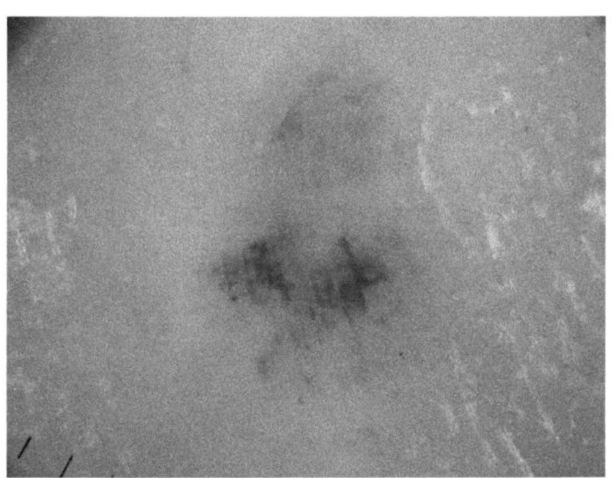

FIGURE 3.53 Another melanoma without a parallel ridge pattern. Again, it can be diagnosed using the BRAAFF algorithm, due to the asymmetry of colors.

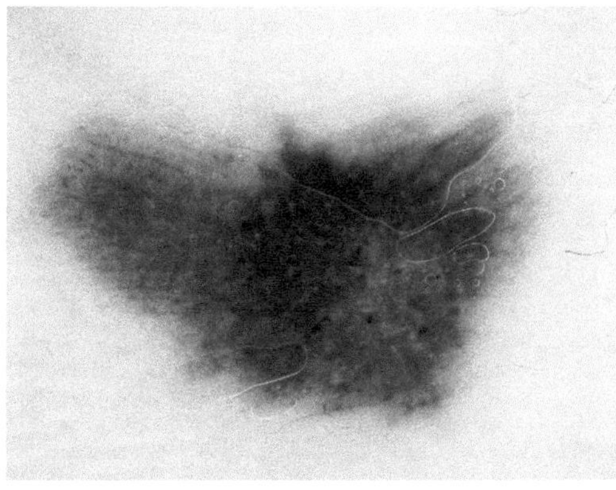

FIGURE 3.54 Plantar melanoma. The detection of pigmentation on the furrows at the periphery of the lesion may lead to misdiagnosis of acral nevus. However, using the BRAAFF algorithm, the asymmetry of the structures and the presence of an eccentric irregular blotch suggest the diagnosis of melanoma.

(Figures 3.57 and 3.58). Not infrequently, nail melanoma expands to the surrounding skin, with the affected cutaneous areas acquiring the characteristics of acral melanoma. The involvement of the proximal nail fold is also known as the "Hutchinson sign" (Figure 3.59).

The differential diagnosis of nail melanoma is mainly composed of subungual nevi, subungual hemorrhage, subungual lentigo, and reactive pigmentation after infection or trauma. Longitudinal melanonychia might also be drug induced or appear in the course of some syndromes, but in the latter scenarios, it will affect more than one nail (Figure 3.60). Nevi also present as longitudinal melanonychia, but they typically develop earlier in life, remain uniform in color, and do not usually cover large parts of the nail plate (Figure 3.61). Congenital nevi represent an exception, since they may cover all the surface of the nail bed and also expand to the surrounding skin (Figure 3.62).

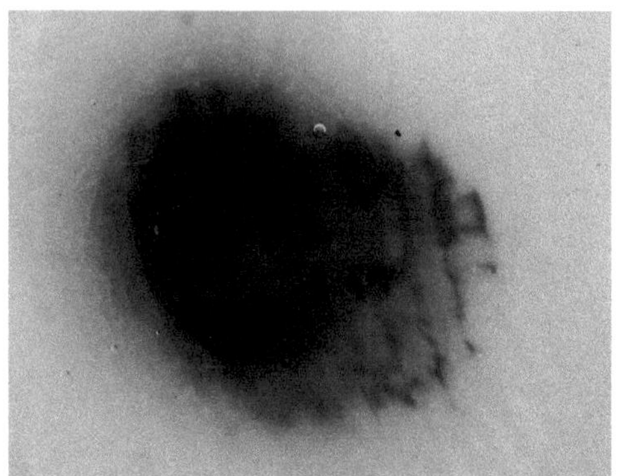

FIGURE 3.55 Plantar melanoma. On the right side of the lesion, a parallel furrow pattern can be seen. However, the evaluation of the lesion using the BRAAFF algorithm reveals asymmetry of structures and an eccentric irregular blotch, suggesting the diagnosis of melanoma.

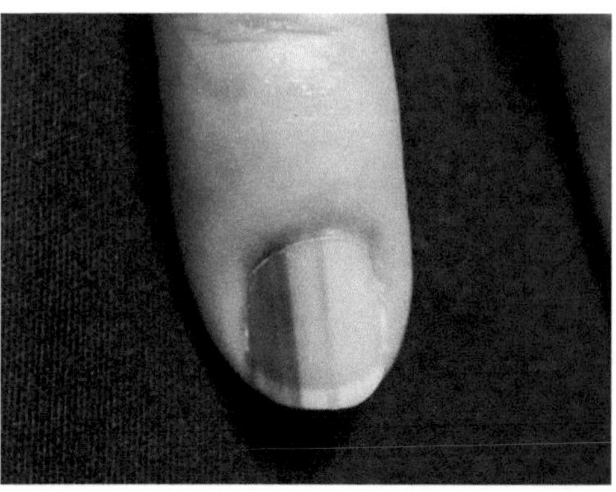

FIGURE 3.56 Longitudinal melanonychia always arises from the proximal nail fold and gradually linearly expands to the distal nailfold.

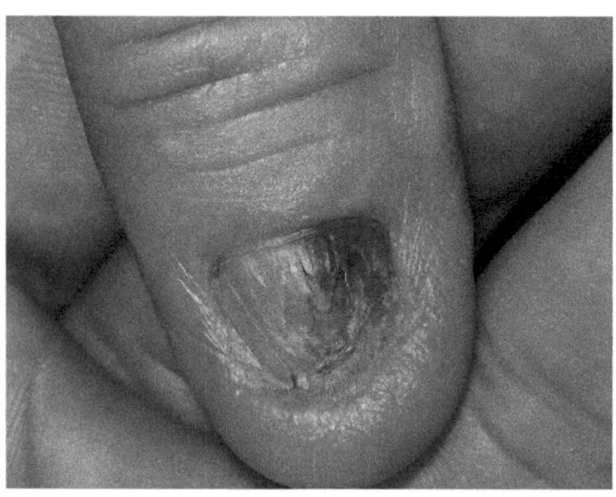

FIGURE 3.57 Onychodystrophia as a result of nail matrix melanoma.

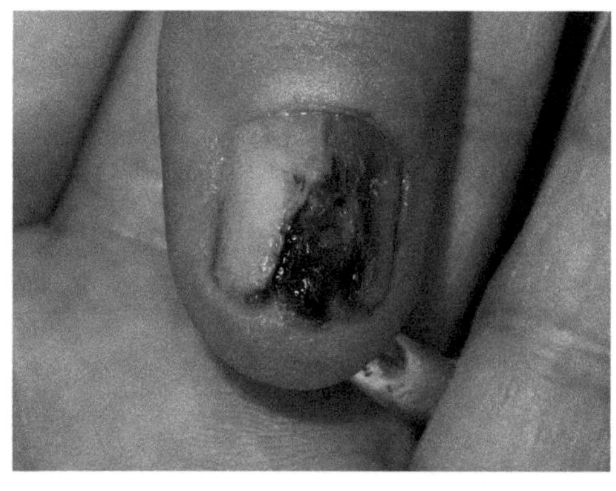

FIGURE 3.58 An advanced melanoma originating from the nail matrix but now expanding to the nail bed, ulcerating, and bleeding.

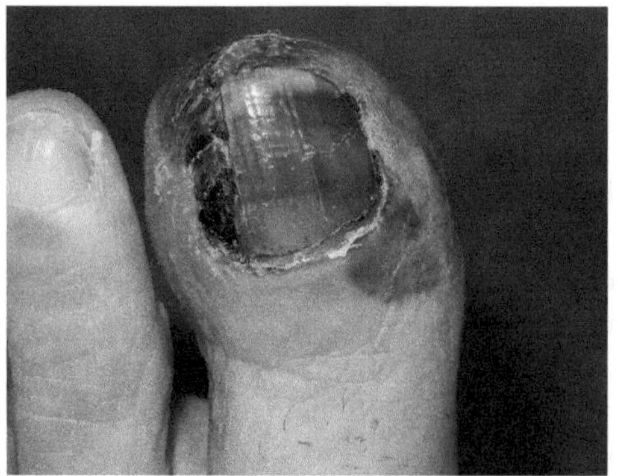

FIGURE 3.59 An advanced melanoma originating from the nail matrix and expanding to the nail bed and the surrounding skin (Hutchinson sign).

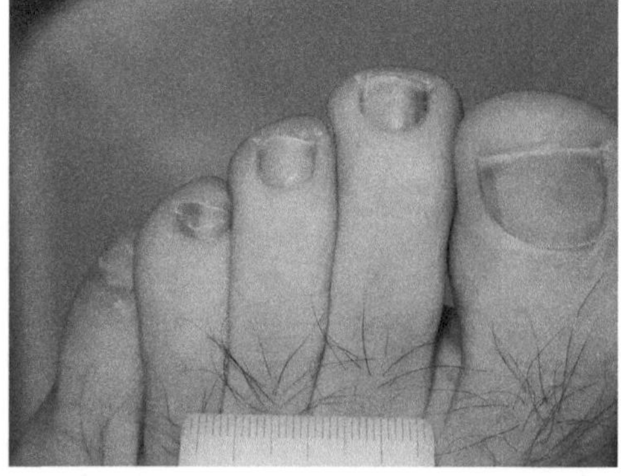

FIGURE 3.60 A drug-induced melanonychia. The fact that two or more nails are affected is highly suggestive of a systemic cause and practically excludes melanoma.

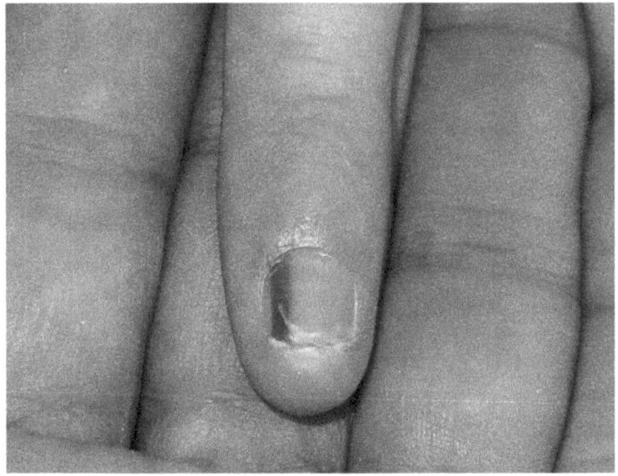

FIGURE 3.61 A nevus of the nail matrix shown projecting as a longitudinal melanonychia that covers less than one-third of the nail plate.

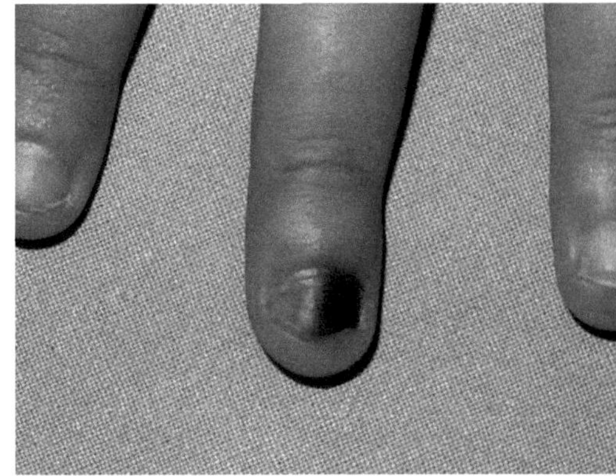

FIGURE 3.62 A congenital subungual nevus covering more than two-thirds of the nail plate.

Dermatoscopic Features

When evaluating dermatoscopically a pigmented nail band, the first task is to determine whether the pigmentation is of melanocytic origin. In melanocytic tumors, the color of the nail band is light or dark brown. The detection of small brown dots or globules along the band also strongly favors a melanocytic tumor. In contrast, subungual lentigo and reactive pigmentation are typified by a gray color of the nail band (Figure 3.63). Subungual hemorrhage is ideally red in color, but longer-standing hemorrhages may dermatoscopically project as brown or black (Figures 3.64 and 3.65). However, most hemorrhages can be recognized by the sharp demarcation of the borders and the presence of satellite blood spots (Figures 3.65 and 3.66). Recognition of a subungual hemorrhage is even easier when it does not arise from the proximal nailfold (Figures 3.67 and 3.68).

If the lesion is assessed as melanocytic, the discrimination between nevus and melanoma is based on the careful dermatoscopic evaluation of the nail band. In nevi, the band consists

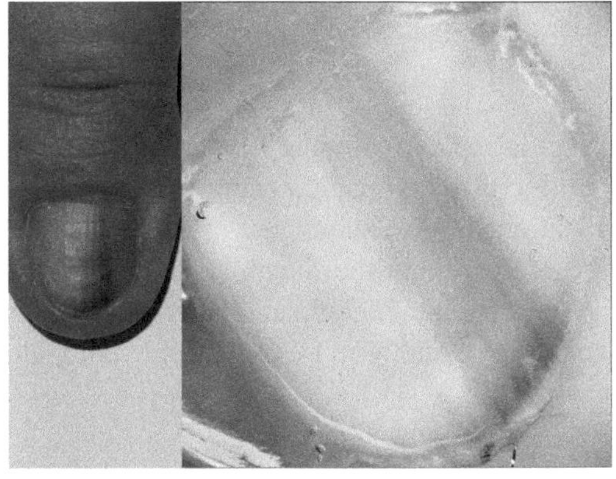

FIGURE 3.63 Gray color of the nail band in dermatoscopy indicates reactive pigmentation or subungual lentigo, minimizing the possibility of a melanocytic tumor.

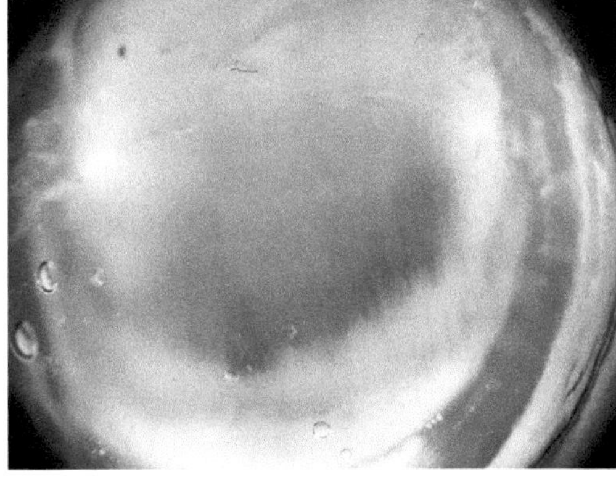

FIGURE 3.64 Subungual hemorrhage: the red color in dermatoscopy enhances the accurate evaluation of the lesion.

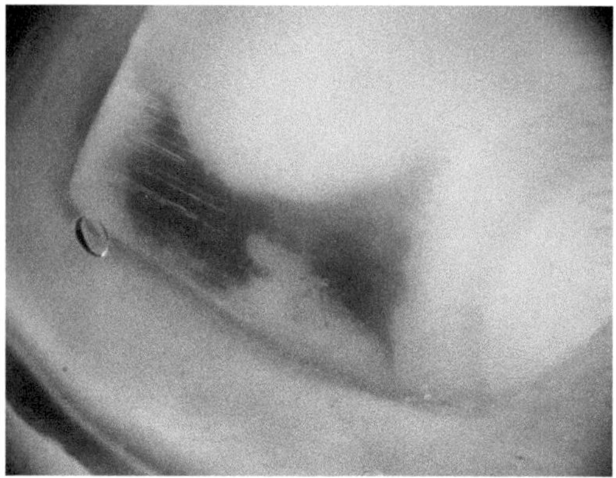

FIGURE 3.65 Subungual hemorrhage. In some parts of the lesion, the color is black, but its sharp demarcation allows for recognition of the hemorrhage.

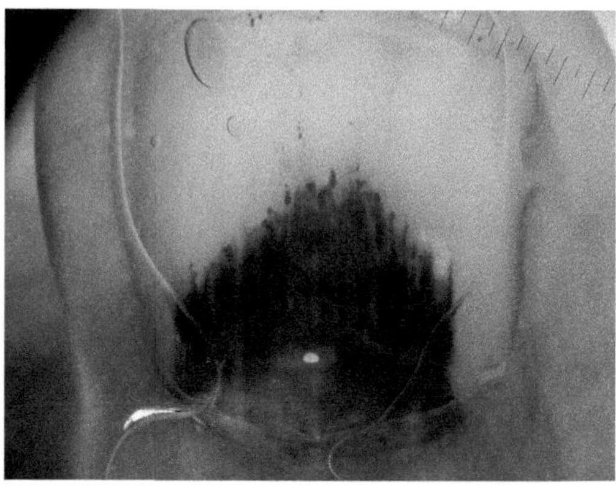

FIGURE 3.66 Subungual hemorrhage. The red globules in the periphery of the lesion are highly indicative of subungual hemorrhage.

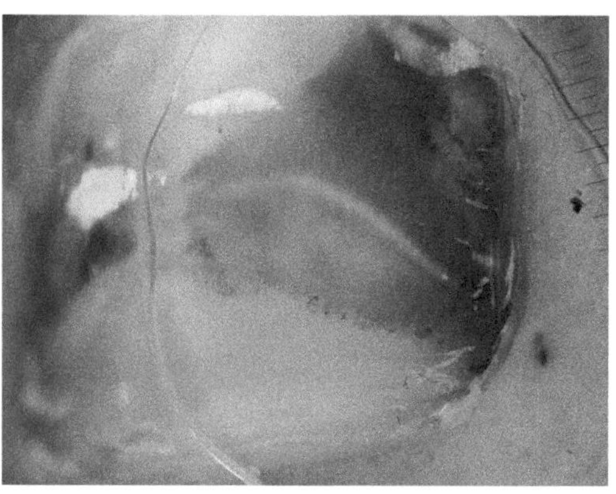

FIGURE 3.67 A subungual hemorrhage that can be easily recognized because of the red color and the fact that it does not arise from the proximal nail fold.

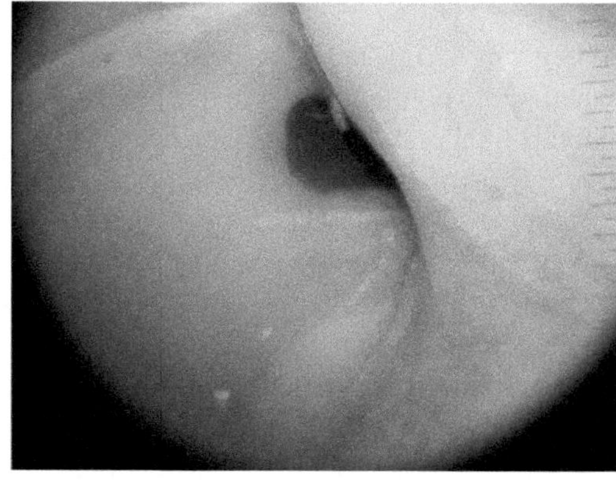

FIGURE 3.68 Subungual hemorrhage: the black color may be misleading, but the fact that the lesion does not arise from the proximal nail fold is highly indicative of subungual hemorrhage.

of parallel thin lines of similar brown hue with regular spacing among them (Figure 3.69). In contrast, the parallel lines in melanoma vary in the intensity of pigmentation and in their thickness and spacing (Figure 3.70). It has to be mentioned that a subungual melanoma might bleed; therefore, the detection of hemorrhage does not exclude the diagnosis of melanoma (Figure 3.71). Furthermore, the pigmented band caused by subungual melanoma is much wider as compared to nevi (with the exception of congenital nevi) and might cover all the nail plate and expand to the surrounding skin (Figure 3.72).

3.1.5 Mucosal Melanoma

Primary melanoma of the mucous membranes is a rare condition and may affect the lips, the gingiva or palate, the nasal mucosa, the vulva, or the glans penis. Although these melanomas also begin as flat pigmented macules, they are often diagnosed at a late stage when they become

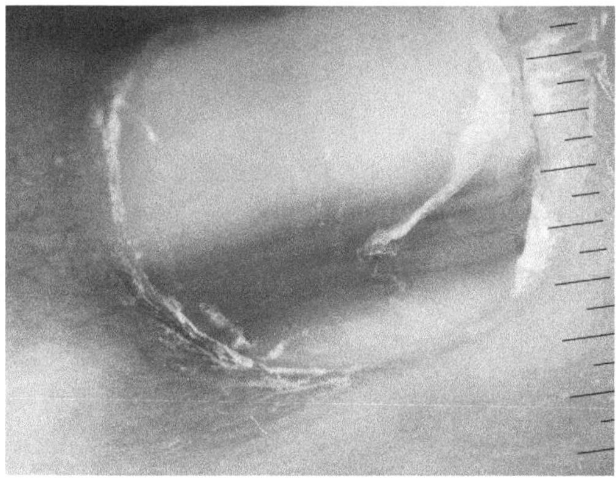

FIGURE 3.69 Subungual nevus. Dermatoscopically, the pigmented band consists of parallel thin lines uniform in color and thickness.

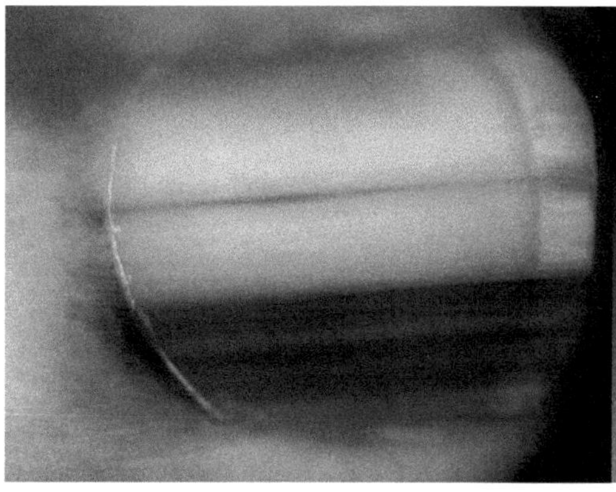

FIGURE 3.70 Subungual melanoma. Dermatoscopically, the parallel lines are characterized by asymmetry in the intensity of pigmentation, thickness, and distance between them.

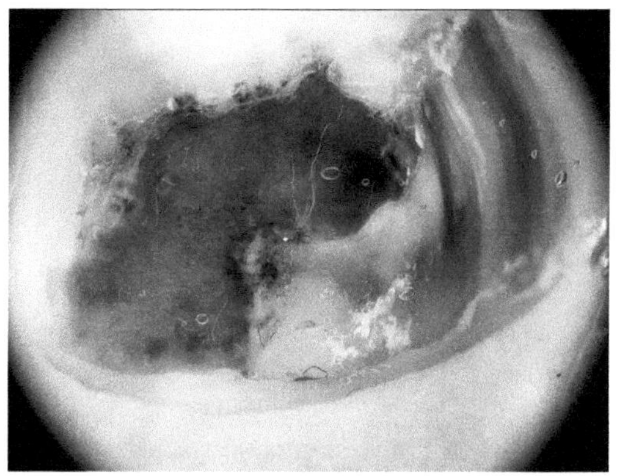

FIGURE 3.71 Subungual melanoma, especially in advanced stages, may bleed. So, the detection of hemorrhage does not exclude a melanoma. In the right side of the lesion, the irregular longitudinal melanonychia can be seen.

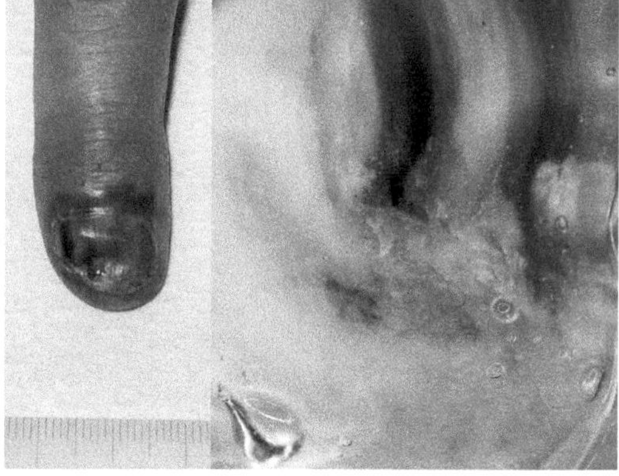

FIGURE 3.72 A subungual melanoma covering all the surface of the nail bed and expanding to the surrounding skin. Dermatoscopy of the periungual skin reveals that the pigmentation is on the ridges.

nodular, asymmetric in shape and color, and ulcerated or bleeding. The main differential diagnoses of mucosal melanoma are the "benign melanotic macules" (melanosis) but also nevi, vascular tumors, and inflammatory and infectious diseases (Figures 3.73 through 3.75). The recognition of benign melanotic macules is based on their multifocal distribution (Figure 3.73) and is much more difficult when there is only a solitary lesion (Figure 3.74).

The dermatoscopic discrimination between melanoma and benign mucosal pigmentations is based on the evaluation of the global pattern of the lesion and the observed colors. Specifically, melanoma usually exhibits a structureless pattern, while benign tumors often exhibit a pattern of globules or lines or circles (Figures 3.76 and 3.77). Furthermore, the detection of gray, blue, or white color should raise the suspicion of melanoma, whereas nevi and benign melanotic macules show typically a light or dark brown coloration (Figures 3.78 and 3.79).

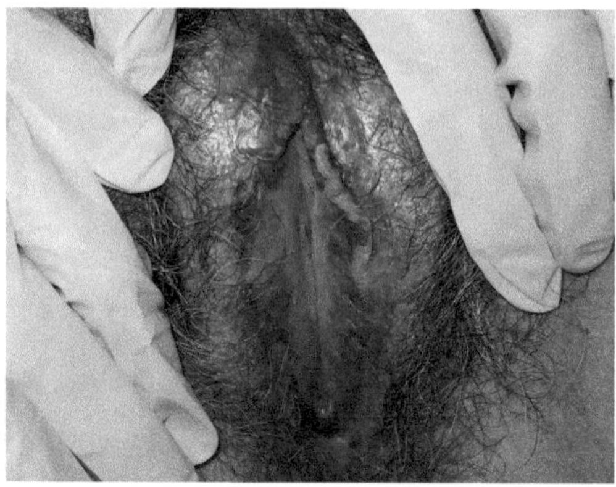

FIGURE 3.73 Melanosis of the mucosa is typically multifocal.

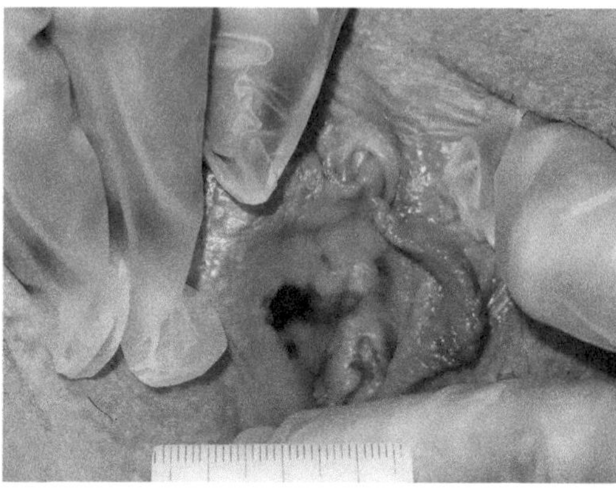

FIGURE 3.74 Benign melanosis: in this case, the clinical differential diagnosis from melanoma is challenging, because the lesion is solitary and peripherally expanding.

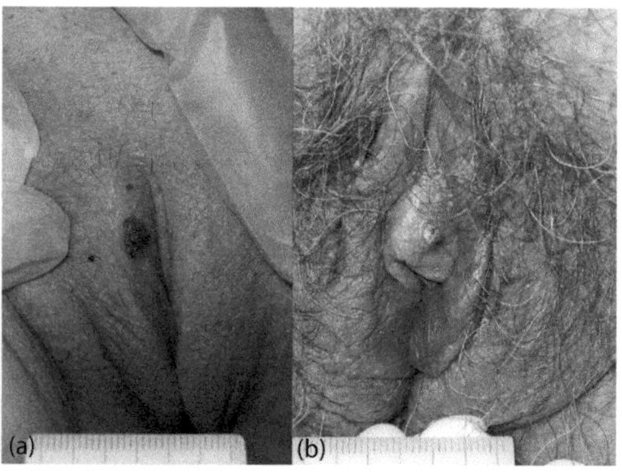

FIGURE 3.75 A nevus (a) and an angiokeratoma (b) on the genital area: both tumors are included in the differential diagnosis of melanoma.

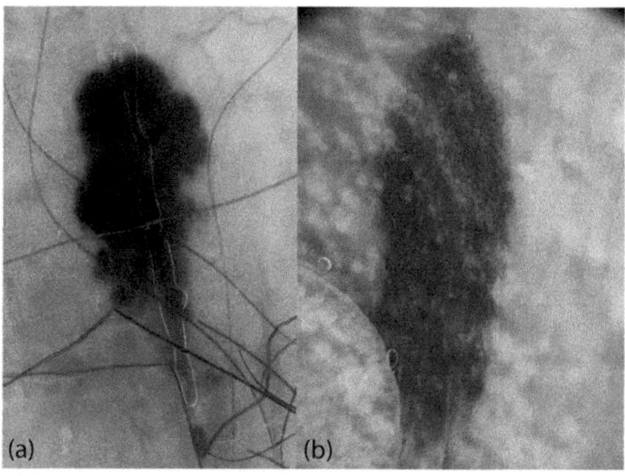

FIGURE 3.76 Most mucosal melanomas dermatoscopically display a structureless pattern (a), whereas most nevi are typified by a globular pattern (b).

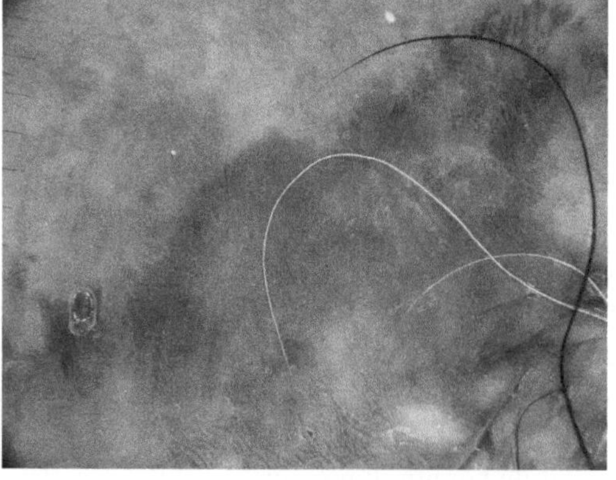

FIGURE 3.77 The parallel lines pattern practically excludes the diagnosis of melanoma and is highly indicative of benign mucosal melanosis.

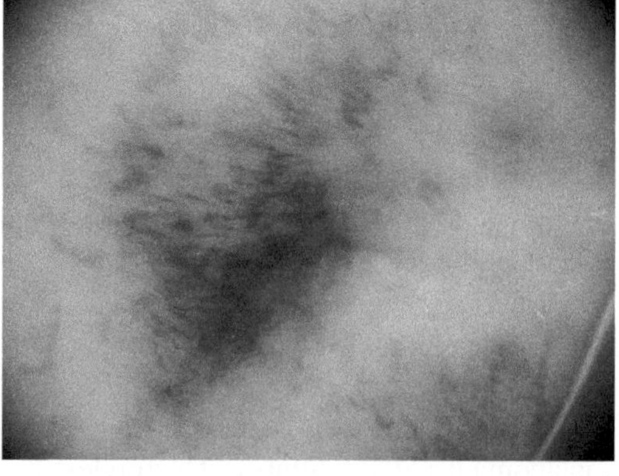

FIGURE 3.78 Melanoma in the lower lip: the dermatoscopic detection of gray color should raise the suspicion of melanoma.

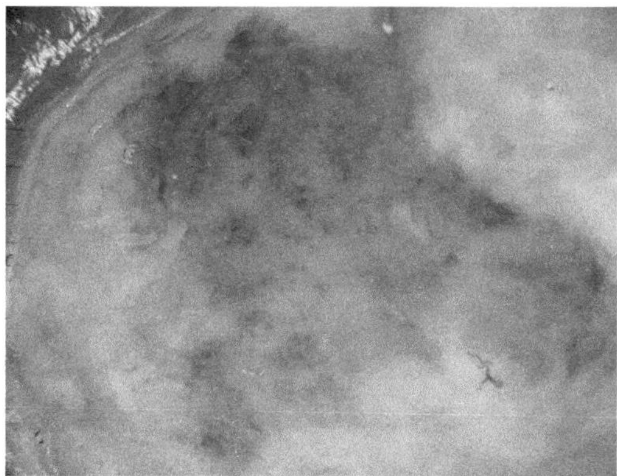

FIGURE 3.79 Benign melanosis: "parallel-line pattern" and brown color as the only color in dermatoscopy.

3.2 Nodular Melanoma

In contrast to conventional melanoma that initially develops as a flat lesion, nodular melanoma originates within the dermis and clinically appears from the very early stages as an elevated tumor with a minimal or no flat component (Figure 3.80). The small papule rapidly enlarges to become a nodule, which later might ulcerate or bleed (Figure 3.81). The most frequent anatomical sites of NM development are the head/neck area, the trunk, and the extremities, but NM may develop on any site of the body surface.

Typically, nodular melanoma is symmetric in shape, well demarcated and uniform in color, which might be black or blue or pink/red (amelanotic nodular melanoma) (Figures 3.80 through 3.83). Effectively, the ABCD clinical rule is completely inefficient for the detection of nodular melanoma. Instead, the EFG clinical criteria (elevation, firmness, growth) are more appropriate, since they reflect the three main characteristics of NM: a nodule of firm consistency that grows rapidly.

Because of its clinical characteristics described earlier, NM often escapes detection until progressing in an advanced stage (Figure 3.84). In addition, NM often develops in "low-risk"

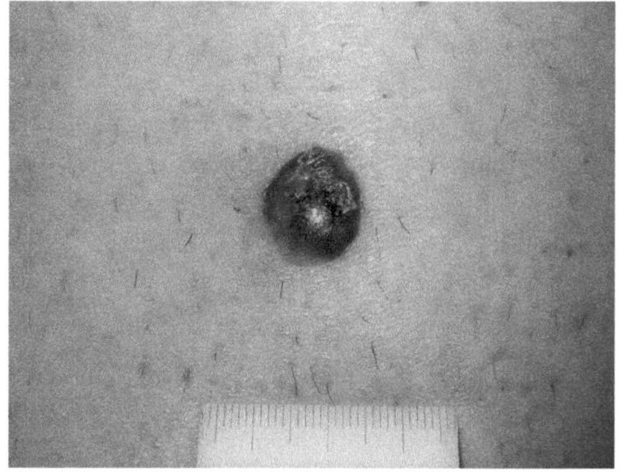

FIGURE 3.80 A nodular melanoma manifesting as a red nodule with a diameter of 1 cm.

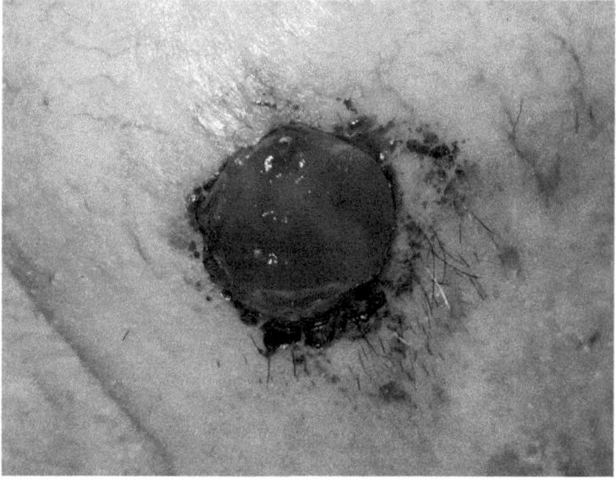

FIGURE 3.81 An advanced nodular melanoma displaying ulceration and hemorrhage.

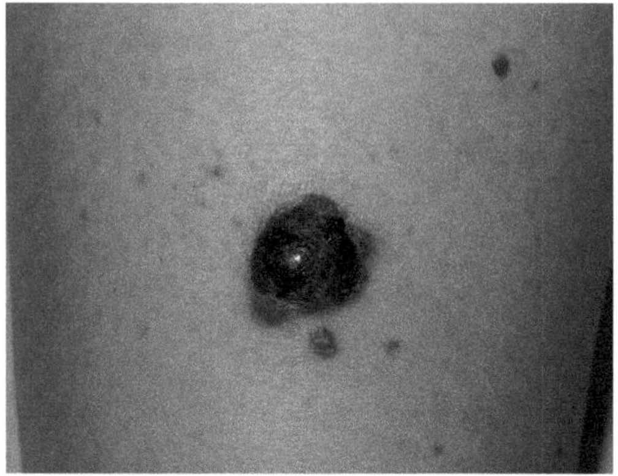

FIGURE 3.82 A nodular melanoma manifesting as a black nodule and a small satellite metastasis below.

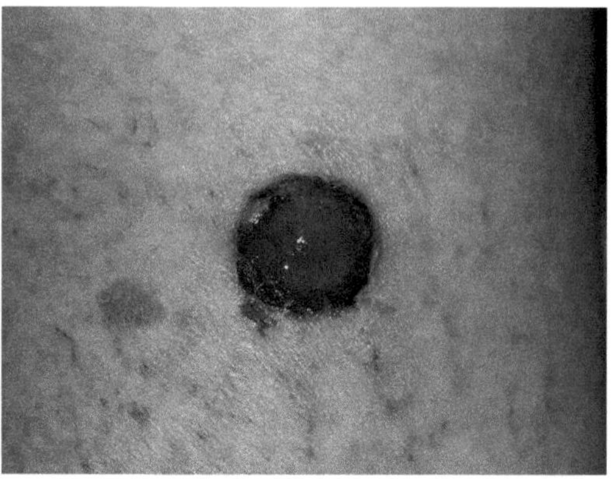

FIGURE 3.83 A nodular amelanotic melanoma with ulceration and bleeding.

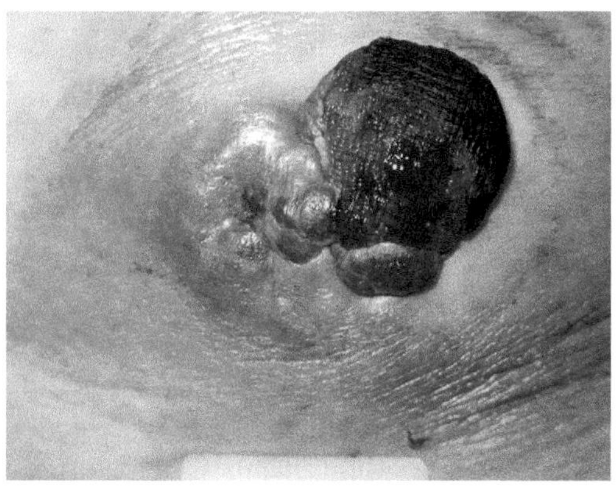

FIGURE 3.84 An advanced nodular melanoma. After surgical removal, the Breslow thickness was 14 mm.

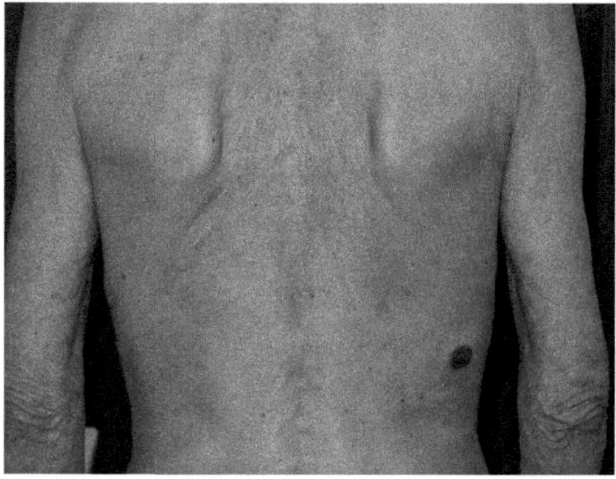

FIGURE 3.85 Nodular melanoma often develops in individuals without risk factors (i.e., with a low nevus count, without family history, etc.).

individuals (i.e., with a low nevus count, without family history, etc.), rendering its diagnosis even more problematic (Figure 3.85). The differential diagnosis of NM is broad, depends on the degree of pigmentation, and consists of dermal and blue nevus, hemangioma, pyogenic granuloma, angiokeratoma, seborrheic keratosis, and other rare neoplasms. A very rare and extremely difficult to recognize subtype is "verrucous melanoma" that might perfectly mimic benign tumors with a verrucous surface (Figure 3.86).

Dermatoscopic Features

The majority of the dermatoscopic structures of conventional melanoma cannot be seen in NM. This is because they correspond to pigment deposition at the level of the dermo-epidermal junction, while the neoplastic cells in NM are located within the dermis. In melanomas containing both a flat and a nodular component, some of the classic melanoma criteria might be present at the flat part of the tumor, significantly enhancing its recognition. In contrast, purely

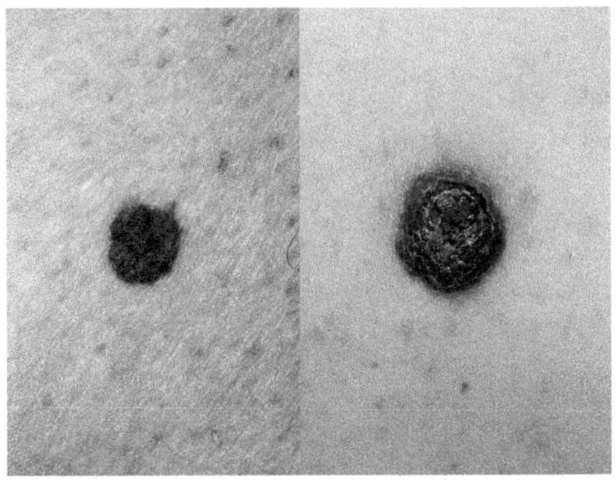

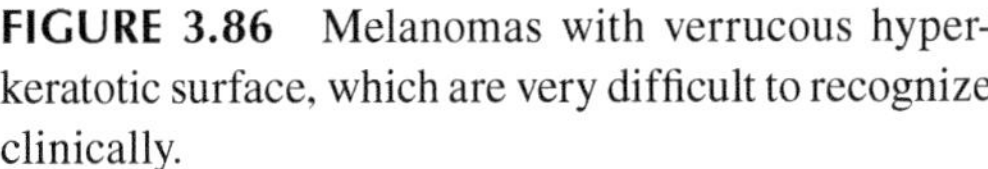

FIGURE 3.86 Melanomas with verrucous hyperkeratotic surface, which are very difficult to recognize clinically.

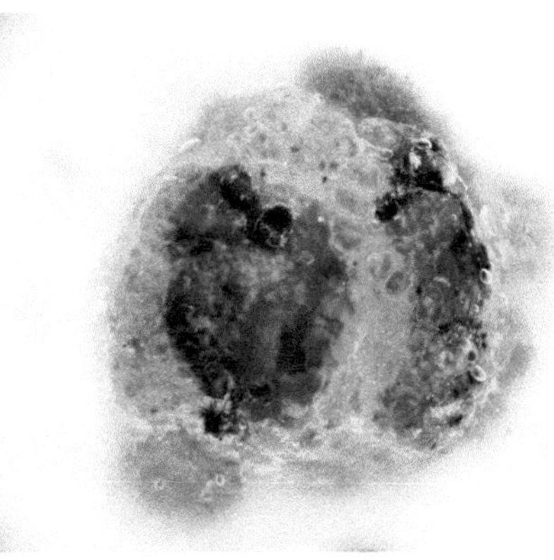

FIGURE 3.87 Nodular melanoma: dermatoscopy reveals blue and black color, without any other melanoma-specific features.

NM rarely exhibits these features, with the exception of blue-white veil and atypical vessels. Accordingly, NM is often difficult to recognize even after dermatoscopic examination.

Three dermatoscopic criteria have been associated with NM, and the detection of any of them in a nodular lesion should warrant immediate excision:

1. The simultaneous presence of blue and black color within the same lesion (blue-black rule), provided that the black color does not correspond to clear-cut comedo-like openings or vascular lacunas (Figures 3.87 through 3.90).
2. An atypical vascular pattern, consisting either of linear irregular vessels or of more than two morphological types of vessels (Figures 3.91 and 3.92).
3. A pink (milky red) dermatoscopic color, even in the absence of any recognizable structure (Figure 3.93).

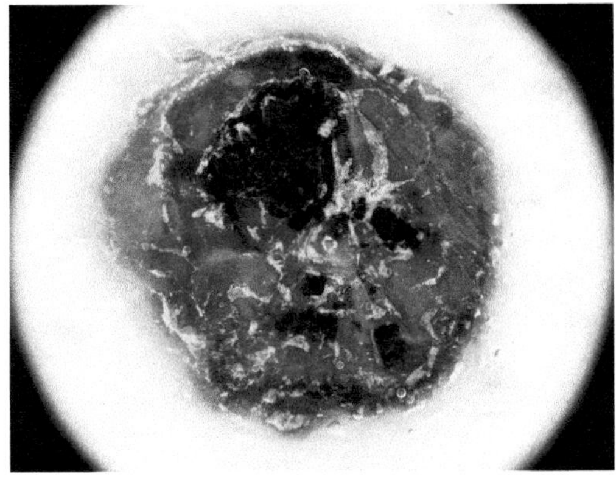

FIGURE 3.88 Nodular melanoma: dermatoscopy reveals blue and black color, without any other melanoma-specific features.

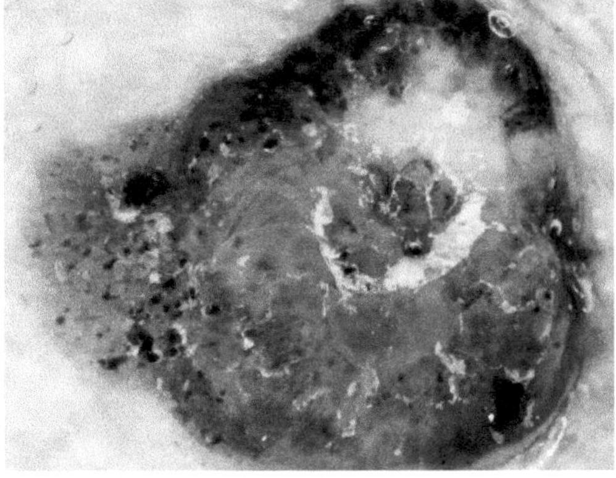

FIGURE 3.89 Nodular melanoma: dermatoscopy reveals blue and black color, without any other melanoma-specific features.

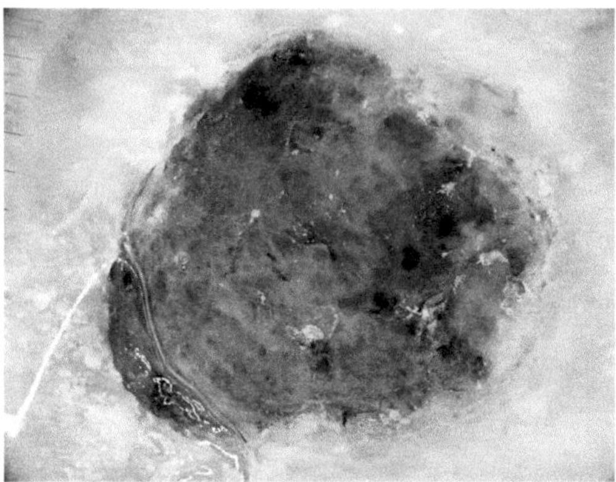

FIGURE 3.90 Nodular melanoma: dermatoscopy reveals blue and black color, without any other melanoma-specific features.

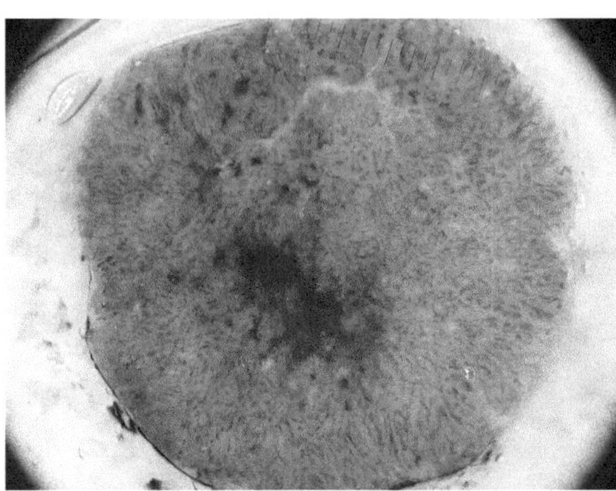

FIGURE 3.91 Nodular melanoma: atypical and irregular linear vessels.

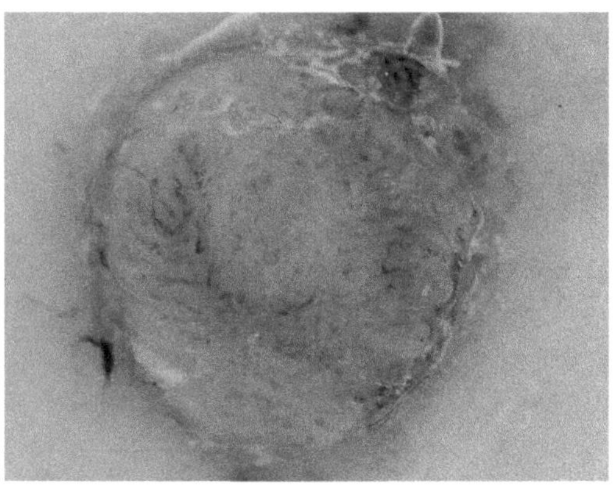

FIGURE 3.92 Nodular melanoma: polymorphous vascular pattern, consisting of atypical linear vessels, dotted and comma vessels.

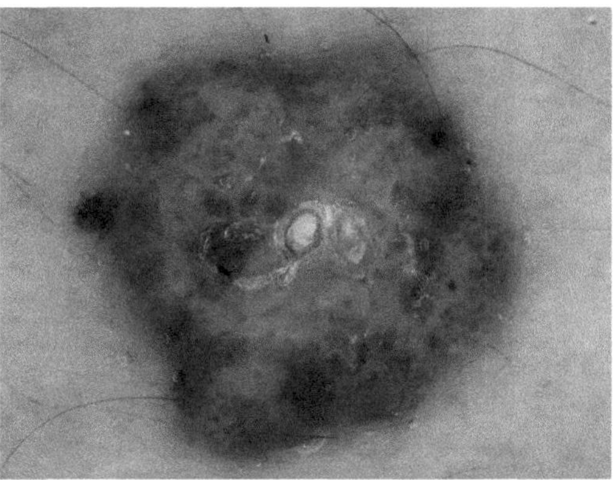

FIGURE 3.93 Milky-red (pink) color is by definition suspicious for melanoma. In this lesion, dotted and glomerular vessels, brown globules, and pigment network on the left side of the lesion can also be seen.

However, in clinical practice, the diagnosis of nodular melanoma cannot be based exclusively on the detection of one of these three criteria. The only safe strategy to minimize the possibility of missing NM is to apply the following rule when evaluating a nodular lesion:

> After clinical and dermatoscopic examination, when a specific and confident diagnosis of a benign tumor (seborrheic keratosis, angioma, dermal nevus) is not feasible, the lesion should be excised to rule out nodular melanoma.

3.3 Amelanotic Melanoma

Amelanotic melanoma does not represent a distinct melanoma subtype, since proportions of both conventional and nodular melanomas are minimally or not at all pigmented. The absence of pigmentation significantly influences the overall clinical appearance of the tumor, rendering its recognition much more difficult.

Amelanotic conventional melanoma is usually a flat tumor with a whitish to pinkish or flesh-colored hue. The tumor might be amelanotic from the very beginning or, more frequently, the lack of pigment represents a result of extensive regression. A possible clue for the recognition of flat amelanotic melanoma is its shiny surface (Figure 3.94). The differential diagnoses include superficial basal cell carcinoma, *in situ* squamous cell carcinoma, regressed nevus, and lichen planus-like keratosis (regressed solar lentigo or seborrheic keratosis).

Amelanotic nodular melanoma almost always lacks pigment during all the stages of its evolution and clinically develops as a rapidly growing pink or red nodule (Figure 3.95). It has to be differentiated from other nonpigmented nodular tumors, including basal cell carcinoma, squamous cell carcinoma, Merkel cell carcinoma, vascular tumors, and other less frequent neoplasms.

Dermatoscopic Features

Considering that the vast majority of the dermatoscopic structures described in the present chapter are brown, black, or blue colored, it is reasonable that they cannot be found in amelanotic melanoma. In hypomelanotic melanoma, dermatoscopy might reveal clinically undetectable pigmentation, significantly enhancing its recognition (Figure 3.96). In contrast, purely amelanotic melanoma is very difficult to diagnose, even with the addition of dermatoscopy.

In the absence of pigment, the only dermatoscopic criteria remaining to be assessed are the vascular structures and the overall color hue.

In the context of flat tumors, dermatoscopy might enhance the discrimination between amelanotic melanoma and other entities based on the evaluation of the vascular pattern. Specifically, the detection of dotted vessels is highly suggestive of a melanocytic tumor (nevus or melanoma), while basal cell carcinoma exhibits linear vessels and actinic keratosis a diffuse perifollicular erythema (strawberry pattern) (Figures 3.97 through 3.99). Intraepidermal carcinoma (Bowen disease) also displays dotted vessels, but they are usually larger in diameter and coiled (glomerular vessels) (Figure 3.100). Certainly, the detection of dotted vessels is insufficient to differentiate between nevus and melanoma, but, at least, it provides the information that the tumor is probably melanocytic. The presence of a second morphological type of vessels within the same lesion (e.g., linear) should be considered a suspicious finding for melanoma. The only other entity that might display a similar dermatoscopic pattern (dotted plus short linear

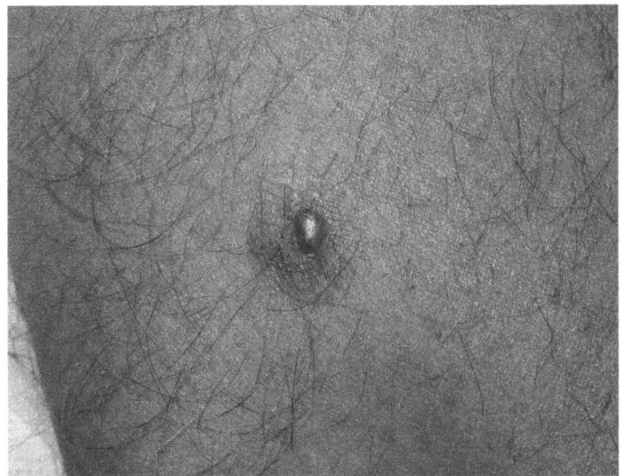

FIGURE 3.94 A useful clinical clue for the recognition of flat amelanotic melanoma is its shiny surface.

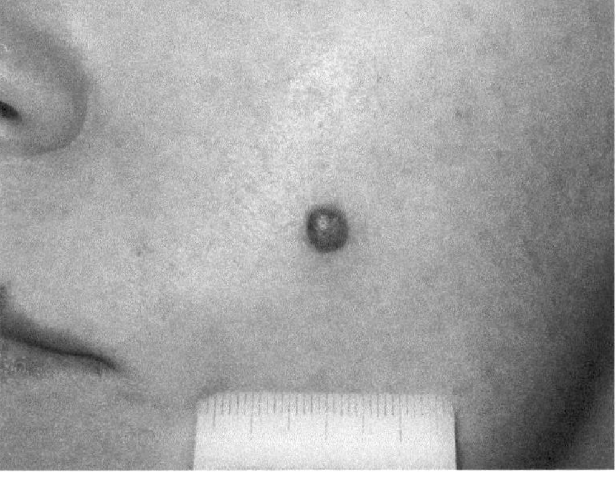

FIGURE 3.95 Amelanotic nodular melanoma usually develops as a rapidly growing pink or red nodule.

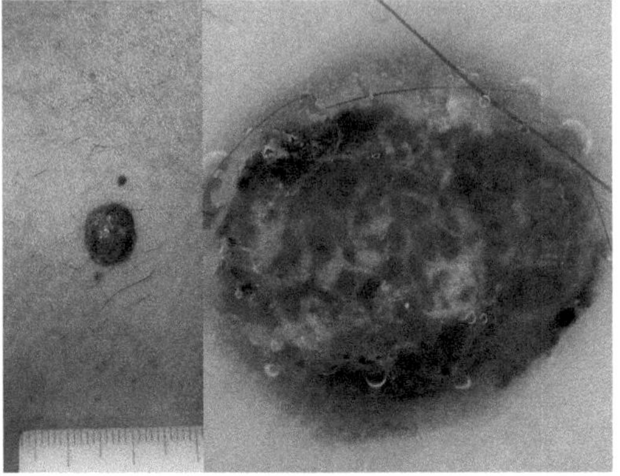

FIGURE 3.96 The dermatoscopic detection of remnants of pigmentation significantly enhances the recognition of this clinically amelanotic melanoma.

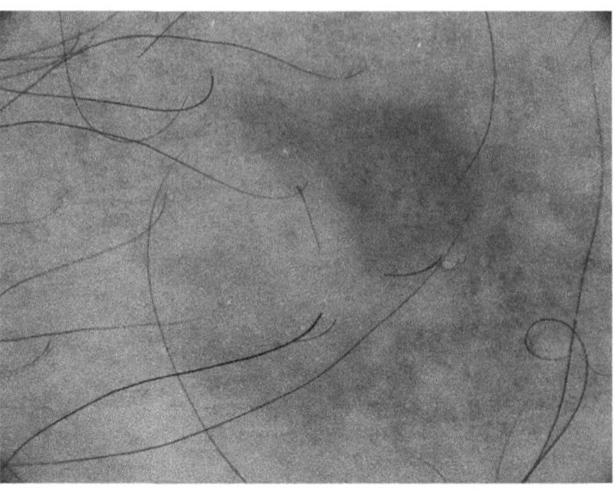

FIGURE 3.97 The dermatoscopic detection of dotted vessels in a flat, nonpigmented lesion is highly suggestive of a melanocytic tumor, with Spitz nevus and melanoma being the most possible diagnoses.

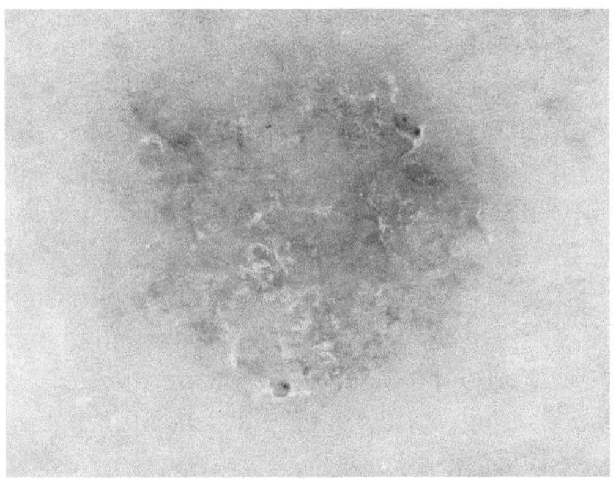

FIGURE 3.98 Superficial basal cell carcinoma is dermatoscopically typified by short linear vessels and multiple erosions.

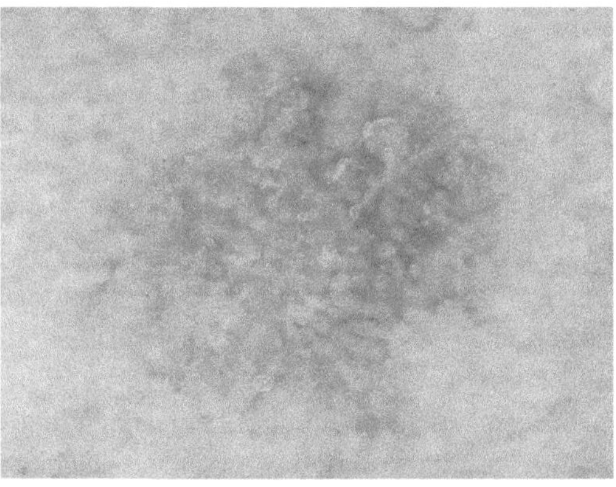

FIGURE 3.99 Actinic keratosis dermatoscopically exhibits a diffuse perifollicular erythema (strawberry pattern).

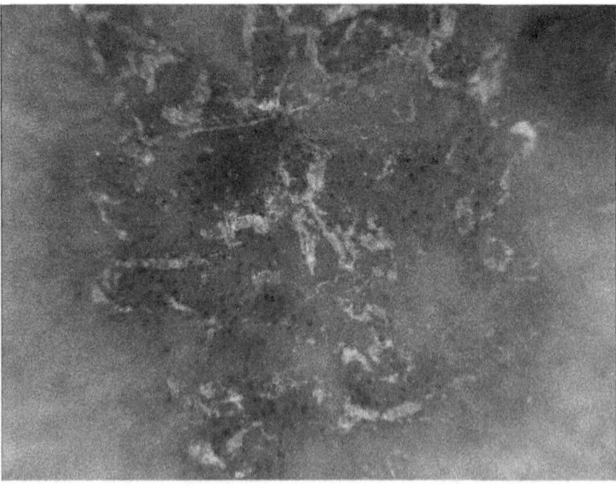

FIGURE 3.100 Intraepidermal carcinoma (Bowen disease) also displays dotted vessels, but they are usually larger in diameter and coiled (glomerular vessels). Also, yellow scales/keratin masses coexist.

vessels) is *lichen planus-like keratosis* (LPLK), which is a SL/SK undergoing regression. The differential diagnosis between flat AM and nonpigmented LPLK is virtually impossible, so lesions displaying the aforementioned pattern should be examined histopathologically (Figures 3.101 and 3.102).

Nodular amelanotic melanoma represents possibly the worst nightmare of clinicians because of its highly unspecific morphology and its unfavorable prognosis. The only two dermatoscopic criteria associated with nodular amelanotic melanoma are atypical vessels (as described for NM earlier) and a pink (milky-red) color (Figure 3.103). These features are highly unspecific, since they can be found in several other tumors including poorly differentiated squamous cell carcinoma, Merkel cell carcinoma, atypical fibroxanthoma, and many others (Figures 3.104 and 3.105). However, given that a dermatoscopic differentiation among these entities is impossible, and considering the aggressive nature of all these tumors, any lesion with such a morphological pattern should be urgently excised.

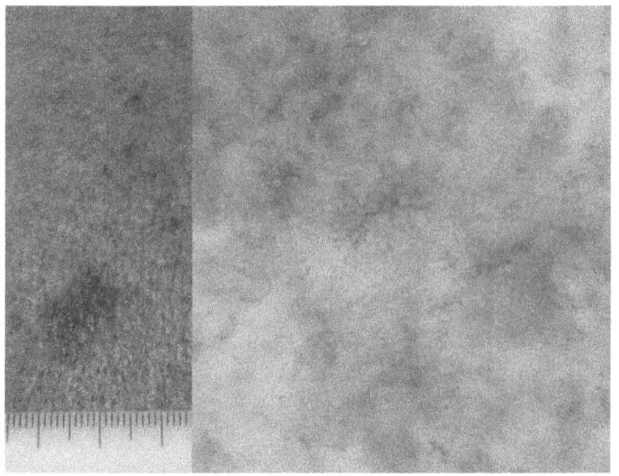

FIGURE 3.101 Flat amelanotic melanoma. The only dermatoscopic clue is the polymorphous vascular pattern, consisting of dotted and short linear vessels. Erosions and keratin masses are absent.

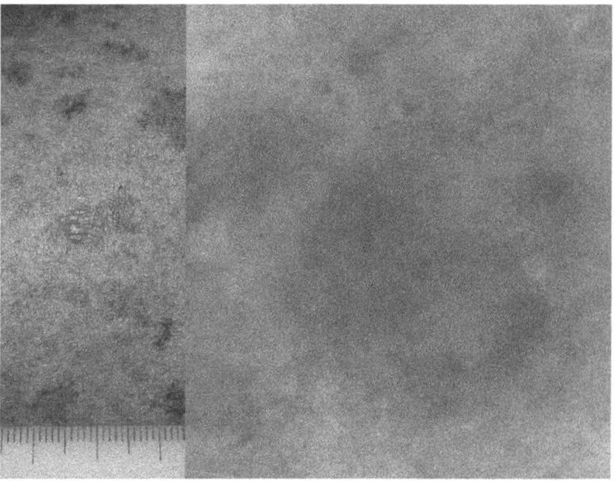

FIGURE 3.102 Lichen planus–like keratosis. The dermatoscopic pattern is very similar to the one seen in flat amelanotic melanoma, since it consists of dotted and short linear vessels. No remnants of the preexisting seborrheic keratosis/solar lentigo can be seen.

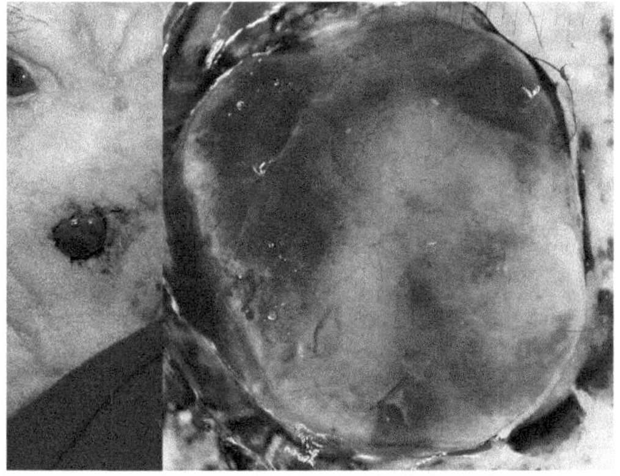

FIGURE 3.103 Nodular amelanotic melanoma. An atypical vascular pattern consisting mainly of linear vessels, which are highly tortuous and varying in diameter.

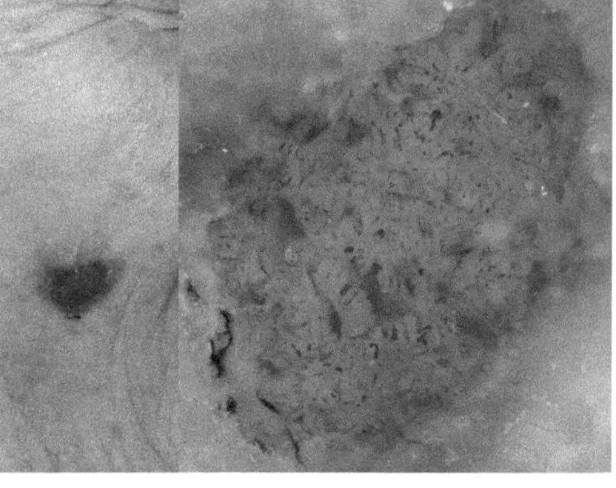

FIGURE 3.104 Poorly differentiated squamous cell carcinoma. The vascular pattern is similar to the previous case of amelanotic melanoma. Some keratin masses can also be seen.

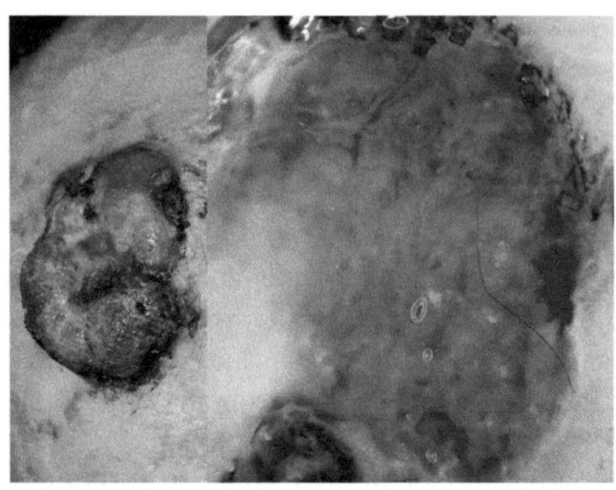

FIGURE 3.105 Dermal sarcoma (also referred to as malignant fibrous histiocytoma). The dermatoscopic vascular pattern is similar to the previous case of amelanotic melanoma.

BIBLIOGRAPHY

Ackerman AB. Mythology and numerology in the sphere of melanoma. *Cancer* 2000;88:491–6.

Ackerman AB, David KM. A unifying concept of malignant melanoma: Biologic aspects. *Hum Pathol.* 1986;17:438–40.

Akay BN, Kocyigit P, Heper AO, Erdem C. Dermatoscopy of flat pigmented facial lesions: Diagnostic challenge between pigmented actinic keratosis and lentigo maligna. *Br J Dermatol.* 2010;163:1212–7.

Altamura D, Menzies SW, Argenziano G et al. Dermatoscopy of basal cell carcinoma: Morphologic variability of global and local features and accuracy of diagnosis. *J Am Acad Dermatol.* 2010;62:67–75.

Argenziano G, Catricalà C, Ardigo M et al. Dermoscopy of patients with multiple nevi: Improved management recommendations using a comparative diagnostic approach. *Arch Dermatol.* 2011;147:46–9.

Argenziano G, Catricalà C, Ardigo M et al. Seven-point checklist of dermoscopy revisited. *Br J Dermatol.* 2011;164:785–90.

Argenziano G, Fabbrocini G, Carli P, de Giorgi V, Sammarco E, Delfino M. Epiluminescence microscopy for the diagnosis of doubtful melanocytic skin lesions. Comparison of the ABCD rule of dermatoscopy and a new 7-point checklist based on pattern analysis. *Arch Dermatol.* 1998;134:1563–70.

Argenziano G, Ferrara G, Francione S, Nola KD, Martino A, Zalaudek I. Dermoscopy—The ultimate tool for melanoma diagnosis. *Semin Cutan Med Surg.* 2009;28:142–8.

Argenziano G, Kittler H, Ferrara G et al. Slow-growing melanoma: A dermoscopy follow-up study. *Br J Dermatol.* 2010;162:267–73.

Argenziano G, Longo C, Cameron A et al. Blue-black rule: A simple dermoscopic clue to recognize pigmented nodular melanoma. *Br J Dermatol.* 2011;165:1251–5.

Argenziano G, Soyer HP, Chimenti S et al. Dermoscopy of pigmented skin lesions: Results of a consensus meeting via the Internet. *J Am Acad Dermatol.* 2003;48:679–93.

Argenziano G, Zalaudek I, Ferrara G et al. Dermoscopy features of melanoma incognito: Indications for biopsy. *J Am Acad Dermatol.* 2007;56:508–13.

Babino G, Lallas A, Longo C, Moscarella E, Alfano R, Argenziano G. Dermoscopy of melanoma and non-melanoma skin cancer. *G Ital Dermatol Venereol.* 2015;150:507–19.

Blum A. Dermoscopy of pigmented lesions of the mucosa and the mucocutaneous junction. *Arch Dermatol.* 2011;147:1181.

Bradford PT, Goldstein AM, McMaster ML, Tucker MA. Acral lentiginous melanoma: Incidence and survival patterns in the United States, 1986–2005. *Arch Dermatol.* 2009;145:427–34.

Braun RP, Baran R, Le Gal F-A et al. Diagnosis and management of nail pigmentations. *J Am Acad Dermatol.* 2007;56:835–47.

Chamberlain AJ, Fritschi L, Kelly JW. Nodular melanoma: Patients' perceptions of presenting features and implications for earlier detection. *J Am Dermatol.* 2003;48:694–701.

Chi Z, Li S, Sheng X et al. Clinical presentation, histology, and prognoses of malignant melanoma in ethnic Chinese: A study of 522 consecutive cases. *BMC Cancer* 2011;11:85.

Clark WH, Elder DE, Van Horn M. The biologic forms of malignant melanoma. *Hum Pathol.* 1986;17:443–50.

Clark WH, From L, Bernardino EA, Mihm MC. The histogenesis and biologic behavior of primary human malignant melanomas of the skin. *Cancer Res.* 1969;29:705–27.

Coit DG, Andtbacka R, Anker CJ et al. Melanoma. *J Natl Compr Canc Netw.* 2012;10:366–400.

Coit DG, Andtbacka R, Anker CJ et al. Melanoma, version 2.2013: Featured updates to the NCCN guidelines. *J Natl Compr Canc Netw.* 2013;11:395–407.

Dalmau J, Abellaneda C, Puig S, Zaballos P, Malvehy J. Acral melanoma simulating warts: Dermoscopic clues to prevent missing a melanoma. *Dermatol Surg.* 2006;32:1072–8.

Forman SB, Ferringer TC, Peckham SJ et al. Is superficial spreading melanoma still the most common form of malignant melanoma? *J Am Acad Dermatol.* 2008;58:1013–20.

Friedman RJ, Rigel DS, Kopf AW. Early detection of malignant melanoma: The role of physician examination and self-examination of the skin. *CA A Cancer J Clin.* 1985;35:130–51.

Gill D, Dorevitch A, Marks R. The prevalence of seborrheic keratoses in people aged 15 to 30 years: Is the term senile keratosis redundant? *Arch Dermatol.* 2000;136:759–62.

Green AC, Baade P, Coory M, Aitken JF, Smithers M. Population-based 20-year survival among people diagnosed with thin melanomas in Queensland, Australia. *J Clin Oncol.* 2012;30:1462–7.

Pock L, Drlik L, Hercogova L. Dermatoscopy of pigmented actinic keratosis – a striking similarity to lentigo maligmant. *Int J Dermatol* 2007;46(4):414-6.

Ishihara K, Saida T, Otsuka F, Yamazaki N; Prognosis and Statistical Investigation Committee of the Japanese Skin Cancer Society. Statistical profiles of malignant melanoma and other skin cancers in Japan: 2007 update. *Int J Clin Oncol.* 2008;13:33–41.

Jaimes N, Braun RP, Thomas L, Marghoob AA. Clinical and dermoscopic characteristics of amelanotic melanomas that are not of the nodular subtype. *J Eur Acad Dermatol Venereol.* 2012;26:591–6.

Kato T, Takematsu H, Tomita Y, Takahashi M, Abe R. Malignant melanoma of mucous membranes. A clinicopathologic study of 13 cases in Japanese patients. *Arch Dermatol.* 1987;123:216–20.

Kittler H. Dermatoscopy: Introduction of a new algorithmic method based on pattern analysis for diagnosis of pigmented skin lesions. *Dermatol Pract Concept.* 2007;13:1.

Koh HK, Michalik E, Sober AJ et al. Lentigo maligna melanoma has no better prognosis than other types of melanoma. *J Clin Oncol.* 1984;2:994–1001.

Lallas A, Argenziano G, Moscarella E, Longo C, Simonetti V, Zalaudek I. Diagnosis and management of facial pigmented macules. *Clin Dermatol.* 2014;32:94–100.

Lallas A, Kyrgidis A, Koga H et al. The BRAAFF checklist: A new dermoscopic algorithm for diagnosing acral melanoma. *Br J Dermatol.* 2015;173:1041–9.

Lallas A, Longo C, Manfredini M et al. Accuracy of dermoscopic criteria for the diagnosis of melanoma *in situ*. *JAMA Dermatol.* 2018;154:414–9.

Lallas A, Moscarella E, Argenziano G et al. Dermoscopy of uncommon skin tumours. *Australas J Dermatol.* 2014;55:53–62.

Lallas A, Pyne J, Kyrgidis A et al. The clinical and dermoscopic features of invasive cutaneous squamous cell carcinoma depend on the histopathological grade of differentiation. *Br J Dermatol.* 2014;172:1308–15.

Lallas A, Sgouros D, Zalaudek I et al. Palmar and plantar melanomas differ for sex prevalence and tumor thickness but not for dermoscopic patterns. *Melanoma Res.* 2014;24:83–7.

Lallas A, Zalaudek I, Apalla Z et al. Management rules to detect melanoma. *Dermatology.* 2013;226:52–60.

Longo C, Moscarella E, Piana S et al. Not all lesions with a verrucous surface are seborrheic keratoses. *J Am Acad Dermatol.* 2014;70:e121–3.

McGovern VJ, Cochran AJ, Van der Esch EP, Little JH, MacLennan R. The classification of malignant melanoma, its histological reporting and registration: A revision of the 1972 Sydney classification. *Pathology.* 1986;18:12–21.

Menzies SW, Ingvar C, Crotty KA, McCarthy WH. Frequency and morphologic characteristics of invasive melanomas lacking specific surface microscopic features. *Arch Dermatol.* 1996;132:1178–82.

Menzies SW, Moloney FJ, Byth K et al. Dermoscopic evaluation of nodular melanoma. *JAMA Dermatol.* 2013;149:699–709.

Nachbar F, Stolz W, Merkle T et al. The ABCD rule of dermatoscopy. High prospective value in the diagnosis of doubtful melanocytic skin lesions. *J Am Dermatol.* 1994;30:551–9.

Oguchi S, Saida T, Koganehira Y, Ohkubo S, Ishihara Y, Kawachi S. Characteristic epiluminescent microscopic features of early malignant melanoma on glabrous skin. A videomicroscopic analysis. *Arch Dermatol.* 1998;134:563–8.

Piraccini BM, Balestri R, Starace M, Rech G. Nail digital dermoscopy (onychoscopy) in the diagnosis of onychomycosis. *J Eur Acad Dermatol Venerol.* 2011;27:509–13.

Pralong P, Bathelier E, Dalle S, Poulalhon N, Debarbieux S, Thomas L. Dermoscopy of lentigo maligna melanoma: Report of 125 cases. *Br J Dermatol.* 2012;167:280–7.

Rigel DS, Carucci JA. Malignant melanoma: Prevention, early detection, and treatment in the 21st century. *CA A Cancer J Clin.* 2000;50:215–36; quiz 237–40.

Rigel DS, Russak J, Friedman R. The evolution of melanoma diagnosis: 25 years beyond the ABCDs. *CA A Cancer J Clin.* 2010;60:301–16.

Saida T, Koga H, Uhara H. Key points in dermoscopic differentiation between early acral melanoma and acral nevus. *J Dermatol.* 2011;38:25–34.

Saida T, Koga H. Dermoscopic patterns of acral melanocytic nevi: Their variations, changes, and significance. *Arch Dermatol.* 2007;143:1423–6.

Saida T, Miyazaki A, Oguchi S et al. Significance of dermoscopic patterns in detecting malignant melanoma on acral volar skin: Results of a multicenter study in Japan. *Arch Dermatol.* 2004;140:1233–8.

Saida T. Malignant melanoma on the sole: How to detect the early lesions efficiently. *Pigment Cell Res.* 2000;13(Suppl 8):135–9.

Schiffner R, Schiffner-Rohe J, Vogt T et al. Improvement of early recognition of lentigo maligna using dermatoscopy. *J Am Dermatol.* 2000;42:25–32.

Scrivener Y, Grosshans E, Cribier B. Variations of basal cell carcinomas according to gender, age, location and histopathological subtype. *Br J Dermatol.* 2002;147:41–7.

Seidenari S, Bassoli S, Borsari S et al. Variegated dermoscopy of *in situ* melanoma. *Dermatology.* 2012;224:262–70.

Stevens NG, Liff JM, Weiss NS. Plantar melanoma: Is the incidence of melanoma of the sole of the foot really higher in blacks than whites? *Int J Cancer.* 1990;45:691–3.

Stolz W, Schiffner R, Burgdorf WHC. Dermatoscopy for facial pigmented skin lesions. *Clin Dermatol.* 2002;20:276–8.

Thomas NE, Kricker A, Waxweiler WT et al. Comparison of clinicopathologic features and survival of histopathologically amelanotic and pigmented melanomas: A population-based study. *JAMA Dermatol.* 2014;150:1306–14.

Tiodorovic-Zivkovic D, Argenziano G, Lallas A et al. Age, gender, and topography influence the clinical and dermoscopic appearance of lentigo maligna. *J Am Acad Dermatol.* 2015;72:801–8.

Tschandl P, Rosendahl C, Kittler H. Dermatoscopy of flat pigmented facial lesions. *J Eur Acad Dermatol Venereol.* 2015; 29:120–7.

Vestergaard ME, Macaskill P, Holt PE, Menzies SW. Dermoscopy compared with naked eye examination for the diagnosis of primary melanoma: A meta-analysis of studies performed in a clinical setting. *Br J Dermatol.* 2008;159:669–76.

Zaballos P, Blazquez S, Puig S et al. Dermoscopic pattern of intermediate stage in seborrhoeic keratosis regressing to lichenoid keratosis: Report of 24 cases. *Br J Dermatol.* 2007;157:266–72.

Zalaudek I, Argenziano G, Leinweber B et al. Dermoscopy of Bowen's disease. *Br J Dermatol.* 2004;150:1112–6.

Zalaudek I, Ferrara G, Leinweber B, Mercogliano A, D'Ambrosio A, Argenziano G. Pitfalls in the clinical and dermoscopic diagnosis of pigmented actinic keratosis. *J Am Acad Dermatol.* 2005;53:1071–4.

Zalaudek I, Kreusch J, Giacomel J, Ferrara G, Catricalà C, Argenziano G. How to diagnose nonpigmented skin tumors: A review of vascular structures seen with dermoscopy: Part II. Nonmelanocytic skin tumors. *J Am Acad Dermatol.* 2010;63:377–86; quiz 387–8.

Zalaudek I, Schmid K, Marghoob AA et al. Frequency of dermoscopic nevus subtypes by age and body site: A cross-sectional study. *Arch Dermatol.* 2011;147:663–70.

4

Benign Nonmelanocytic Skin Tumors

4.1 Epithelial Skin Tumors

4.1.1 Solar Lentigo

Solar lentigos (SLs, synonyms: actinic lentigo, senile lentigo) typically present as multiple, variably large (up to a few centimeters), light to dark brown, bizarrely outlined macules on chronically sun-exposed body sites, such as the face, dorsum of the hands, and extensor surface of the forearms (Figure 4.1). They are commonly seen in severely sun damaged skin of elderly individuals, but their appearance at a younger age is not uncommon. In most cases, there are no diagnostic difficulties from a clinical point of view. However, occasionally, there might be a clinical overlap with lentigo maligna (LM), which also arises on chronically sun-damaged skin. In such cases, dermatoscopy may enhance the accurate diagnosis.

The dermatoscopic features of SL are site dependent, with extra facial lesions frequently displaying densely arranged, roundish to oval brown circles, remnants of a fine pigment network (Figure 4.2). Additional features include curved, parallel, brown lines (fingerprint-like structures) (Figure 4.3) or a structureless brown pattern with a sharp convex-concave demarcation ("moth-eaten") (Figure 4.4).

SLs on the face are dermatoscopically typified by a light to dark brown pseudonetwork with sharp demarcation. The pseudonetwork is a result of a structureless brown pigmentation, which is interrupted by numerous nonpigmented follicular openings (Figure 4.5). When parallel curved lines, brown elongated circles (fingerprint-like structures or fat fingers), and sharp demarcation (jelly sign or "moth-eaten" borders) are additionally seen along with the brown pseudonetwork, then the diagnosis of SL is significantly facilitated. The dermatoscopic discrimination from LM is based on the detection of one or more of the aforementioned characteristic features of SL, as well as by the absence of gray structures (gray dots, gray globules, asymmetric follicular openings, rhomboidal structures, and gray circles surrounding the follicular openings). Regressing SL, also known as lichen planus–like keratosis (LPLK), is much more difficult to discriminate from LM, because it displays gray color, which represents a highly confounding feature (Figure 4.6).

4.1.2 Ink-Spot Lentigo

Ink-spot lentigo is a heavily pigmented reticulated type of SL. It typically develops as a solitary, irregularly outlined black macule on the shoulders of individuals with fair skin and a history of severe sunburns. On the surrounding skin, multiple, additional, brown freckles (solar freckles) or solar lentigos are usually seen. Because of its irregular shape and strikingly black color, ink-spot lentigo may mimic melanoma and might raise false concerns. Dermatoscopy significantly facilitates the recognition of ink-spot lentigo by revealing a unique pattern, consisting of a dark

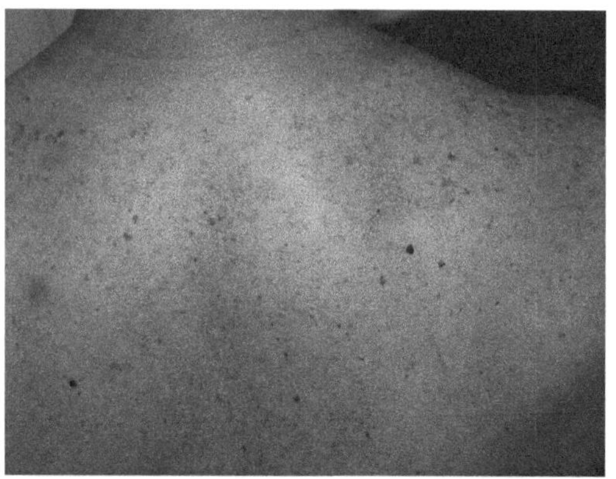

FIGURE 4.1 Clinical image of typical solar lentigos.

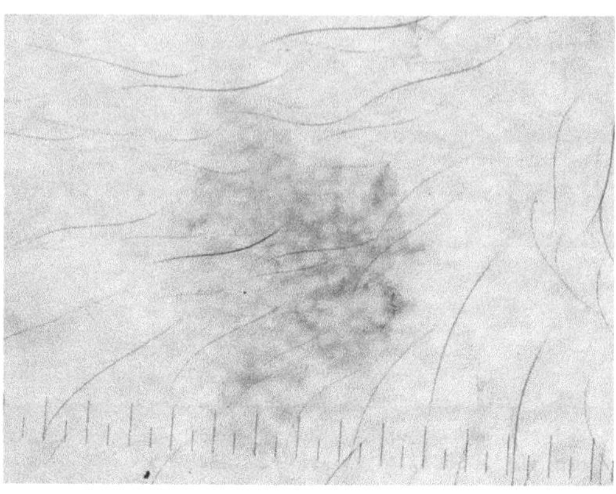

FIGURE 4.2 A solar lentigo on the back, dermatoscopically typified by a delicate reticular brown pattern.

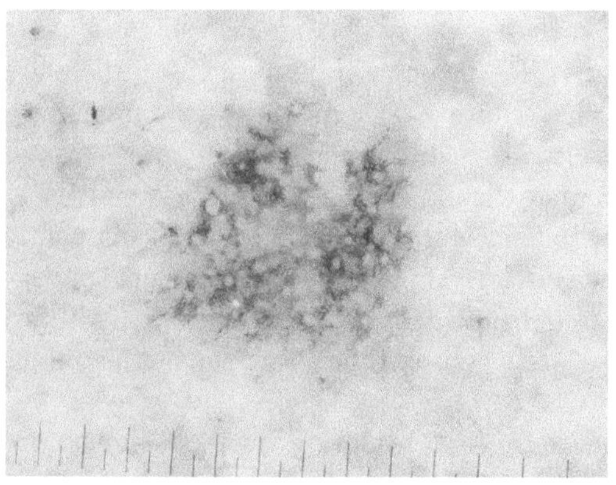

FIGURE 4.3 A solar lentigo dermatoscopically displaying curved, parallel, brown lines (fingerprint-like structures).

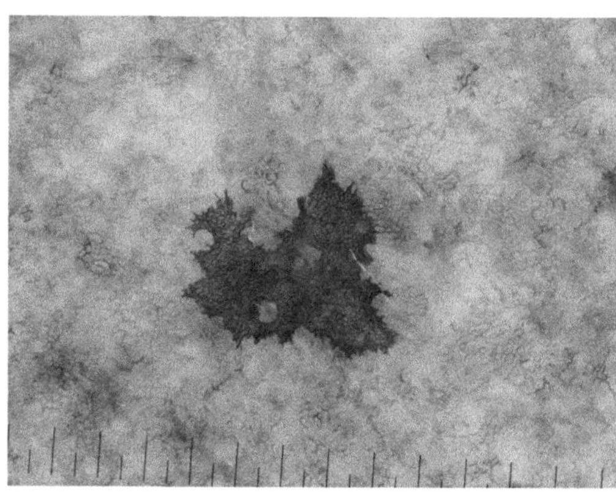

FIGURE 4.4 A solar lentigo with sharp "moth-eaten" demarcation. Brown fingerprint-like structures and reticular pattern are observed on the surrounding skin.

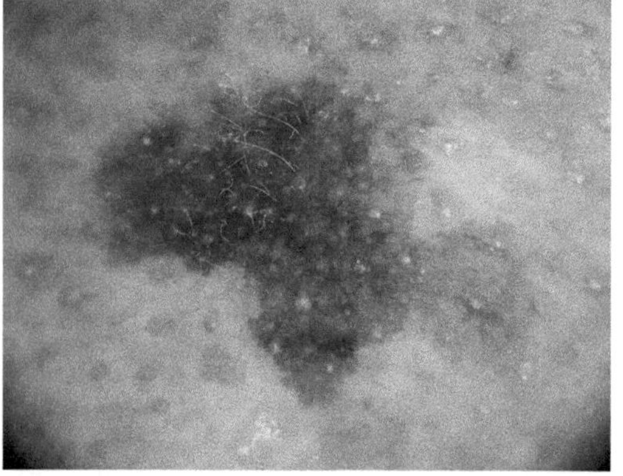

FIGURE 4.5 Pseudonetwork of a facial solar lentigo, consisting of a structureless brown pigmentation, interrupted by numerous nonpigmented follicular openings.

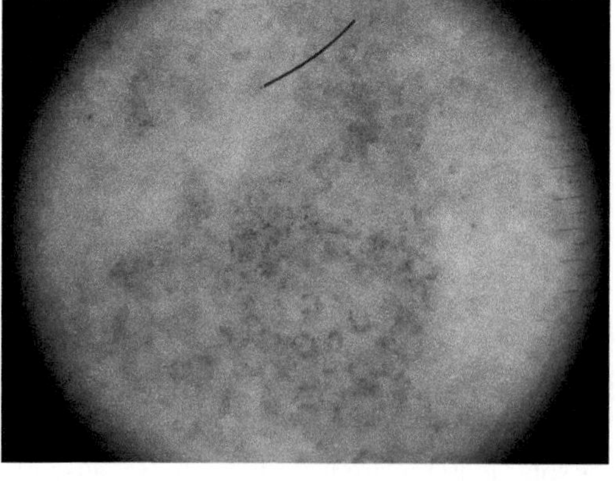

FIGURE 4.6 Gray structures (gray circles, gray dots, and gray/brown lines) seen with dermatoscopy are highly suspicious of melanoma *in situ*.

brown to black interrupted (broken-up) pigment network with thick lines and wide meshes (Figure 4.7).

4.1.3 Seborrheic Keratosis

Seborrheic keratosis (SK) is a common, benign, epithelial skin tumor that can develop anywhere on the body except on palms and soles. SKs appear as solitary or multiple, slightly raised to nodular, well-demarcated lesions with a keratotic, papillomatous, or smooth surface (Figures 4.8 and 4.9). The color of SKs varies from yellowish to opaque brown-black or gray. Sharp demarcation, dull and verrucous surface, and prominent follicular openings represent useful clinical signs that allow a straightforward diagnosis in most cases. At times, irritated SKs or peculiar histopathologic variants such as melanoacanthoma or clonal SK may cause diagnostic difficulties.

The most common dermatoscopic features of SK are multiple milia-like cysts (Figure 4.10), multiple comedo-like openings (Figure 4.11), a cerebriform (brain-like) pattern (Figure 4.12), and sharp demarcation of the border (Figure 4.13). In irritated SK, hairpin vessels (Figure 4.14) and thick dotted vessels, each one surrounded by a whitish halo, represent the predominant

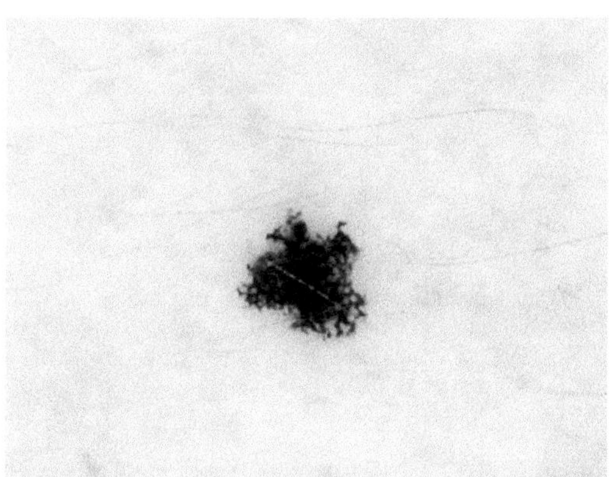

FIGURE 4.7 Dermatoscopic image of an ink-spot lentigo displaying a dark brown/black interrupted pigment network.

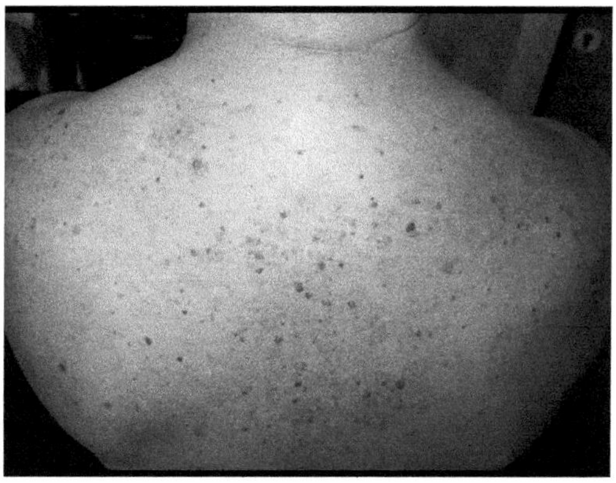

FIGURE 4.8 Clinical image of classical seborrheic keratoses.

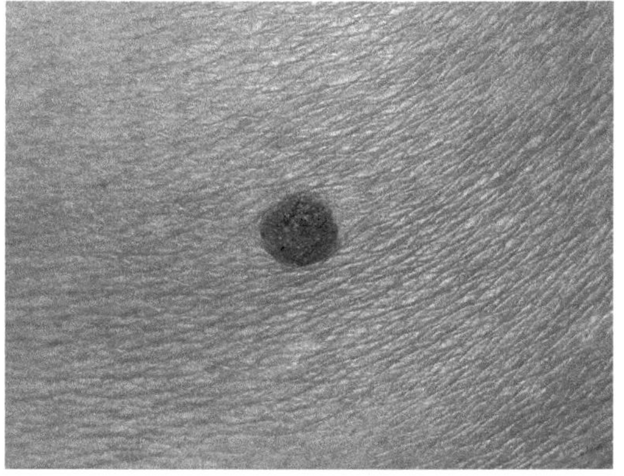

FIGURE 4.9 Clinical close-up image of a classical seborrheic keratosis.

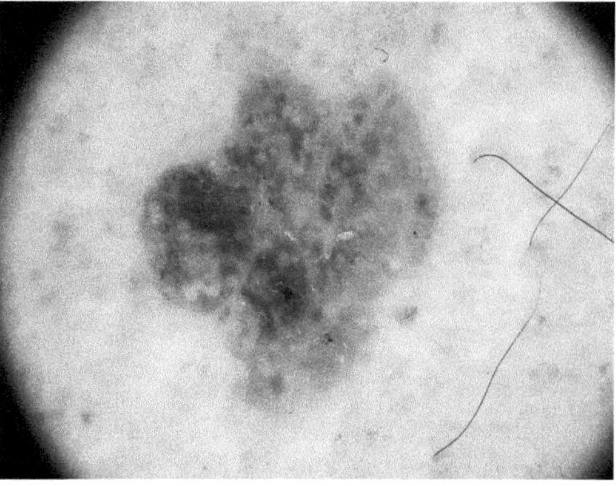

FIGURE 4.10 Multiple milia-like cysts in a classical seborrheic keratosis.

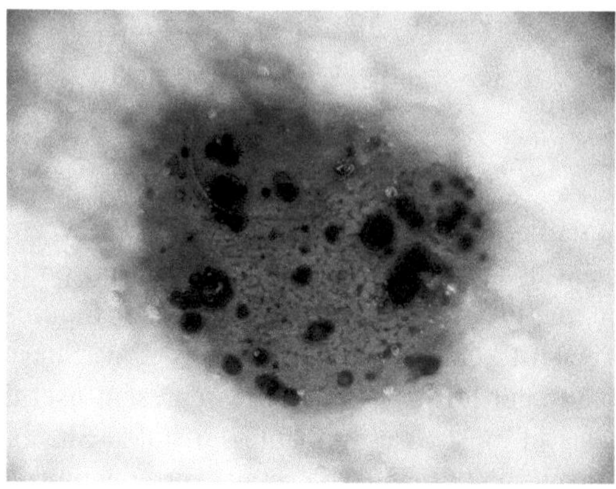

FIGURE 4.11 Comedo-like openings in a classical seborrheic keratosis.

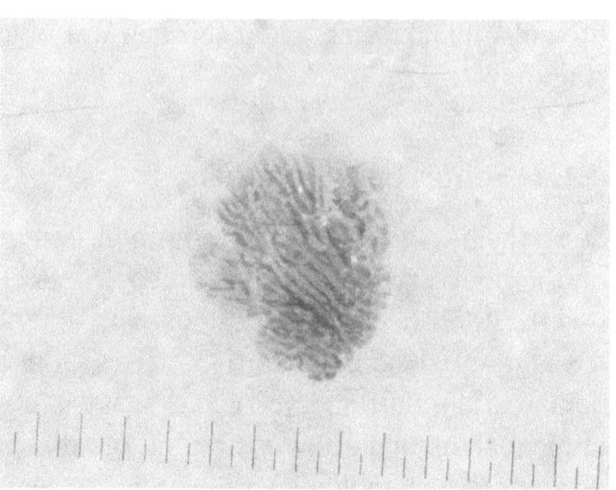

FIGURE 4.12 Cerebriform pattern in a classical seborrheic keratosis.

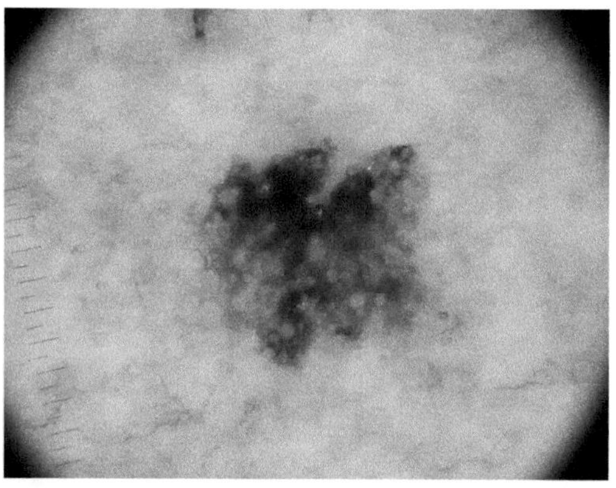

FIGURE 4.13 Sharp demarcation of the borders in a seborrheic keratosis.

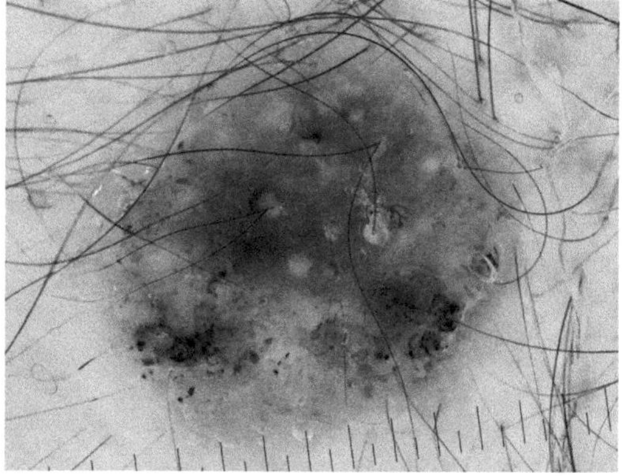

FIGURE 4.14 Irritated seborrheic keratosis with hairpin vessels and thick dotted vessels surrounded by whitish halos.

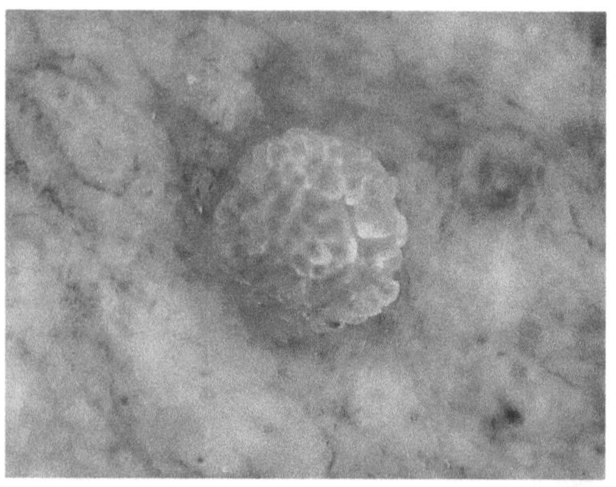

FIGURE 4.15 Capillary loops in common warts.

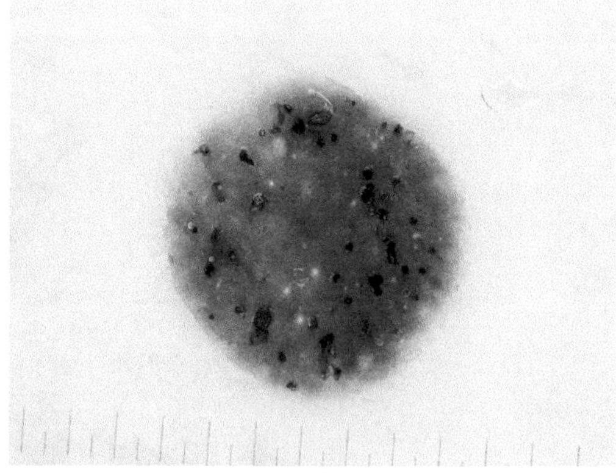

FIGURE 4.16 Acanthotic type of seborrheic keratosis with multiple milia-cysts and comedo-like openings.

feature. These vessels correspond to long capillary loops and can be seen in other keratinizing tumors such as squamous cell carcinoma and common warts (Figure 4.15). Among various histopathologic variants of SK, acanthotic, reticulated, and verrucous subtypes are the most common ones. Each one of them displays a distinctive dermatoscopic pattern, consisting of different combinations of the previously mentioned criteria.

Acanthotic Type

Acanthotic type is the most common subtype of SKs. Its color varies from yellow to light-brown to black-gray. Dermatoscopy reveals multiple milia-like cysts and comedo-like openings (Figure 4.16). Moreover, a brain-like (cerebriform) appearance is very common in acanthotic SK, especially when located on the face. Hairpin vessels, exophytic papillary structures, and a peripheral delicate pigment network may also be seen. Fingerprinting, a sharp demarcation, and a moth-eaten border represent additional characteristics of initial SK developing from SL.

Reticulated Type

Reticulated SK usually presents as a small (<6 mm), slightly raised, uniform colored, and sharply demarcated lesion. Dermatoscopically, it exhibits a network-like structure, composed of densely aligned, brown, round or oval circles or thick reticular lines (Figure 4.17). However, the network-like structure of an SK dermatoscopically differs from the classic network of a melanocytic tumor, since the former is characterized by a striking sharp demarcation, while the latter has the tendency to fade toward the periphery.

Keratotic Type

Dermatoscopy of SK of this type reveals only white to yellow horn masses that impede the visualization of underlying structures (Figure 4.18). As melanoma may sometimes acquire a similar pattern, histopathologic examination of any solitary lesion with this pattern is generally recommended.

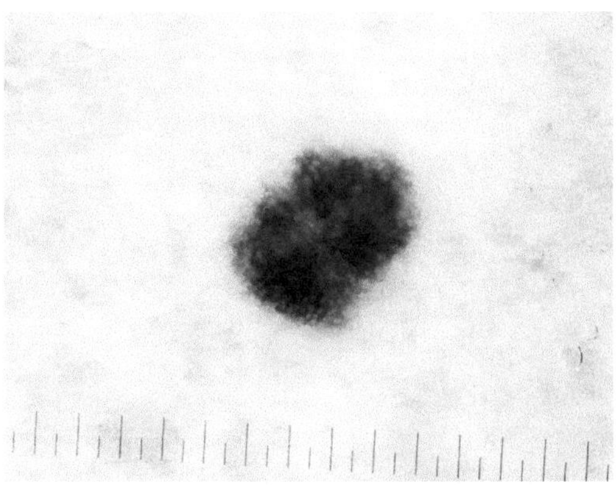

FIGURE 4.17 Reticulated seborrheic keratosis with densely aligned thick lines.

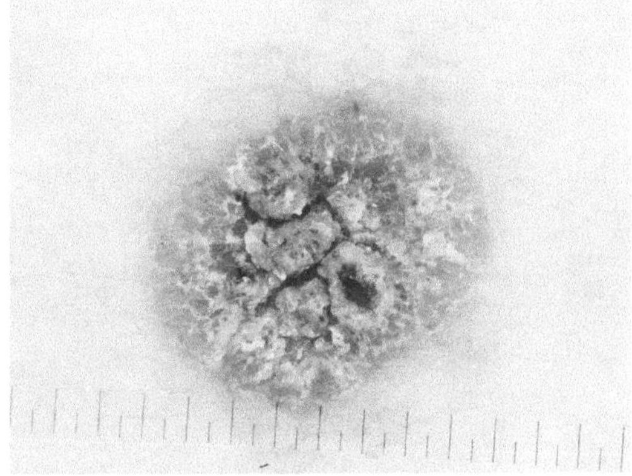

FIGURE 4.18 Keratotic seborrheic keratosis with white to yellow horn mass that impedes the visualization of underlying structures.

4.1.4 Lichen Planus–Like Keratosis

LPLK refers to an SL or an SK undergoing spontaneous regression. Clinically, LPLK is typically a flat gray to gray-brown macule. The main differential diagnosis of LPLK is regressive melanoma, and a confident diagnosis of LPLK is feasible only if remnants of the preexisting benign lesion (SK or SL) are still maintained. If not, a diagnostic biopsy is strongly recommended to rule out melanoma.

Dermatoscopically, LPLK is characterized by diffuse brownish-gray granules, which might coalesce to form globules, streaks, or even rhomboidal structures (Figure 4.19). However, as these features are commonly observed also in regressed melanoma or lentigo maligna, a lesion dermatoscopically characterized by regression (i.e., localized or diffuse gray granules) should always be biopsied, unless parts of a preexisting SL or SK are clearly evident.

4.2 Vascular Tumors

The pigmentation in vascular tumors is caused by hemoglobin. Therefore, the dermatoscopic hallmark of all vascular tumors is a mixture of red-purple-blue or black-colored, well-circumscribed, round to oval structures, known as lacunas.

4.2.1 Cherry Angioma

Cherry angiomas are very frequently found vascular tumors, dermatoscopically typified by red to purple lacunas (globules), which are well-circumscribed, round to oval structures, histopathologically corresponding to dilated, blood-filled vessels in the papillary dermis. A white veil or white lines are frequently seen among the lacunas (Figure 4.20). Most cherry angiomas are very easy to recognize clinically. A few cherry angiomas might be morphologically equivocal for a macroscopic aspect, and dermatoscopy will usually reveal a lacunar pattern and solve the diagnostic uncertainty (Figure 4.21).

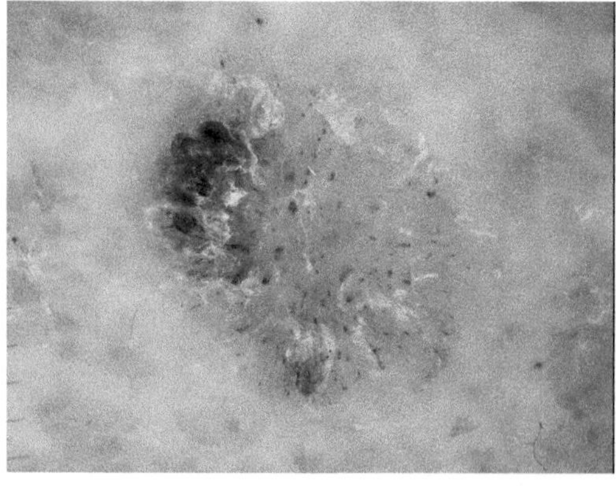

FIGURE 4.19 Nearly fully regressed lichen planus–like keratosis with diffuse brownish-gray granules in dermatoscopy. A remaining part of the preexisting seborrheic keratosis can also be seen.

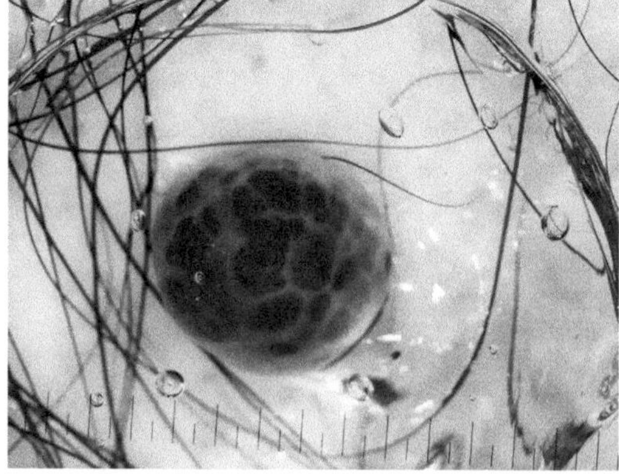

FIGURE 4.20 Cherry hemangioma with typical red to purple lacunas and globules. White lines are seen among these structures.

4.2.2 Angiokeratoma

Angiokeratoma dermatoscopically displays more commonly red-purple or purple-blue lacunas or structureless areas and sharply demarcated black lacunas, frequently associated with whitish-yellowish keratotic areas. The black globules correspond to congealed blood in the stratum corneum of thrombosed vascular lacunas (Figure 4.22).

4.2.3 Pyogenic Granuloma

In contrast to hemangioma or angiokeratoma, pyogenic granuloma rarely shows black or purple-blue globules. Instead, it is dermatoscopically characterized by bright red structureless areas combined with white intersecting lines and a whitish peripheral rim (collarette) (Figure 4.23). Taking into account that amelanotic melanoma may mimic pyogenic granuloma from a clinical and dermatoscopic aspect, the diagnosis of pyogenic granuloma should always be histopathologically confirmed.

4.2.4 Subcorneal and Subungual Hemorrhage

Subcorneal hemorrhage (also called black heel due to the striking black color of congealed hemoglobin in the stratum corneum) is usually caused by trauma, typically developing on the heels of young athletes (Figure 4.24) and less frequently on the palms. Similarly, subungual hemorrhage occurs following a nail trauma. Clinically, subcorneal and subungual hemorrhages appear as asymptomatic, well-demarcated, homogeneous, red-black macules.

Dermatoscopy typically reveals a sharply demarcated dark red to black structureless pigmentation (Figure 4.25). Moreover, satellite red-black dots or globules are often present, facilitating the accurate diagnosis. Subcorneal hemorrhage may occasionally exhibit a parallel ridge pattern, which is considered as a dermatoscopic criterion indicative of early acral melanoma. In this scenario, the positive scratch test (i.e., removal of pigmentation by scratching the stratum corneum) with a needle or scalpel is a helpful tip that often will reveal the subcorneal hemorrhage (Figure 4.26).

Concerning the nails, subungual hemorrhage does not arise from the proximal nail fold and does not linearly expand to the distal nail plate, as does longitudinal melanonychia. Instead, subungual hemorrhage is dermatoscopically seen as a sharply demarcated red to black

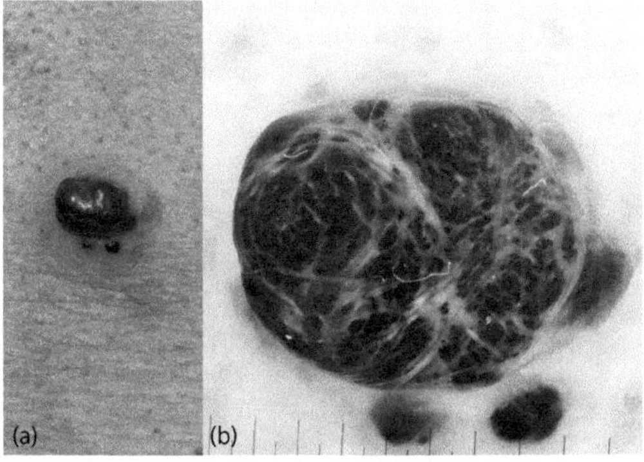

FIGURE 4.21 Clinical image of an atypical hemangioma (a). Dermatoscopy reveals the typical pattern of a hemangioma and confirms the diagnosis (b).

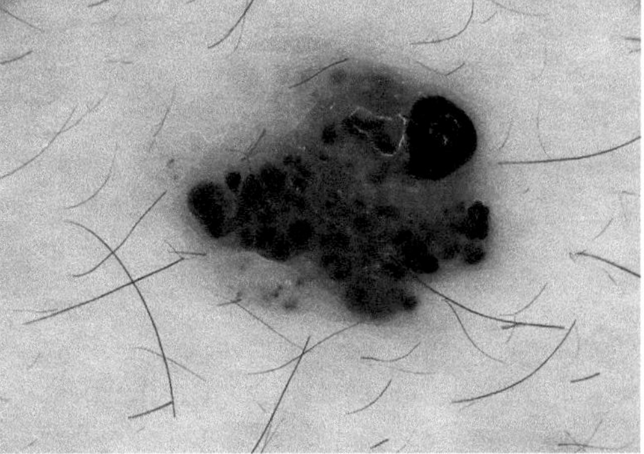

FIGURE 4.22 Congealed blood in an angiokeratoma, dermatoscopically seen as black globules. Blue-purple lacunas are also seen.

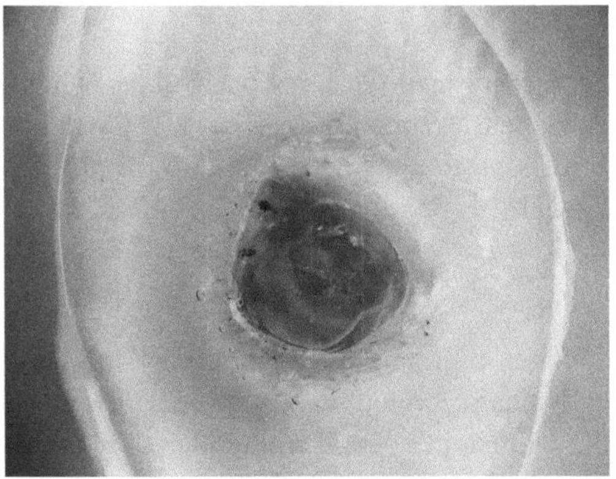

FIGURE 4.23 Dermatoscopic image of pyogenic granuloma displaying bright red structureless areas associated with white intersections (white lines).

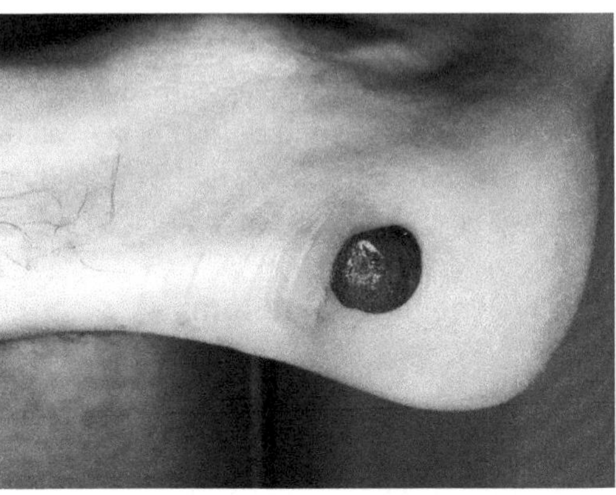

FIGURE 4.24 Clinical image of a subcorneal hemorrhage on a young man's heel (black heel) presenting as a sharply circumscribed, homogeneous, red-black macule.

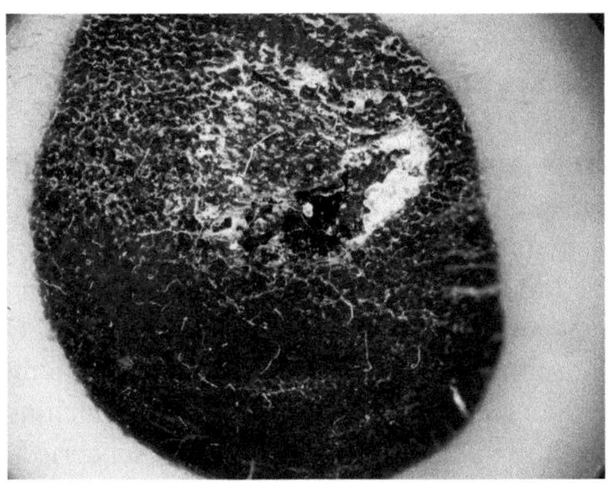

FIGURE 4.25 A subcorneal hemorrhage dermatoscopically presenting as black structureless pigmentation.

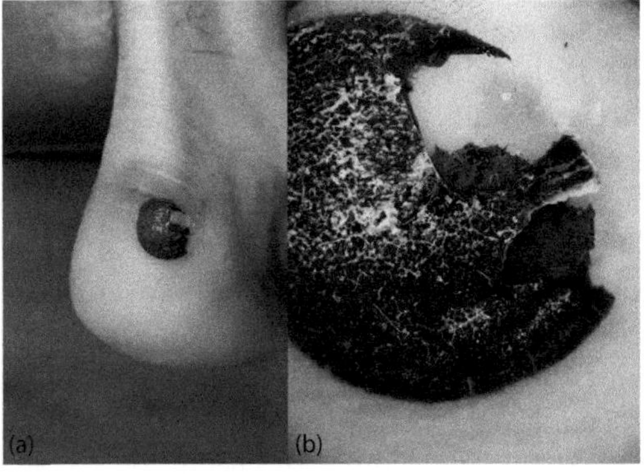

FIGURE 4.26 Clinical (a) and dermatoscopic (b) images of the hemorrhage shown in Figure 4.25 after the scratch test with a scalpel that revealed the hemorrhage.

structureless color partially covering the nail plate. The presence of a roundish border at the proximal end and streaks or lines along with blood spots at the distal end are helpful additional clues to recognize subungual hemorrhage (Figures 4.27 and 4.28).

4.3 Tumors of the Fibrous Tissue

4.3.1 Dermatofibroma

Dermatofibroma (DF) is a very common benign skin tumor. It is considered to represent a reaction to various causes, such as injuries, insect bites, or ruptured follicles. It usually develops on the lower legs but may appear anywhere on the body. Clinically, DF is a firm plaque or nodule with a diameter ranging from 0.5 mm to 1 cm and color varying from light-brown to dark-brown, purple, red, or yellow (Figure 4.29). A characteristic and useful clinical sign for its recognition is the dimple-like depression (dimple or flag sign) following lateral compression of the lesion, after which the skin dimples (Figure 4.30).

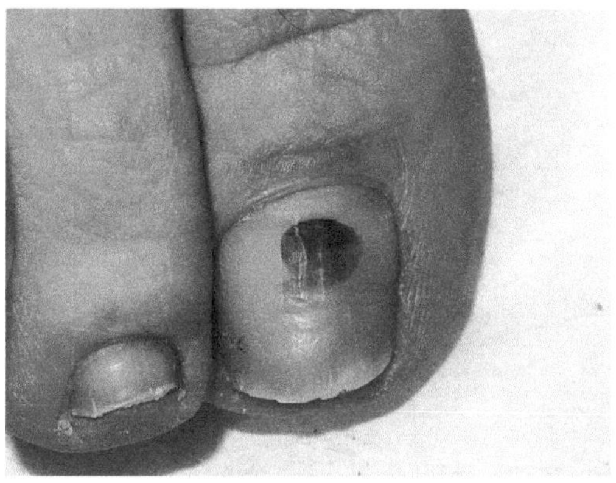

FIGURE 4.27 Clinical image of subungual hemorrhage.

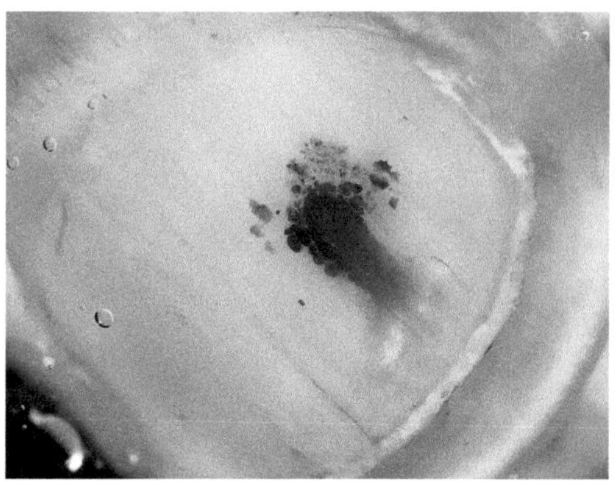

FIGURE 4.28 Dermatoscopy of a subungual hemorrhage that covers only a part of the nail plate reveals a red structureless area and satellite blood spots.

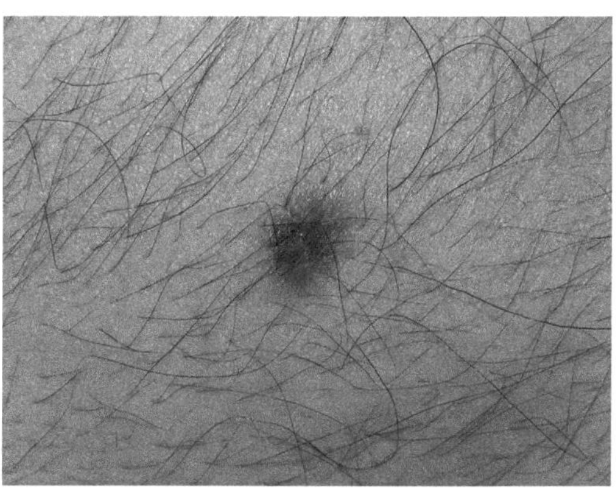

FIGURE 4.29 Clinical image of a dermatofibroma.

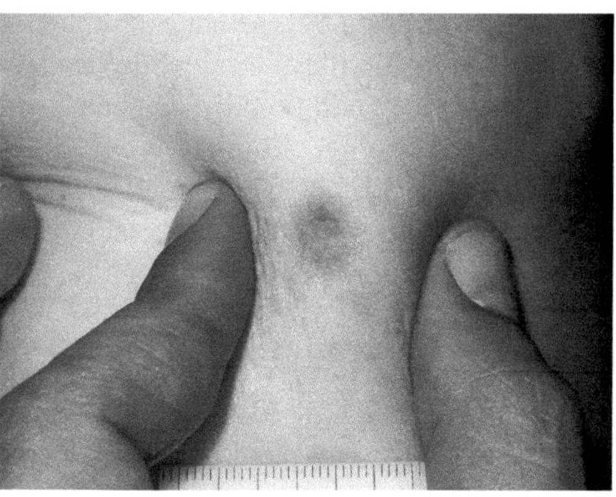

FIGURE 4.30 Dimple or flag sign following lateral compression of the lesion.

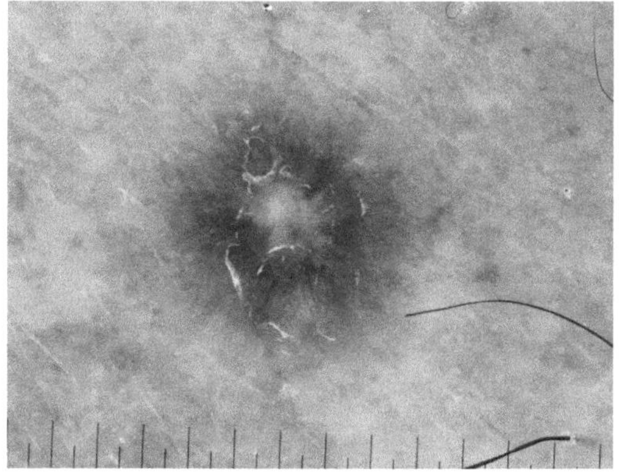

FIGURE 4.31 Dermatofibroma with a central white (scar-like) patch, surrounded by a delicate, light-brown pigment network.

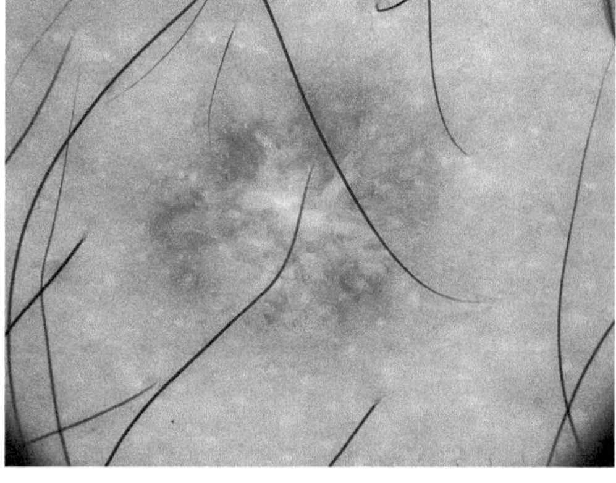

FIGURE 4.32 A dermatofibroma dermatoscopically displaying small, roundish, light-brown globules within the central white patch.

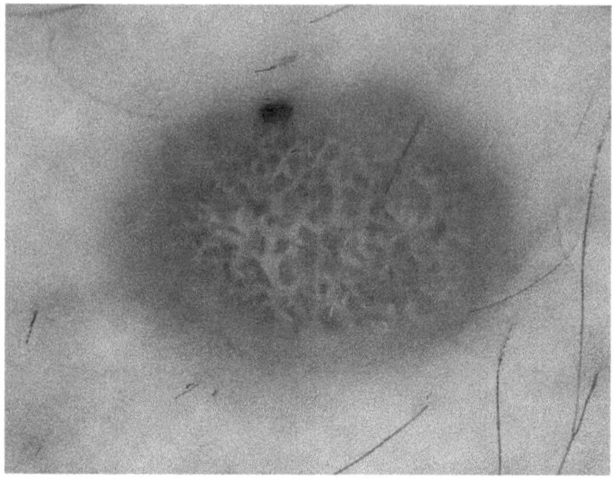

FIGURE 4.33 A dermatofibroma dermatoscopically typified by central white network lines surrounding vascular structures.

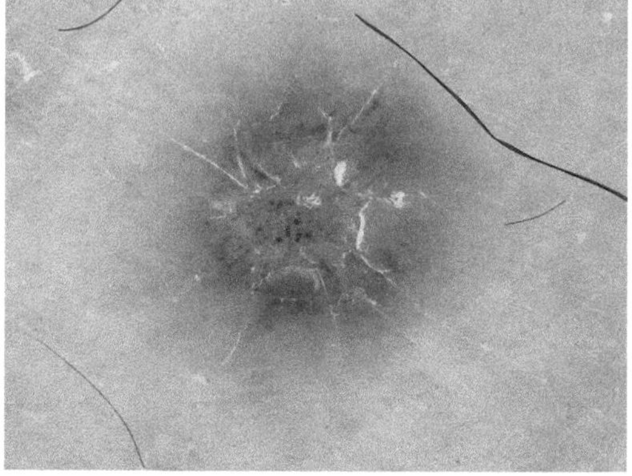

FIGURE 4.34 A dermatofibroma dermatoscopically displaying dotted and short linear vessels within the central whitish part.

The most frequent dermatoscopic pattern of DF consists of a central white (scar-like) patch, which is surrounded by a delicate, regular, usually light-brown pigment network (Figure 4.31). Sometimes, within the central white patch, several, small, roundish to oval globules of light-brown color may additionally be seen or even a white network, albeit rarely. The latter is more frequently observed in large DFs. A reddish halo around the lesion may also be found. Approximately 50% of DFs may also exhibit vascular structures, with erythema and dotted vessels being the most common vascular findings (Figures 4.32 through 4.34).

4.4 Common Adnexal Tumors

Adnexal tumors are divided on three main categories according to their origin: follicular, sebaceous, and sweat gland tumors. Several distinct adnexal tumors do exist, most of them benign in nature. Dermatoscopically, it has been proposed that many adnexal tumors are typified by features similar to the ones seen in basal cell carcinoma. Most descriptions of the dermatoscopic morphology of adnexal tumors are based on case reports and will not be mentioned in the current book.

4.4.1 Sebaceous Hyperplasia

Sebaceous hyperplasia clinically appears as solitary or more often as multiple, red-yellowish, umbilicated papules and may mimic nodular basal cell carcinoma (Figure 4.35).

Dermatoscopically, it is characterized by a whitish umbilicated, polylobular or structureless center, surrounded by elongated, scarcely branching vessels (crown vessels) (Figure 4.36).

4.4.2 Eccrine Poroma

Eccrine poroma is a sweat gland tumor with many distinct histopathologic subtypes. Dermatoscopically, it has been characterized as "the great mimicker," since it practically can assimilate all the frequent benign and malignant tumors. Eccrine poroma may be pigmented or nonpigmented. When pigmented, it may simulate melanoma or basal cell carcinoma as it may exhibit dermatoscopic features more commonly observed in the last tumors, namely brown or blue-gray pigmentation (Figures 4.37 and 4.38). Non-pigmented variants may mimic basal cell carcinoma or may display a polymorphous vascular pattern consisting of coiled, hairpin or linear vessels, thus mimicking amelanotic melanoma (Figure 4.39).

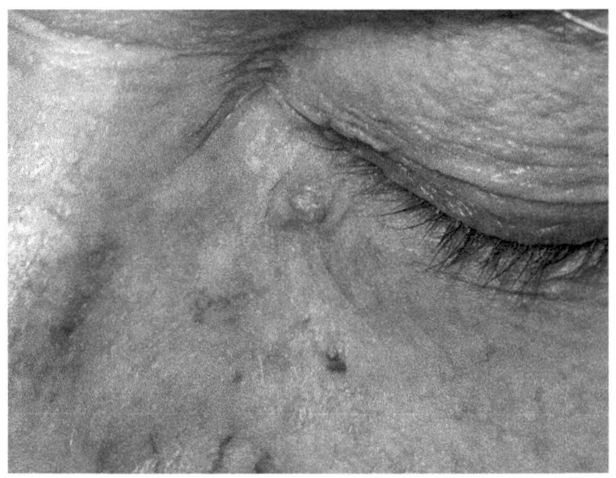

FIGURE 4.35 Clinical image of sebaceous hyperplasia similar to nodular basal cell carcinoma.

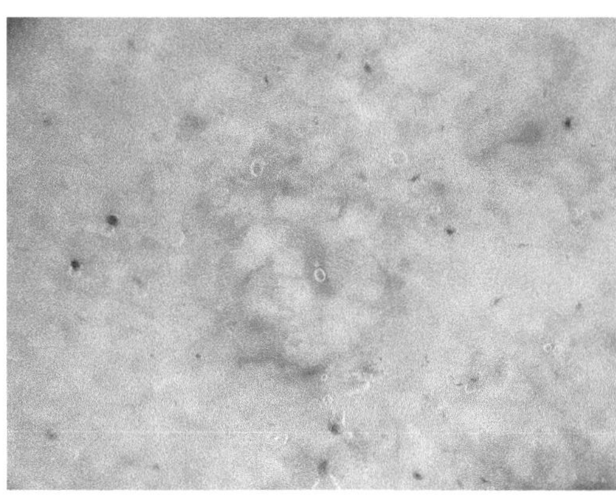

FIGURE 4.36 Dermatoscopy of sebaceous hyperplasia reveals a whitish umbilicated, polylobular center, surrounded by elongated, scarcely branching vessels (crown vessels).

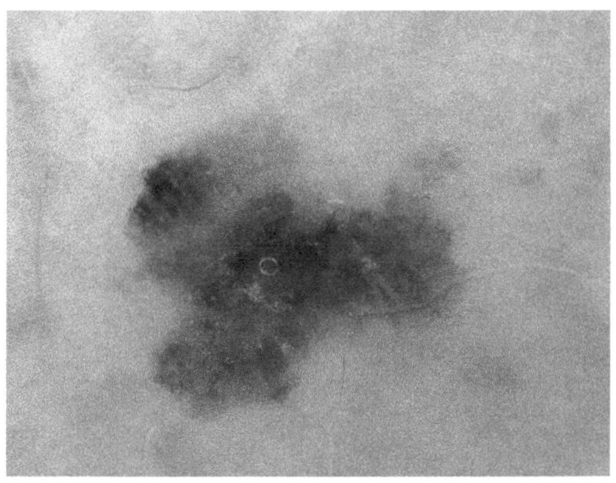

FIGURE 4.37 Pigmented eccrine poroma with diffuse brown pigmentation simulating melanoma.

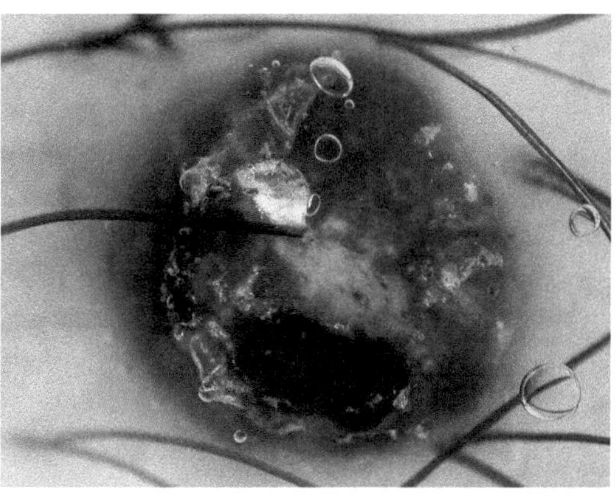

FIGURE 4.38 Pigmented eccrine poroma with blue-gray pigmentation simulating nodular basal cell carcinoma.

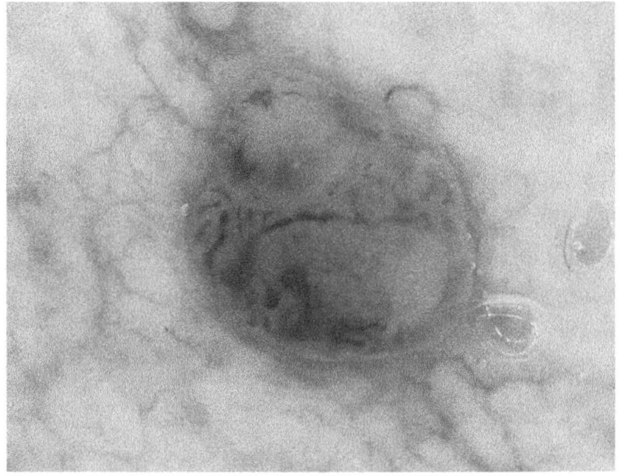

FIGURE 4.39 Nonpigmented eccrine poroma with linear and hairpin vessels simulating amelanotic melanoma.

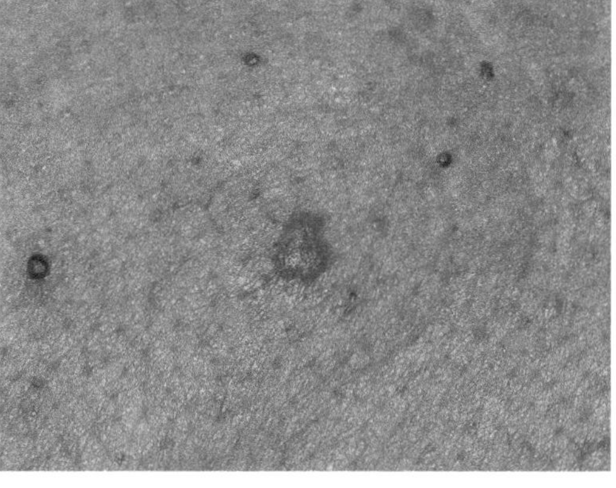

FIGURE 4.40 A clear cell acanthoma clinically manifesting as a pink-red nodule on the trunk.

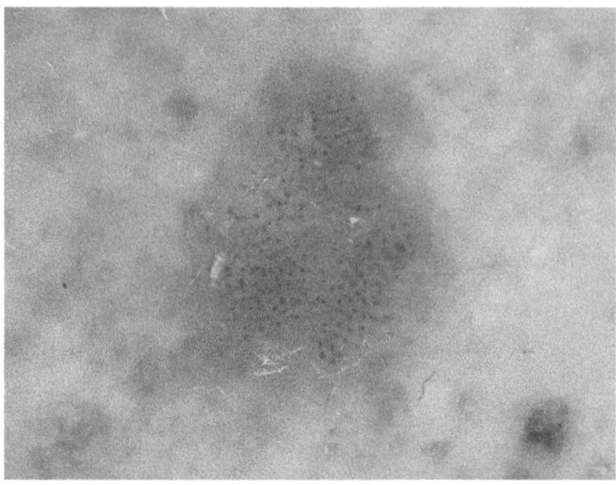

FIGURE 4.41 Dermatoscopy reveals red dots distributed linearly like strings of pearls forming polygons, a pattern that is pathognomonic for clear cell acanthoma.

4.5 Clear Cell Acanthoma

Clear cell acanthoma (CCA) is a benign tumor with a not fully elucidated pathogenesis. Although it was considered a benign epidermal tumor, recent evidence rather suggests that it is a reactive inflammatory dermatosis. Clinically, it appears as a red-purple nodule (Figure 4.40) more often on the lower extremities. Differential diagnosis includes benign and malignant skin tumors as well as inflammatory skin diseases. Dermatoscopically, it is characterized by the presence of dotted and sometimes glomerular vessels arranged linearly like strings of pearls. This unique dermoscopic pattern is almost pathognomonic and allows a straightforward diagnosis (Figure 4.41).

BIBLIOGRAPHY

Argenziano G, Soyer HP, De Giorgi V et al. *Dermoscopy: An Interactive Atlas*. Milan, Italy: EDRA; 2000.

Braun RP, Rabinovitz HS, Krischer J et al. Dermoscopy of pigmented seborrheic keratosis: A morphological study. *Arch Dermatol*. 2002;138:1556–60.

Lallas A, Moscarella E, Argenziano G et al. Dermoscopy of uncommon skin tumours. *Australas J Dermatol*. 2014;55(1):53–62.

Nicolino R, Zalaudek I, Ferrara G et al. Dermoscopy of eccrine poroma. *Dermatology*. 2007;215(2):160–3.

Nishikawa Y, Kaneko T, Takiyoshi N et al. Dermoscopy of eccrine poroma with calcification. *J Dermatol Case Rep*. 2009;3(3):38–40.

Sahin MT, Ozturkcan S, Ermertcan AT et al. A comparison of dermoscopic features among lentigo senilis/initial seborrheic keratosis, seborrheic keratosis, lentigo maligna and lentigo maligna melanoma on the face. *J Dermatol*. 2004;31:884–9.

Shalom A, Schein O, Landi C et al. Dermoscopic findings in biopsy-proven poromas. *Dermatol Surg*. 2012;38(7 Pt 1):1091–6.

Stolz W, Schiffner R, Burgdorf WH. Dermatoscopy for facial pigmented skin lesions. *Clin Dermatol*. 2002;20:276–8.

Tiodorovic-Zivkovic D, Lallas A, Longo C, Moscarella E, Zalaudek I, Argenziano G. Dermoscopy of clear cell acanthoma. *J Am Acad Dermatol*. 2015;72:S47–9.

Wolf IH. Dermoscopic diagnosis of vascular lesions. *Clin Dermatol*. 2002;20:273–5.

Zaballos P, Ara M, Puig S et al. Dermoscopy of sebaceous hyperplasia. *Arch Dermatol.* 2005;141(6):808.

Zaballos P, Marti E, Cuellar F et al. Dermoscopy of lichenoid regressing seborrheic keratosis. *Arch Dermatol.* 2006;142:410.

Zaballos P, Puig S, Llambrich A et al. Dermoscopy of dermatofibromas: A prospective morphological study of 412 cases. *Arch Dermatol.* 2008;144(1):75–83.

Zalaudek I, Kreusch J, Giacomel J et al. How to diagnose nonpigmented skin tumors: A review of vascular structures seen with dermoscopy: Part II. Nonmelanocytic skin tumors. *J Am Acad Dermatol.* 2010;63(3):377–86; quiz 387–8.

5

Malignant Nonmelanocytic Tumors

5.1 Basal Cell Carcinoma

Basal cell carcinoma (BCC) is the most common type of skin cancer accounting for approximately 80% of nonmelanoma skin cancers, and its incidence has doubled over the last few years. Although BCC is observed in people of all races and skin types, it is most often found in light-skinned individuals, particularly among those with very fair skin color and red or blond hair.

It has been well established that dermatoscopy has a significant role in BCC diagnosis with a diagnostic accuracy ranging from 95% to 99%. The dermatoscopic pattern of BCC is a result of different combinations of well-known criteria, which are as follows:

Nonpigmented Structures

- *Arborizing vessels*: Stem vessels of large diameter, branching irregularly into finest terminal capillaries. Their color is bright red, being perfectly in focus due to their location on the surface of the tumor.
- *Superficial fine telangiectasia*: Short, fine, focused linear vessels with very few branches.
- *Ulceration*: One or more large structureless areas of red to black-red color.
- *Multiple small erosions*: Small brown-red to brown-yellow crusts.
- *Shiny white-red structureless areas*: Translucent to opaque white to red areas.
- *White shiny structures (blotches/strands)*: White shiny clods or larger structureless areas with a shiny, bright color which can be seen only with polarized dermatoscopy.

Pigmented Structures

- *Leaf-like areas*: Translucent brown to gray/blue peripheral bulbous extensions that never arise from pigmented networks or from adjacent confluent pigmented areas.
- *Spoke-wheel areas*: Well-circumscribed radial projections, usually tan but sometimes blue or gray, meeting at an often darker (dark brown, black, or blue) central axis.
- *Concentric structures*: Irregularly shaped globular-like structures with different colors (blue, gray, brown, black) and a darker central area. They possibly represent variations or "precursors" of the spoke-wheel areas.
- *In-focus dots*: Loosely arranged, well-defined small gray dots, which appear sharply in focus.
- *Multiple blue-gray globules*: Numerous, loosely arranged, round to oval well-circumscribed structures, which are smaller than the nests.

- *Blue-gray ovoid nests*: Well-circumscribed confluent or near confluent pigmented ovoid or elongated configurations, larger than globules, and not intimately connected to pigmented tumor body.

5.1.1 Dermatoscopy and Histopathologic Subtype

Dermatoscopy not only enhances the diagnostic accuracy but also allows for the prediction of the histopathologic subtype of BCC, as each one of them displays a specific dermatoscopic pattern consisting of a combination of the aforementioned criteria.

Nonpigmented Basal Cell Carcinoma

The dermatoscopic hallmark of nodular-cystic BCC is the large, focused, bright red, and branching arborizing vessels, usually combined with a translucent pinkish background and ulceration (Figures 5.1 through 5.3).

Both infiltrative and sclerodermiform (morpheaform) BCC dermatoscopically display arborizing vessels and ulceration. However, the vessels are usually finer, more scattered, and

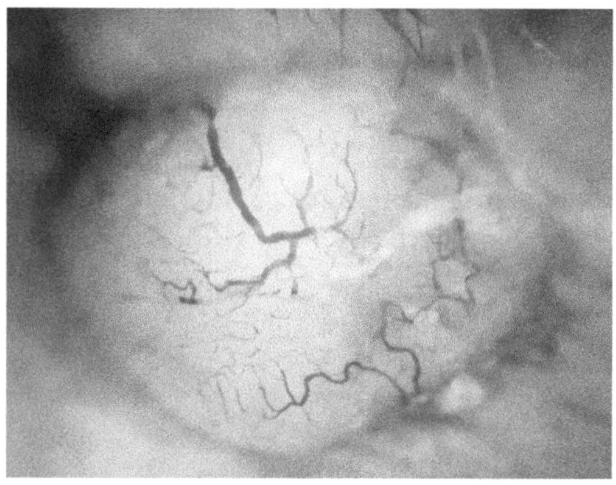

FIGURE 5.1 The typical focused, linear branching vessels on nodular basal cell carcinoma in a translucent, pinkish background.

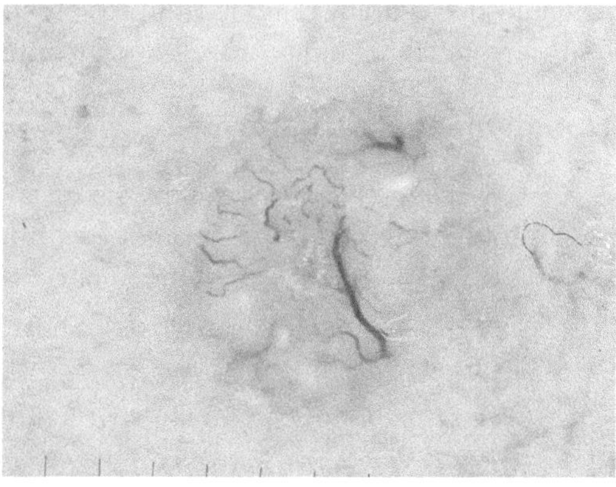

FIGURE 5.2 Another example of classical arborizing vessels of nodular basal cell carcinoma.

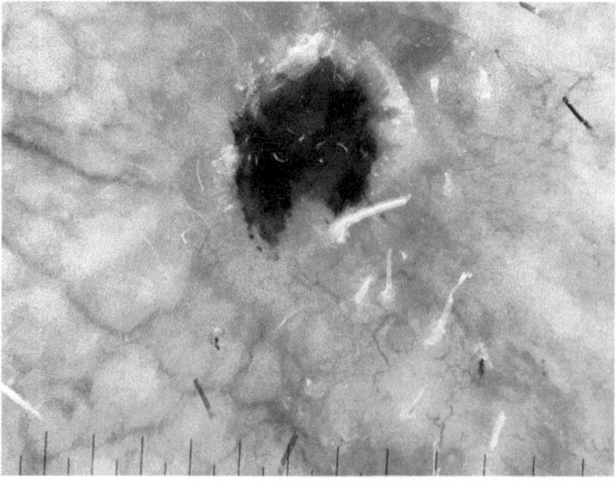

FIGURE 5.3 A nodular basal cell carcinoma with linear branching arborizing vessels in a translucent background and an ulceration at the upper part.

have fewer branches as compared to the vessels of nodular BCC. In addition, dermatoscopy may also reveal white-red structureless areas in infiltrative BCC and white structureless areas and/or white shiny blotches/strands in sclerodermiform BCC, histopathologically corresponding to the underlying fibrosis (Figure 5.4).

Superficial BCC dermatoscopically displays a shiny white to red, translucent, or opaque structureless background and, occasionally, short fine telangiectasias with relatively few ramifications. Multiple small superficial erosions represent a frequent additional feature (Figure 5.5). The dermatoscopic pattern of superficial BCC may vary according to the anatomical location. Specifically, superficial BCCs located on the limbs may exhibit dotted and/or glomerular vessels (instead of the typical telangiectasias as described previously), often combined with white shiny blotches/strands (Figures 5.6 and 5.7).

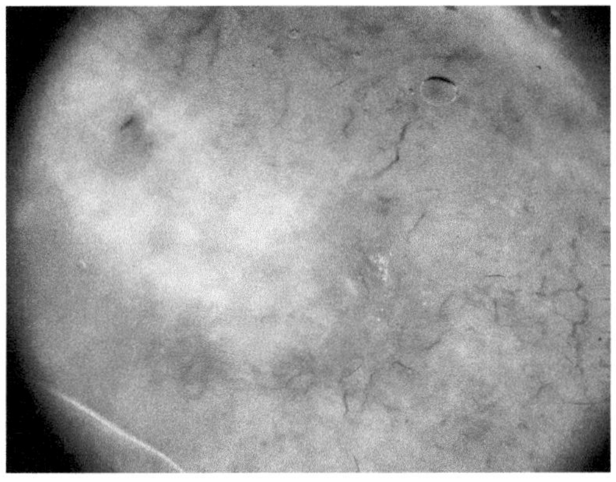

FIGURE 5.4 Dermatoscopic image of sclerodermiform BCC with branching vessels, white structureless areas, and white shiny blotches/strands.

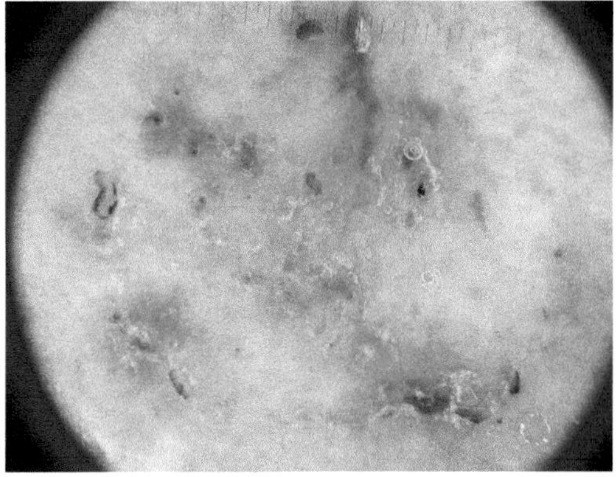

FIGURE 5.5 Superficial basal cell carcinoma dermatoscopically characterized by a white-red background and multiple small erosions and fine telangiectasias.

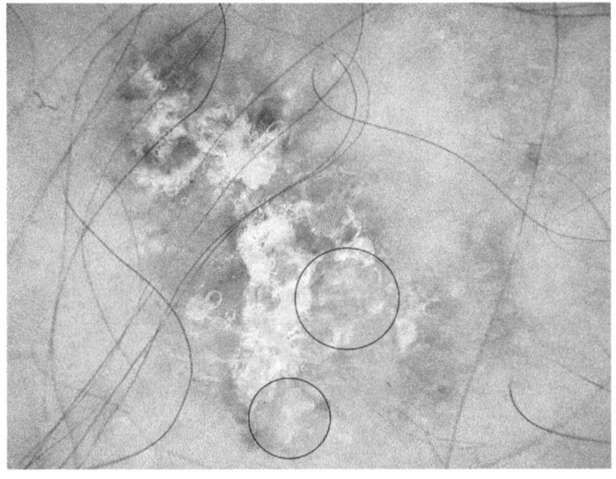

FIGURE 5.6 Dermatoscopy of a superficial basal cell carcinoma on the lower leg revealing glomerular vessels, white scales, and white shiny blotches/strands (black circles).

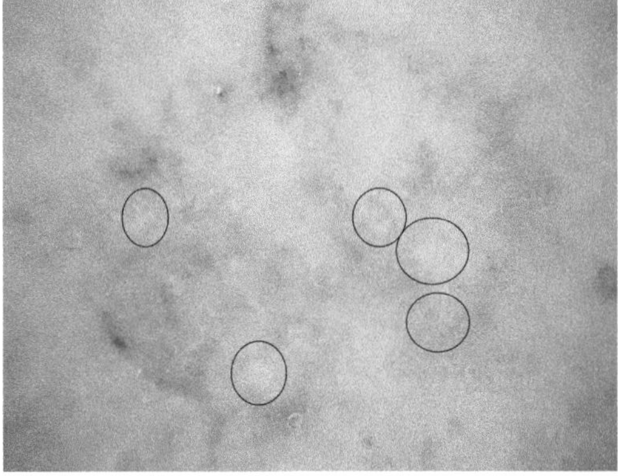

FIGURE 5.7 A superficial basal cell carcinoma on the lower leg dermatoscopically typified by dotted vessels, a small erosion at the upper part of the lesion, and multiple white, shiny blotches/strands (black circles).

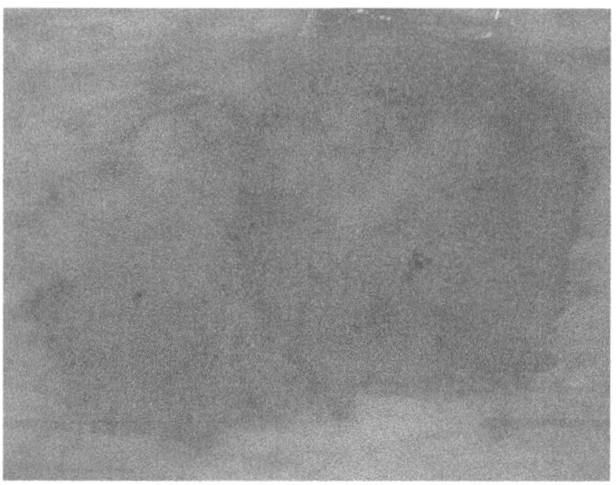

FIGURE 5.8 A fibroepithelioma of Pinkus dermatoscopically characterized by dotted vessels at the periphery and linear vessels in the center.

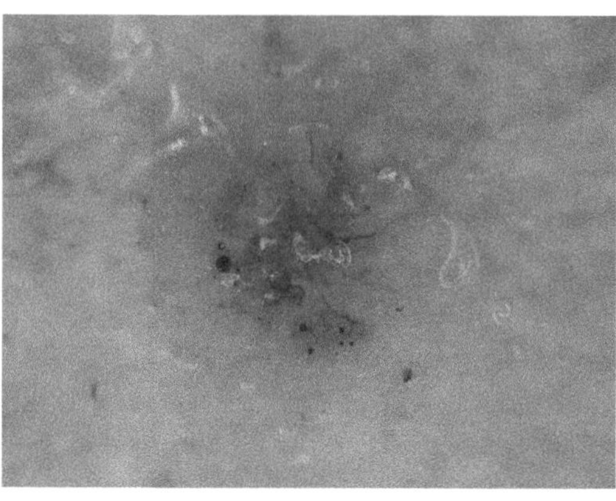

FIGURE 5.9 A pigmented nodular basal cell carcinoma dermatoscopically displaying arborizing vessels and blue-gray dots and globules.

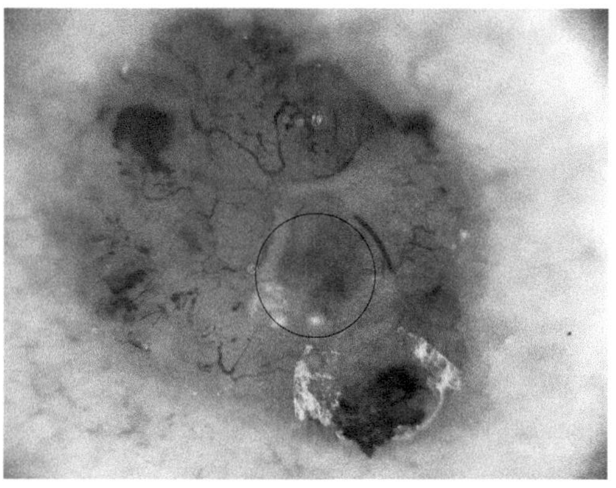

FIGURE 5.10 Dermatoscopy of a nodular basal cell carcinoma revealing arborizing vessels, ulceration, and a large blue-gray ovoid nest (black circle).

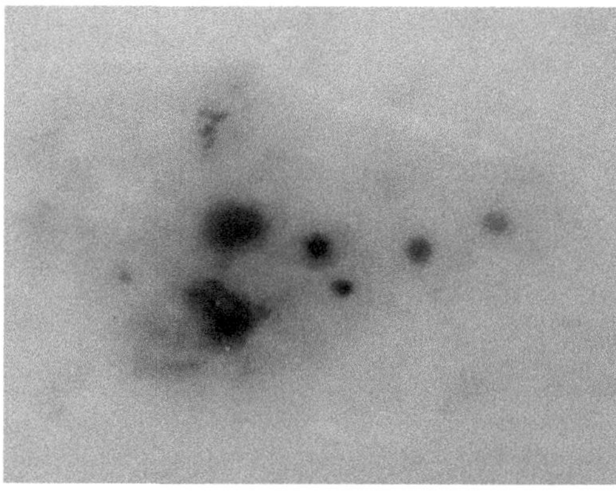

FIGURE 5.11 Multiple blue globules and nests as the only dermatoscopic feature of a basal cell carcinoma.

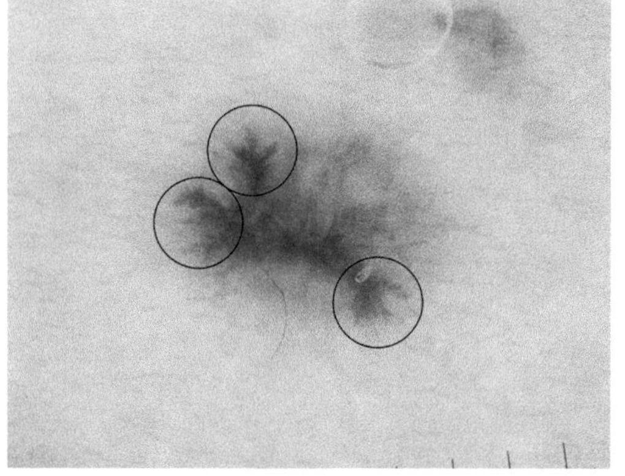

FIGURE 5.12 A pigmented superficial basal cell carcinoma with peripheral light brown leaf-like areas (circles).

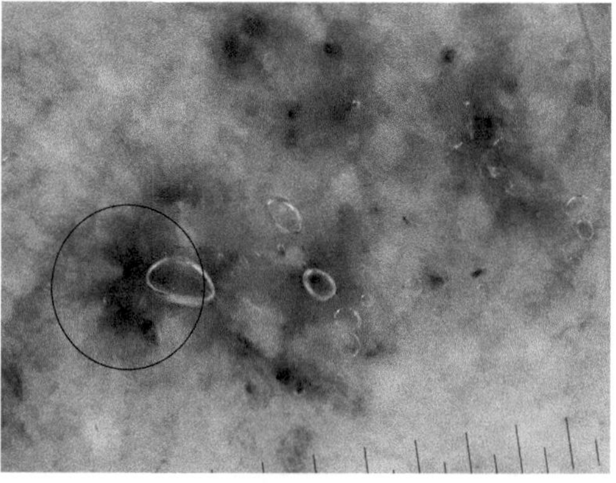

FIGURE 5.13 A superficial basal cell carcinoma dermatoscopically displaying multiple small erosions and leaf-like areas (circle).

Fibroepithelioma of Pinkus, a rare variant of BCC, is dermatoscopically characterized by a white-pinkish background along with fine arborizing vessels in the center and dotted vessels at the periphery (Figure 5.8).

Pigmented Basal Cell Carcinoma

The dermatoscopic findings of pigmented BCCs vary again according to the histopathologic subtype. Specifically, pigmented nodular BCC exhibits loosely arranged blue-gray dots/globules and/or blue-gray ovoid nests indicating the tumor depth, since these blue-colored structures correspond to basaloid nests deeper in the dermis. These features are often (but not necessarily) combined with arborizing vessels (Figures 5.9 through 5.11).

When pigmented, both infiltrative and sclerodermiform BCC exhibit blue-gray ovoid nests, multiple blue-gray dots/globules, and in-focus dots indicating their nonsuperficial nature.

Pigmented superficial BCC is dermatoscopically typified by peripheral light brown to grayish leaf-like areas (linear projections converging to a common base) or spoke-wheel areas, composed of a central darker globule surrounded by lighter, peripheral linear projections (Figures 5.12 through 5.14). A similar feature is the "concentric structure," which is an oval area with a darker center and is considered to represent the early phase of a spoke-wheel area (Figure 5.14). These light brown to grayish structures seen in superficial BCC indicate that the pigmentation is located at the level of the dermo-epidermal junction. Mixed tumors (with a superficial and nodular component) exist, and the dermatoscopic features seen in each component vary accordingly (Figure 5.15).

Table 5.1 summarizes the dermatoscopic criteria of BCC according to histopathologic subtype. From a macroscopic aspect, BCC often mimics benign skin tumors such as dermal nevus, common wart, sebaceous hyperplasia, or seborrheic keratosis (Figure 5.16). By revealing one or more of the criteria summarized in the table, dermatoscopy usually allows for the early recognition of BCC (Figure 5.17). Therefore, every skin lesion, even those that are clinically "innocent," should be examined with the dermatoscope.

In patients with Gorlin–Goltz syndrome, dermatoscopy also facilitates recognition of the characteristic palmar pits by revealing linearly arranged dotted vessels (Figure 5.18).

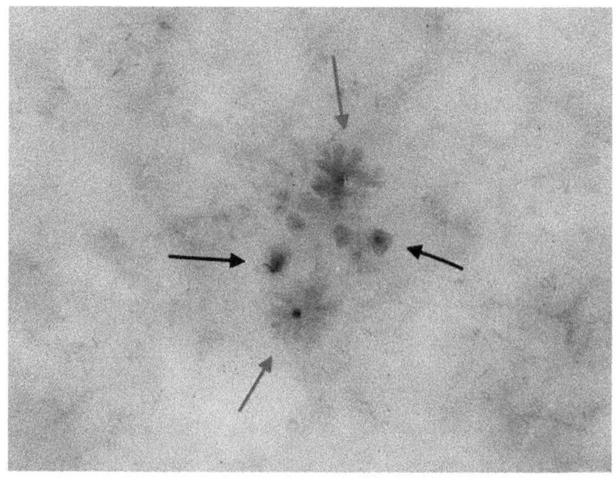

FIGURE 5.14 Spoke-wheel areas (red arrows) and concentric structures (black arrows) in a superficial basal cell carcinoma.

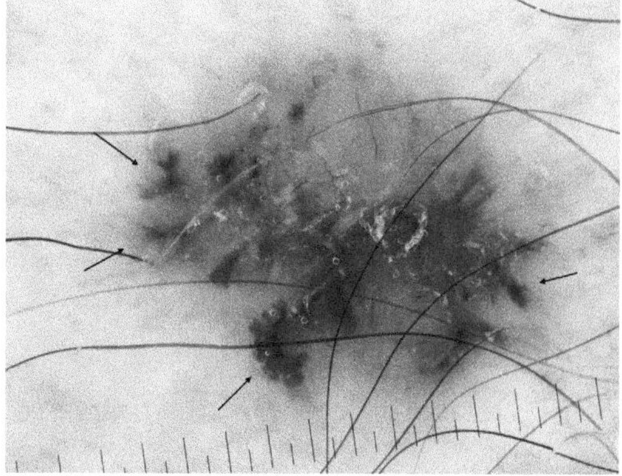

FIGURE 5.15 Dermatoscopy of a mixed basal cell carcinoma reveals arborizing vessels and blue color in the center, corresponding to the nodular component, and brown-colored leaf-like areas at the periphery, corresponding to the superficial component (arrows).

TABLE 5.1

Dermatoscopic Criteria of Basal Cell Carcinoma (BCC) According to the Histopathologic Subtype and the Presence or Absence of Pigmentation

Type of BCC	Dermatoscopic Criteria
Superficial	
Nonpigmented	Superficial fine telangiectasia Multiple small erosions Shiny white-red structureless areas Dotted vessels with or without white, shiny blotches/strands (when located on the limbs)
Pigmented	Maple leaf–like areas Spoke-wheel areas Concentric structures Multiple brown dots
Nodular	
Nonpigmented	Arborizing vessels Ulceration Pinkish, translucent background
Pigmented	Blue-gray ovoid nests Multiple blue-gray dots/globules
Morpheaform	
Nonpigmented	Arborizing vessels[a] Ulceration Whitish background
Pigmented	Blue-gray ovoid nests Multiple blue-gray dots/globules
Fibroepithelioma of Pinkus	White-pinkish background Fine arborizing vessels in the center Dotted vessels at the periphery
Basosquamous carcinoma	
Nonpigmented	Arborizing vessels Keratin masses White structureless areas Superficial scale Ulceration/blood crusts Blood spots in keratin masses
Pigmented	Blue-gray ovoid nests Multiple blue-gray dots/globules

[a] Usually finer, more scattered, and with fewer branches compared to the vessels of nodular BCC.

5.1.2 Dermatoscopy and Response to Treatment

Clinicians may also use dermatoscopy to evaluate the response of basal cell carcinoma to treatment and monitoring for possible recurrence. Specifically, it has been reported that the presence of any pigmented structure, ulceration/small erosions, or arborizing vessels, indicates residual disease (Figure 5.19). In contrast, their disappearance is associated with complete response (Figure 5.20). Reappearance of one or more of the latter criteria during follow-up suggests tumor recurrence. Finally, lesions in which white/red structureless areas and/or

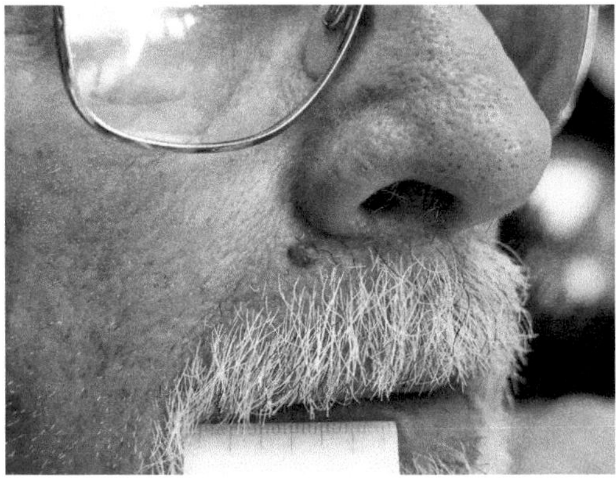

FIGURE 5.16 Clinical image of a nodular basal cell carcinoma that could be clinically diagnosed as a dermal nevus or seborrheic keratosis.

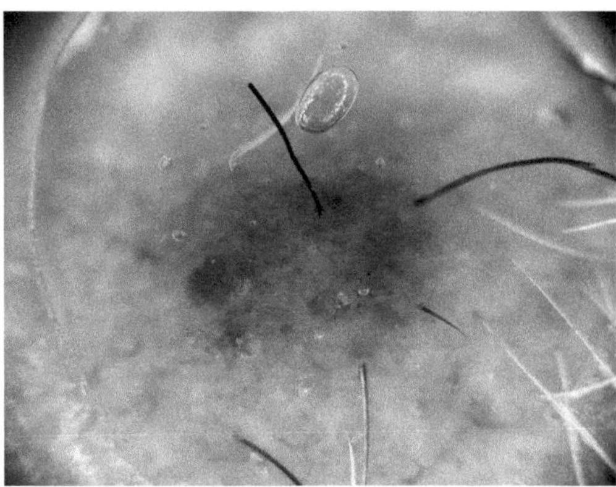

FIGURE 5.17 Dermatoscopy of the previous tumor reveals arborizing vessels and blue-gray dots and nests, suggesting the diagnosis of basal cell carcinoma.

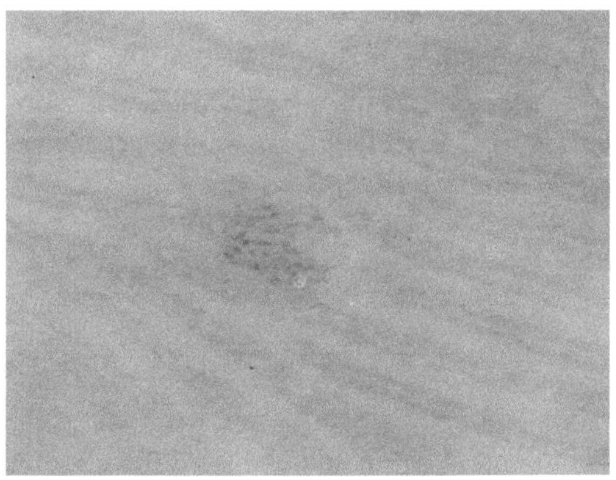

FIGURE 5.18 Dermatoscopic image of palmar pits with the characteristic vessels in Gorlin–Goltz syndrome.

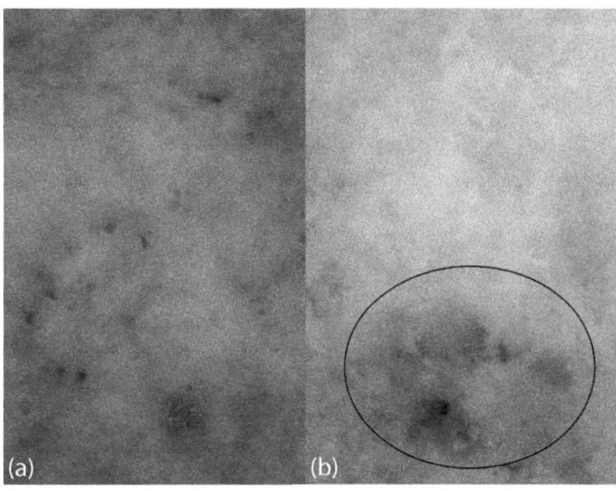

FIGURE 5.19 A basal cell carcinoma before (a) and after (b) treatment with imiquimod. The presence of pigmented structures (circle) is pathognomonic of residual disease.

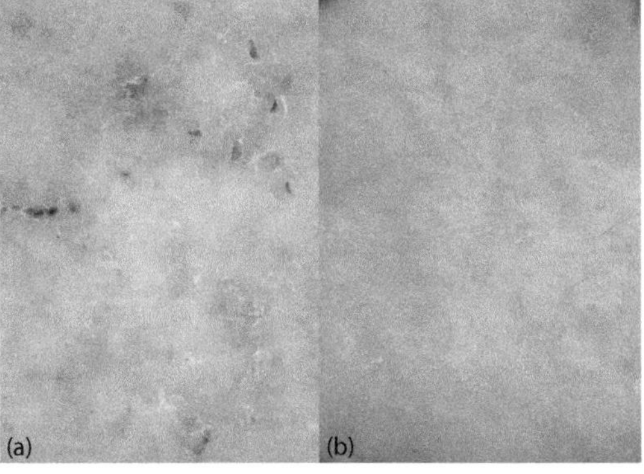

FIGURE 5.20 A basal cell carcinoma before (a) and after (b) treatment with imiquimod. The disappearance of all dermatoscopic criteria is highly suggestive of complete tumor clearance.

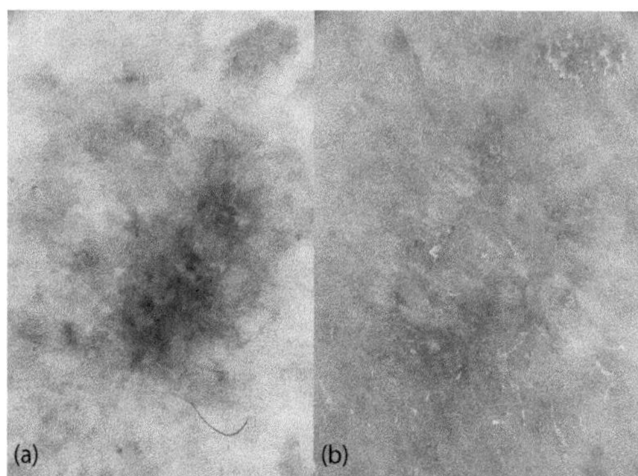

FIGURE 5.21 A basal cell carcinoma before (a) and after (b) treatment with imiquimod. Post-treatment dermatoscopy reveals short linear vessels and white color. These features are not very informative since they might either correspond to residual disease or be treatment induced.

superficial fine telangiectasias are observed after treatment should be closely monitored in order to recognize early recurrence (Figure 5.21).

Dermatoscopy is also useful in the accurate determination of the tumor margins before surgical excision, thus increasing the possibility of clear margins. This is because dermatoscopy might detect a subclinical tumor expansion by revealing BCC-associated criteria at the periphery of the lesion, which might be assessed as uninvolved with the naked eye.

5.2 Keratinocyte Skin Cancer

The term *keratinocyte skin cancer* refers to different stages in the progression of malignant neoplasms of epidermal keratinocytes, which show squamous phenotypic differentiation, namely, actinic keratosis, intraepidermal carcinoma, and invasive squamous cell carcinoma (SCC).

5.2.1 Actinic Keratosis

Actinic keratoses (AKs) are the most common neoplasms within the spectrum of keratinocyte skin cancer. They are defined as the earliest form of SCC (squamous cell carcinoma *in situ*). AKs rarely develop as single lesions. Usually, multiple lesions affect an entire field of chronically sun-damaged skin (Figure 5.22). This led to the concept of "field cancerization," which refers to the presence of genetically altered cell clones in normal-appearing skin contiguous to fields of neoplastic cells, which have the potential for clonal expansion and, therefore, lead to constant and consequent development of new tumors within this field.

According to their thickness, AKs are clinically classified into three grades (grades I, II, and III); grade I AKs are slightly palpable (better felt than seen), grade II refers to moderately thick AKs (easily felt and seen), and grade III AKs, which are very thick, hyperkeratotic, and/or obvious (Figures 5.23 through 5.25). Each grade corresponds to a different dermatoscopic pattern. Grade I AKs are dermatoscopically characterized by red pseudonetwork and discrete white scales (Figure 5.26). Grade II AKs are dermatoscopically typified by the "strawberry pattern," which consists of an erythematous background intermingled by white to yellow, keratotic, and enlarged follicular openings (resembling the surface of a strawberry) (Figures 5.27 and 5.28).

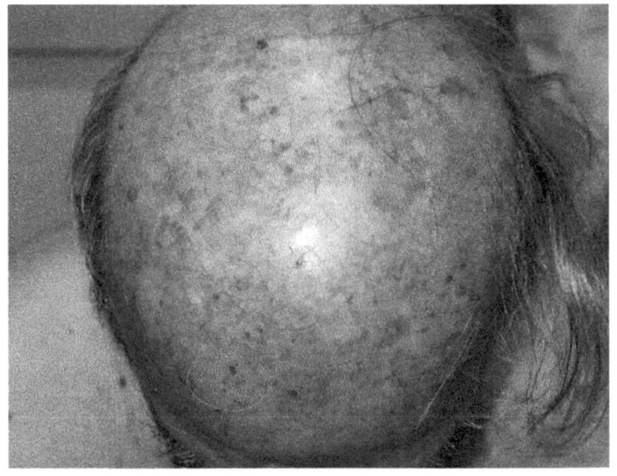

FIGURE 5.22 Multiple actinic keratoses in a cancerized field.

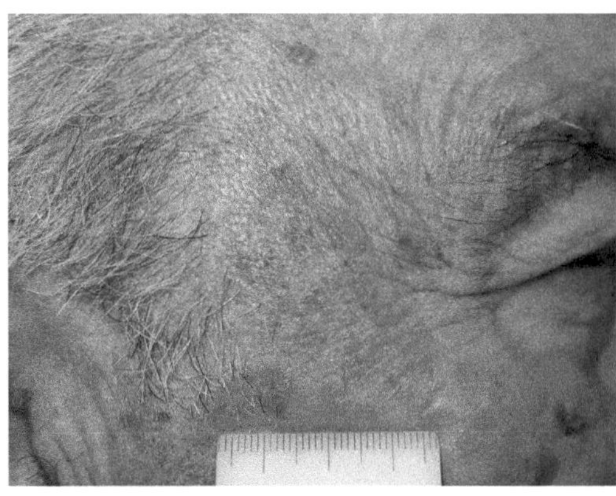

FIGURE 5.23 Clinical image of a grade I actinic keratosis. Only a slight erythema is visible.

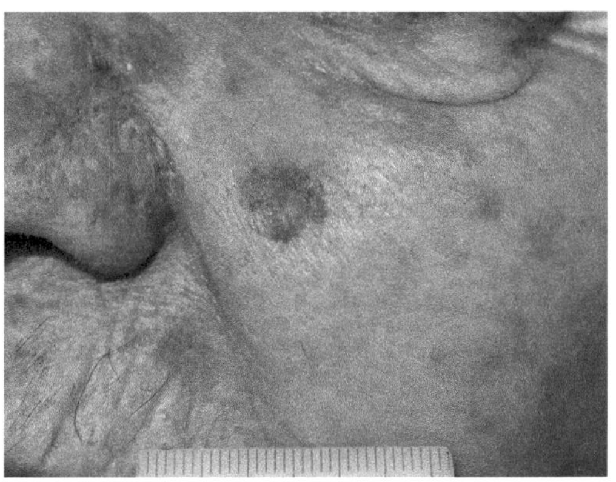

FIGURE 5.24 Clinical image of a grade II actinic keratosis typified by intense erythema and slight scaling.

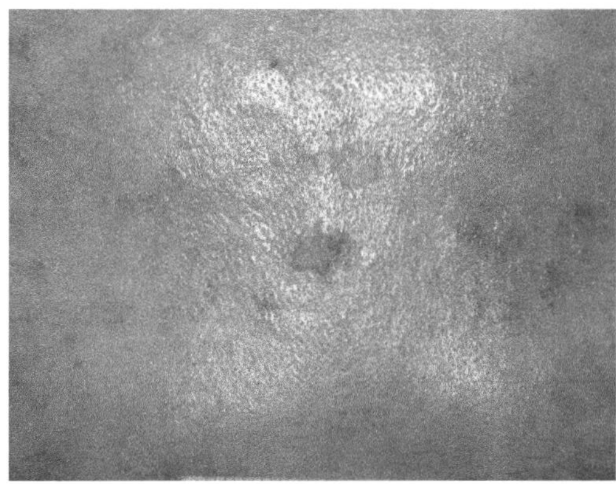

FIGURE 5.25 Clinical image of a grade III actinic keratosis with a hyperkeratotic surface.

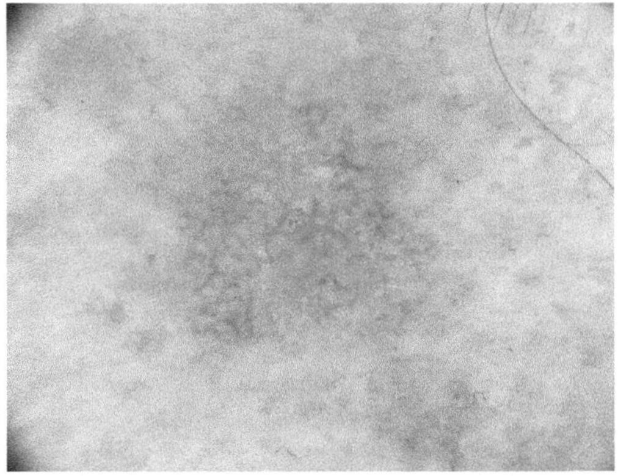

FIGURE 5.26 Dermatoscopy of a grade I actinic keratosis revealing a red pseudonetwork and discrete white scales.

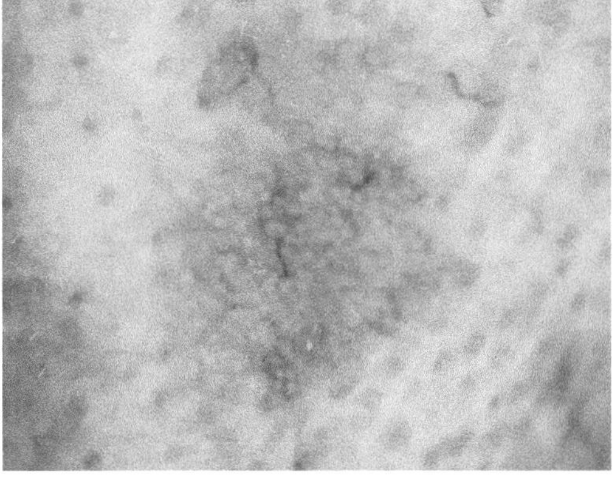

FIGURE 5.27 A grade I–II actinic keratosis dermatoscopically displaying a red background interrupted by white follicular openings (strawberry pattern).

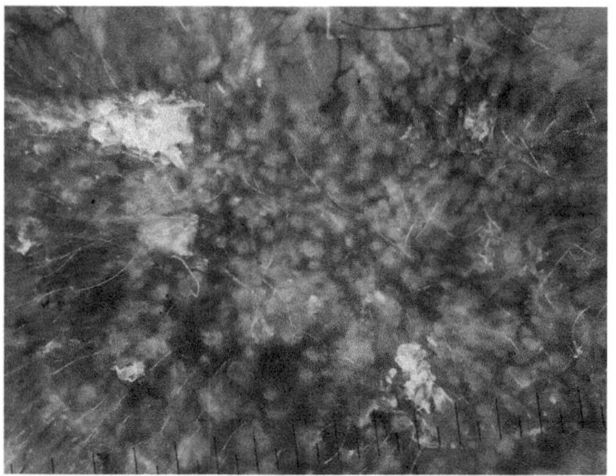

FIGURE 5.28 A grade II actinic keratosis dermatoscopically typified by a classic strawberry pattern.

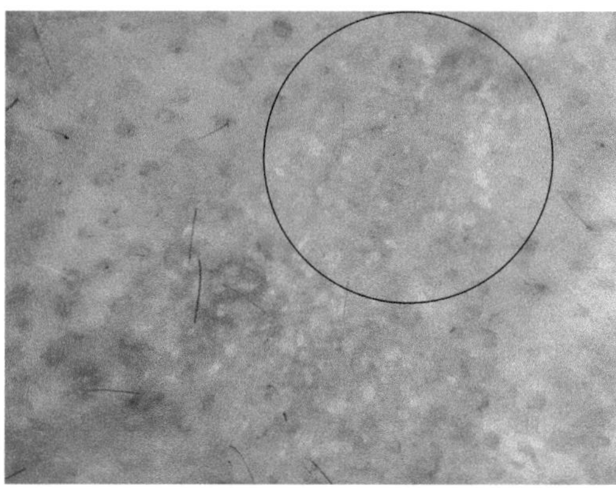

FIGURE 5.29 Rosettes in actinic keratosis seen only with polarized dermatoscopy (circle).

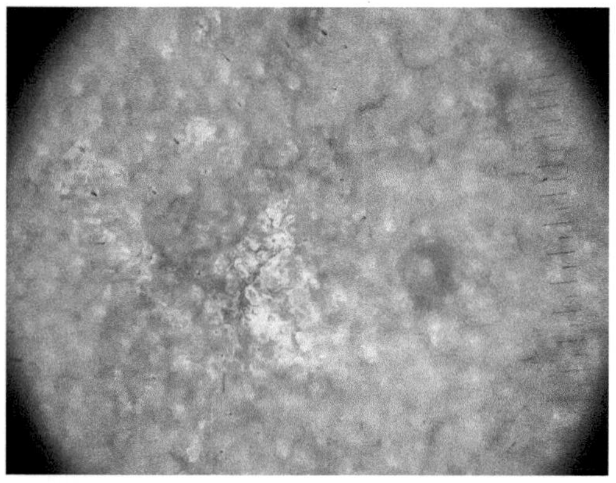

FIGURE 5.30 Dermatoscopy of a grade II–III actinic keratosis, revealing a strawberry pattern in some parts of the lesion, while other areas are covered by thick scales.

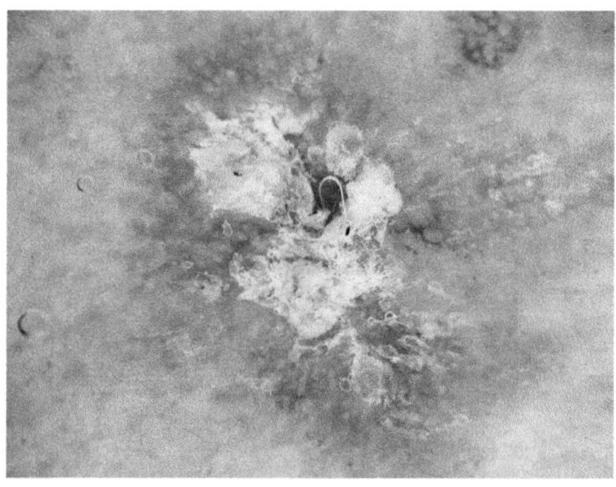

FIGURE 5.31 A grade III actinic keratosis covered by thick scales in the center. At the periphery, a red background and white follicular openings can be seen.

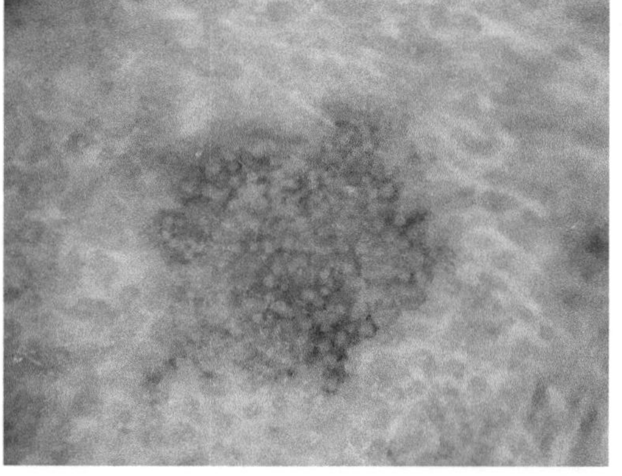

FIGURE 5.32 The typical dermatoscopic pattern of pigmented actinic keratosis consists of white and enlarged follicles and brown color in between them (brown pseudonetwork).

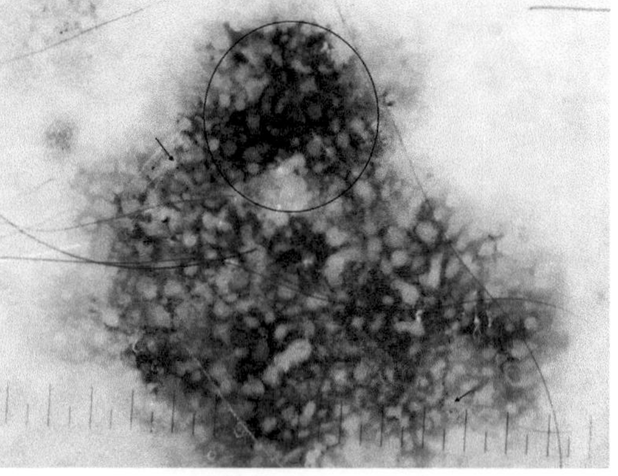

FIGURE 5.33 A pigmented AK dermatoscopically displaying gray dots (arrows), rhomboid structures (circle), asymmetrical pigmented follicular openings, and enlarged hair follicles.

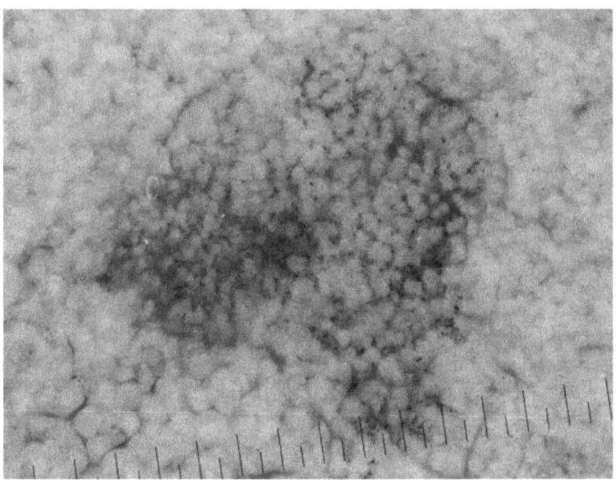

FIGURE 5.34 Gray dots at the outline of the follicles of a pigmented AK.

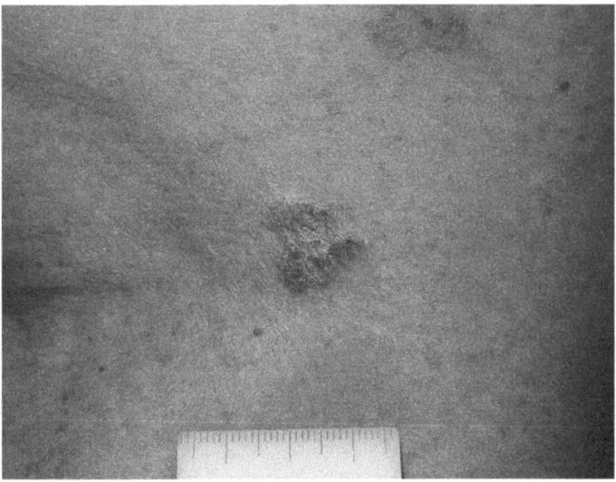

FIGURE 5.35 Clinical image of Bowen disease.

With polarized dermatoscopy, inside the white follicles of AK, four white dots in a square are often seen (rosettes) (Figure 5.29). Grade III AKs exhibit either enlarged follicular openings filled with keratotic plugs over a scaly and white-yellow background or white-yellow structureless areas due to hyperkeratosis (Figures 5.30 and 5.31). The diagnostic sensitivity and specificity of dermatoscopy in the diagnosis of AK have been reported to reach 98% and 95%, respectively.

As far as pigmented AKs are concerned, the most common dermatoscopic finding is a brown-gray "pseudonetwork" consisting of brown lines that surround the enlarged hair follicles (Figure 5.32). Red pseudonetwork and scales may additionally be seen, facilitating the diagnosis. Moreover, pigmented AK may exhibit gray dots (annular-granular pattern) and asymmetrically pigmented follicular openings, features commonly seen also in lentigo maligna (LM), rendering their discrimination sometimes very difficult (Figures 5.33 and 5.34). The differential diagnosis between pigmented AK and LM is separately discussed in Chapter 9.

5.2.2 Intraepidermal Carcinoma or Bowen's Disease

Bowen disease (BD) is a SCC *in situ* with full-epidermal thickness dysplasia. Clinically, BD usually manifests as a slow-growing solitary erythematous patch or plaque with a well-demarcated scaly surface (Figure 5.35).

Dermatoscopy of BD reveals dotted and/or glomerular (coiled) vessels, white to yellow scales, and a red-yellow background (Figure 5.36). At the magnification of the handheld dermatoscope (×10), glomerular vessels usually project as large-diameter red dots, while at higher magnifications their coiled morphology becomes apparent (Figure 5.37). Both dotted and glomerular vessels can be observed within the same lesion and are usually arranged in small, densely packed clusters or groups or linearly at the periphery (Figure 5.38).

In addition to the aforementioned criteria, dermatoscopy of pigmented BD might reveal brown-gray structureless areas and small brown globules/dots arranged either in a patchy distribution or in peripheral lines (Figure 5.39). Dermatoscopy was also shown to be useful for monitoring pigmented BD treated with local therapies. Disappearance of disease-specific dermatoscopic criteria is associated with complete response and histopathologic clearance of the tumor.

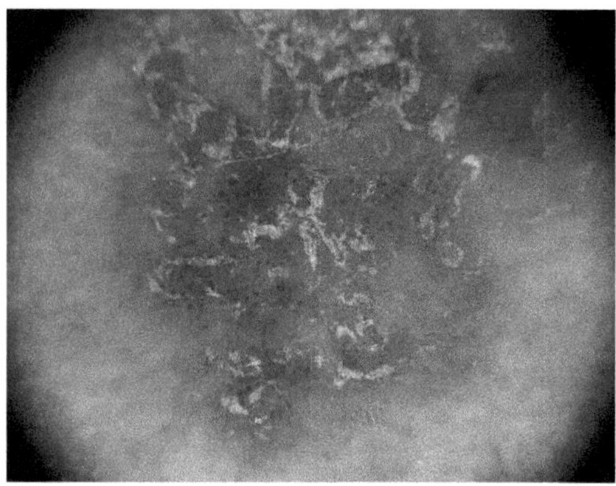

FIGURE 5.36 Dermatoscopic image of Bowen disease displaying white surface scales and dotted and glomerular vessels distributed in clusters.

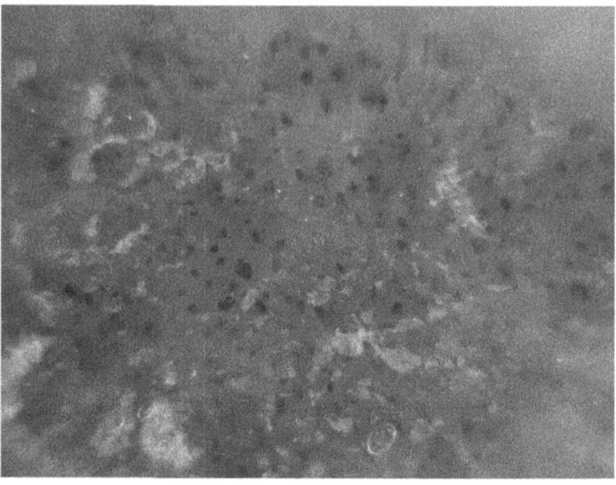

FIGURE 5.37 Glomerular vessels at high magnification.

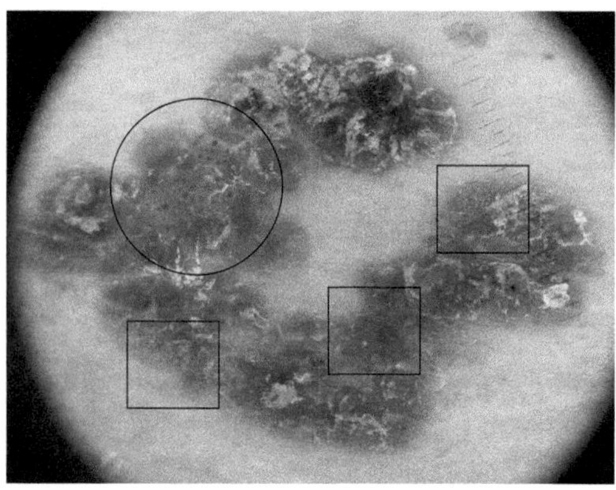

FIGURE 5.38 Clusters of dotted vessels (squares) and a cluster of glomerular vessels (circle) in Bowen disease.

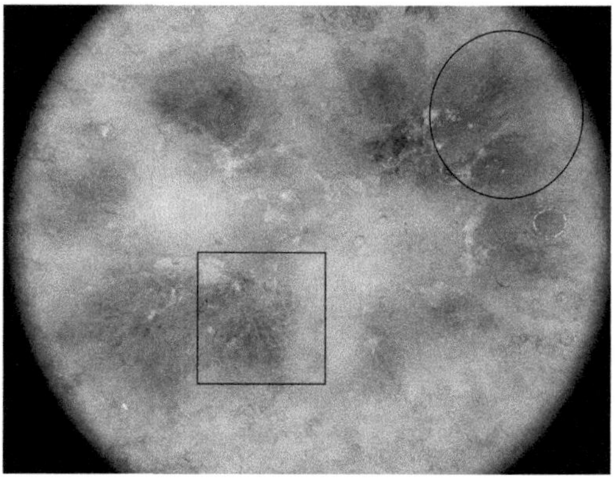

FIGURE 5.39 Pigmented Bowen disease dermatoscopically typified by brown globules and dots distributed in clusters (square) and in peripheral lines (circle).

5.2.3 Squamous Cell Carcinoma

Squamous cell carcinoma (SCC) is a malignant tumor that arises from the keratinizing cells of the epidermis or its appendages and is the second most common skin cancer after BCC. It is locally invasive and has the potential to metastasize, mainly to the regional lymph nodes, but also to distant organs. If detected and treated early, SCC has a 95% cure rate. In contrast, when neglected, it may cause local tissue destruction and may metastasize with a very poor prognosis.

Clinically, SCC usually manifests as an indurated, hyperkeratotic nodule, often with central ulceration and keratin mass (Figure 5.40), or as an ulcerated papule, nodule, or plaque, without evidence of keratinization (Figure 5.41). Typically, SCC develops within a severely sun-damaged field among several neighboring AKs.

Similar to BCC, the dermatoscopic pattern of SCC depends on histopathologic parameters, with the grade of differentiation being the major of them. The dermatoscopic criteria of SCC can be divided into two categories: (a) vascular structures and (b) criteria associated with keratinization. In general, the more differentiated the tumor is, the more evident the structures related to keratinization are. On the contrary, poorly differentiated SCC tends to lack these

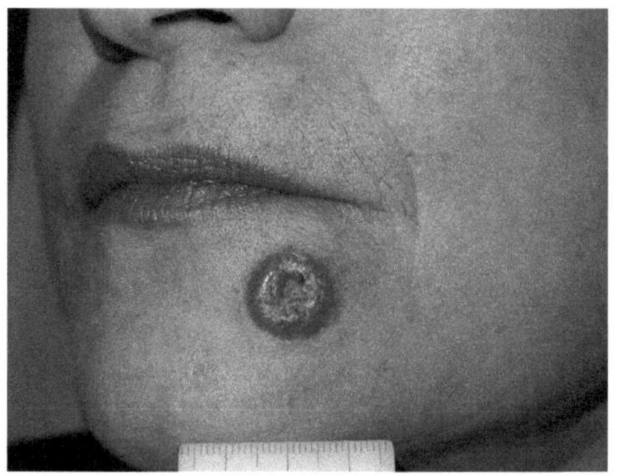

FIGURE 5.40 A squamous cell carcinoma developing as a centrally ulcerated nodule.

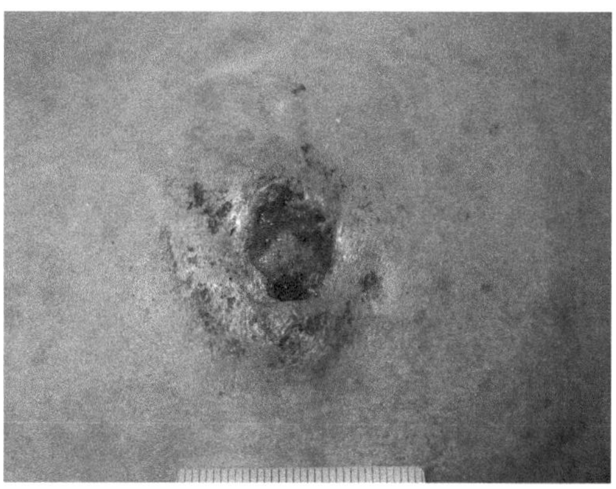

FIGURE 5.41 A squamous cell carcinoma developing as an indurated and ulcerated plaque.

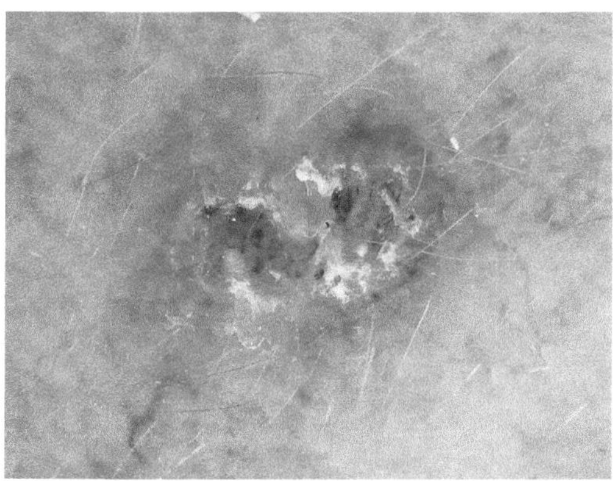

FIGURE 5.42 White-yellow scales in a squamous cell carcinoma.

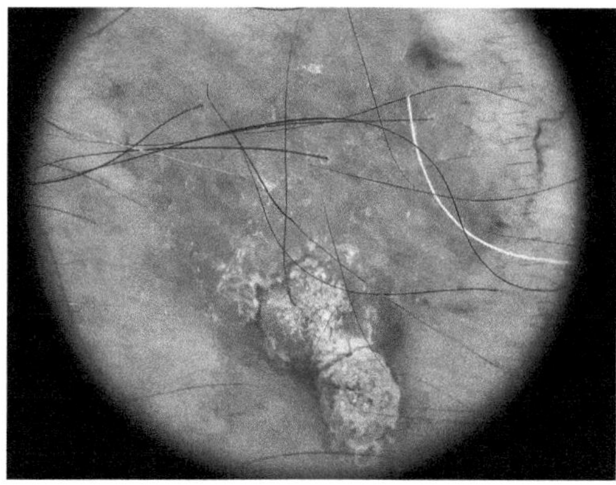

FIGURE 5.43 Amorphous white-yellow keratin mass in a squamous cell carcinoma.

criteria and exclusively display vascular structures. Ulceration or bleeding is also frequently seen in SCC.

Keratinization-associated criteria (may be observed either alone or combined): white-yellow scales (Figure 5.42), white-yellow amorphous keratin masses (Figure 5.43), white structureless areas (Figure 5.44), white halos surrounding vessels (Figure 5.45), and white circles surrounding follicles, also known as targetoid follicular openings (Figure 5.46). The latter feature is considered as the most specific for SCC and histopathologically corresponds to the hyperplastic epithelium of the enlarged follicular openings.

Vascularization-associated criteria: Several different morphologic types of vessels may be observed, including dotted and/or glomerular vessels, hairpin vessels, and linear-irregular vessels (Figures 5.47 through 5.49). Blood spots within keratin masses is another peculiar dermatoscopic feature of SCC (Figure 5.50).

Well-Differentiated Squamous Cell Carcinoma

Well-differentiated SCC is dermatoscopically typified by white structureless areas, keratin masses, peripheral hairpin vessels and/or linear vessels, white halos surrounding vessels, and white circles surrounding follicles (Figure 5.51).

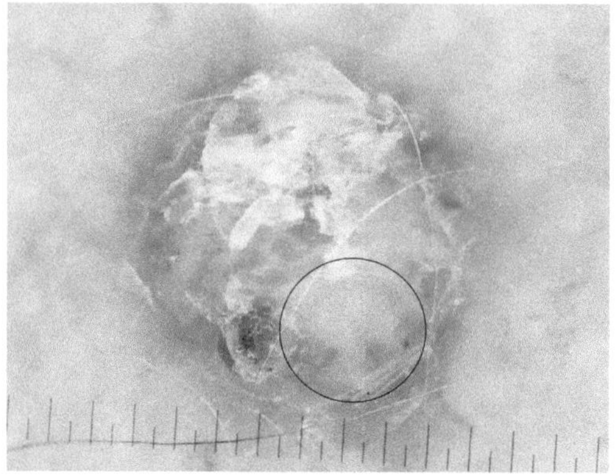

FIGURE 5.44 White structureless areas in a squamous cell carcinoma (circle).

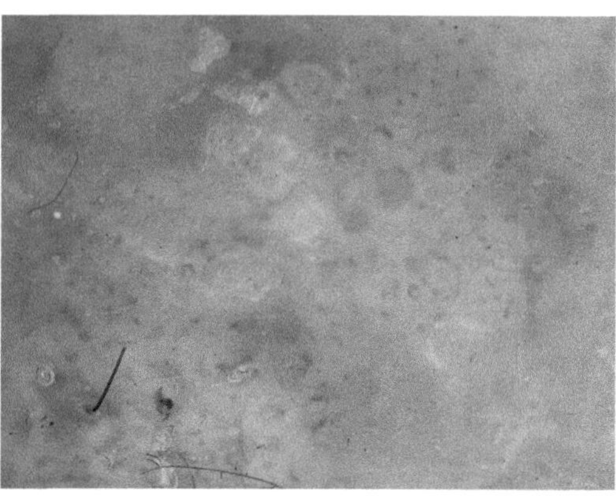

FIGURE 5.45 White halos surrounding vessels in a squamous cell carcinoma.

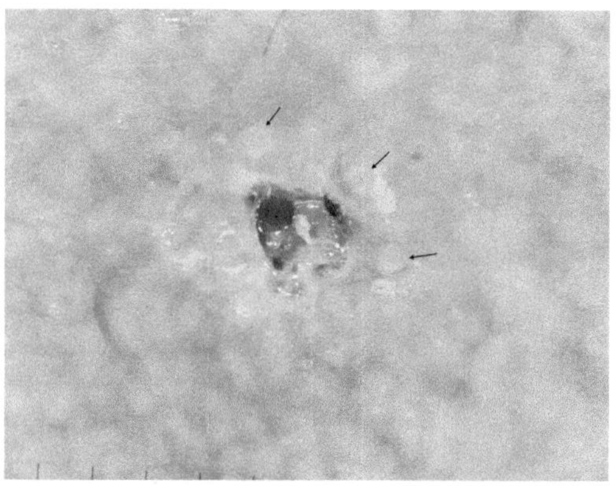

FIGURE 5.46 White circles surrounding follicular openings in a squamous cell carcinoma (arrows).

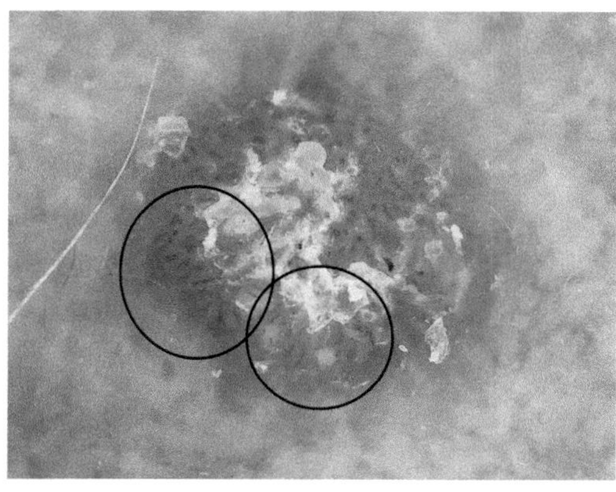

FIGURE 5.47 Hairpin vessels in a squamous cell carcinoma (circles).

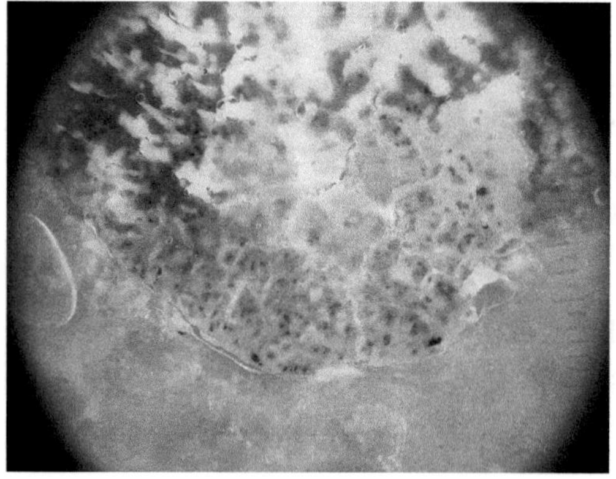

FIGURE 5.48 Dotted and glomerular vessels in a squamous cell carcinoma.

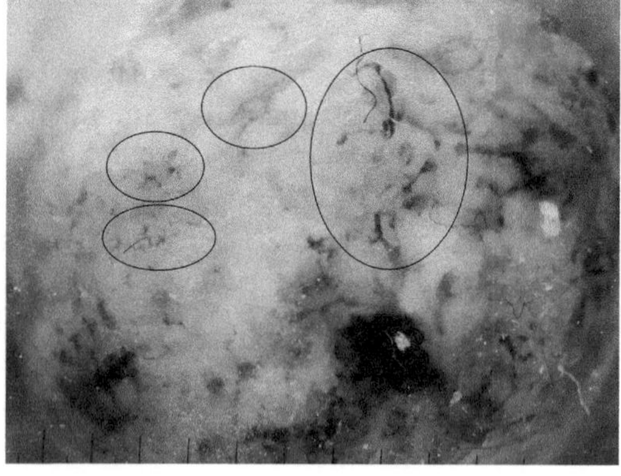

FIGURE 5.49 Linear-irregular vessels in a squamous cell carcinoma (circles).

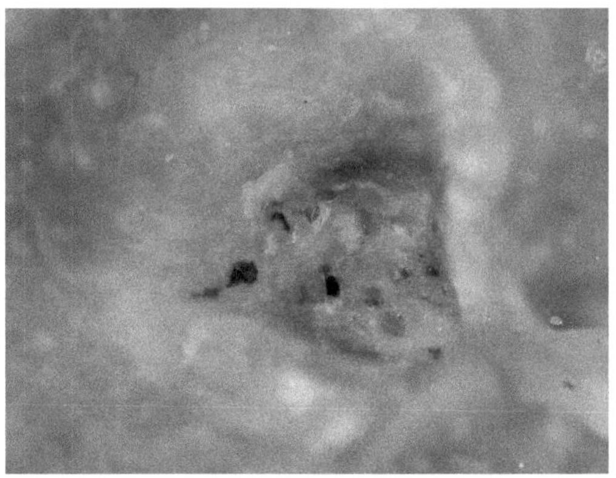

FIGURE 5.50 Blood spots in keratin masses in a squamous cell carcinoma.

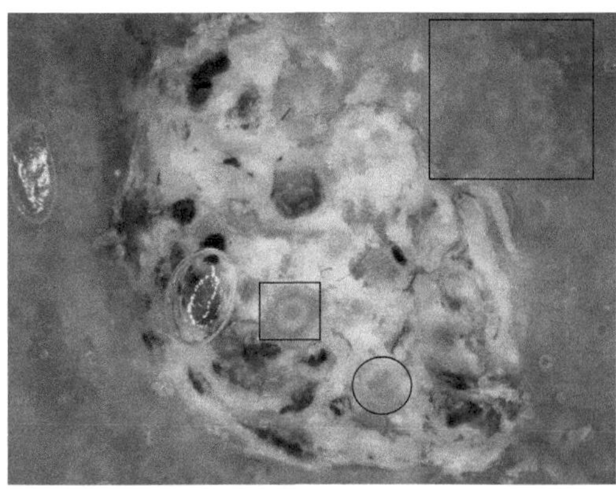

FIGURE 5.51 A typical example of well-differentiated squamous cell carcinoma, dermatoscopically displaying amorphous keratin masses, white circles surrounding follicles (squares), and white halos surrounding vessels (circle).

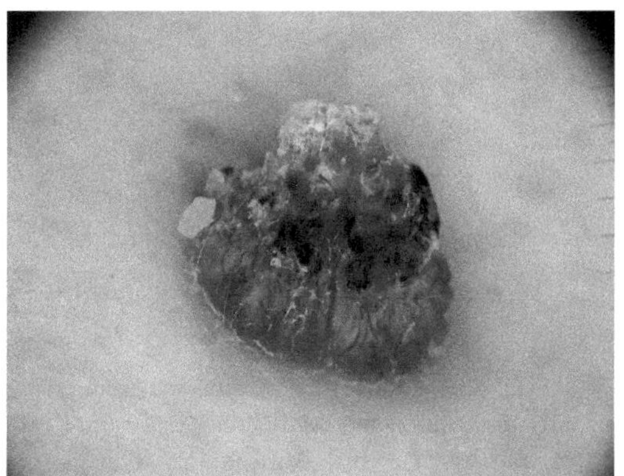

FIGURE 5.52 Dermatoscopy of keratoacanthoma typically reveals a central keratin mass and hairpin vessels at the periphery, usually surrounded by white color.

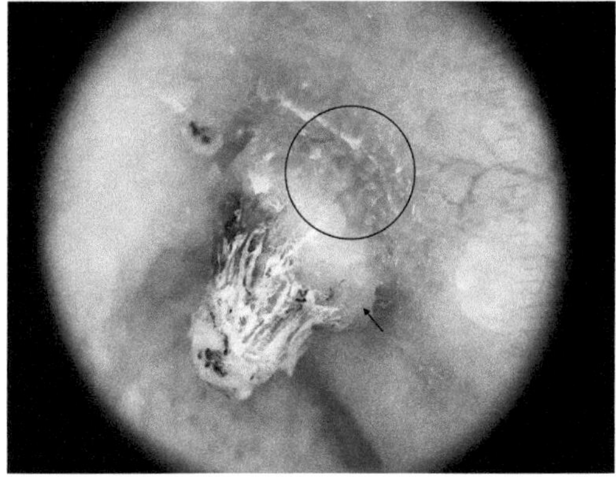

FIGURE 5.53 A keratoacanthoma displaying a central keratin mass, peripheral hairpin vessels (arrow), and white circles surrounding follicles at the periphery (circle).

Keratoacanthoma is considered as a subtype of well-differentiated SCC. It is dermatoscopically typified by a large, central, white-to-yellow keratin mass and hairpin vessels at the periphery, usually surrounded by a white halo (Figure 5.52). White circles surrounding follicles can additionally be seen at the periphery (Figure 5.53).

Poorly Differentiated Squamous Cell Carcinoma

Poorly differentiated SCC lacks signs of keratinization and usually presents as an ulcerated plaque with polymorphous vessels (linear, dotted, glomerular). As a result, the dermatoscopic predominant color is red instead of white (Figure 5.54).

5.2.4 Dermatoscopic Model of the Progression from Actinic Keratosis into Squamous Cell Carcinoma

The progression from AK into invasive SCC is dermatoscopically characterized by an evident increase in vascularization and keratinization structures. As a rule, the vascular structures in AK are not predominant. AKs dermatoscopically display perifollicular erythema, and if vessels are present, they are usually small and linear (Figure 5.55). When the full epidermis is involved (Bowen disease), dotted/glomerular vessels initially appear (Figure 5.56), followed by hairpin and linear-irregular vessels in case of infiltration of the dermis (invasive SCC) (Figure 5.57). Similarly, keratinization is increased as the tumor progresses. The scarce white scales of grade I AK gradually evolve into diffuse yellow-whitish opaque scales, followed by the development of white structureless areas or a central mass of keratin, white halos, white circles, and ulceration (Figure 5.58).

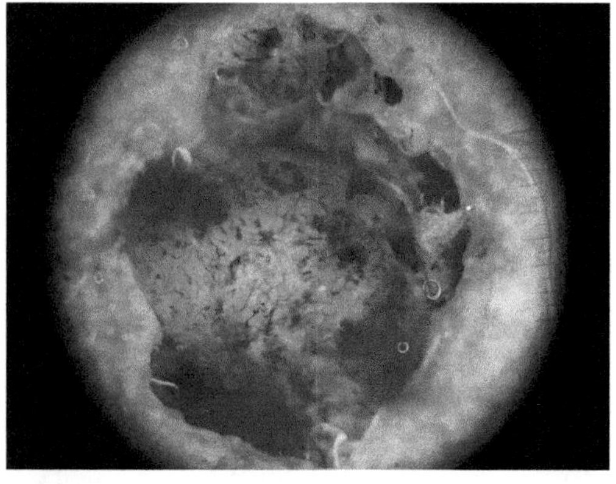

FIGURE 5.54 A poorly differentiated squamous cell carcinoma with linear irregular vessels and ulceration. Red color is predominant.

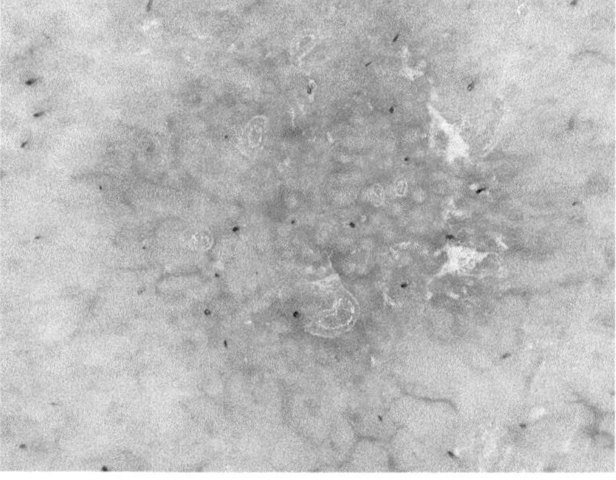

FIGURE 5.55 In actinic keratosis, vessels are usually not seen at all, or, if present, they are few, short, and linear in between the hair follicles (red pseudonetwork).

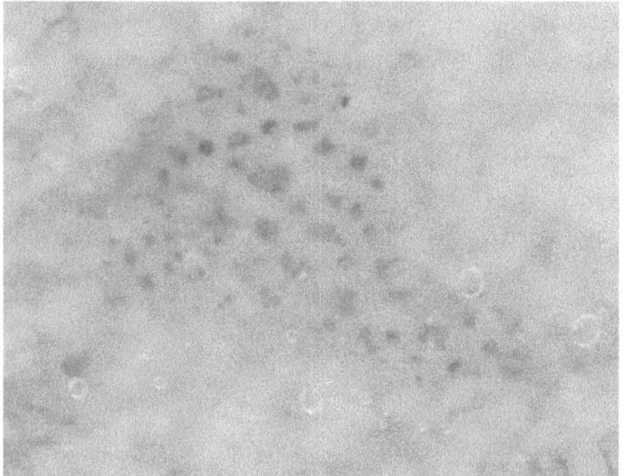

FIGURE 5.56 The appearance of dotted and glomerular vessels indicates a full-thickness involvement of the epidermis (Bowen disease).

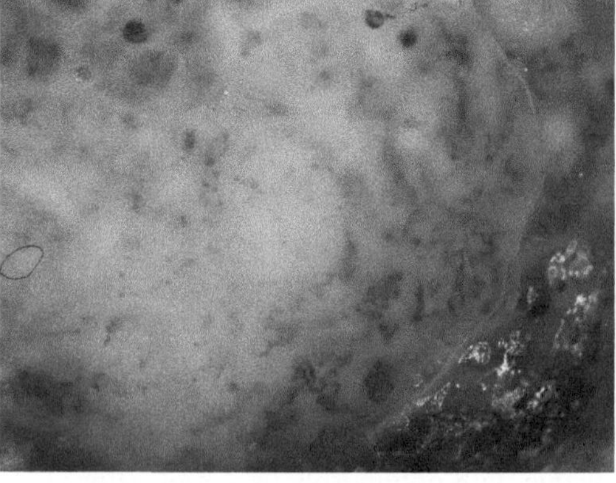

FIGURE 5.57 The appearance of linear irregular vessels indicates invasion of the dermis.

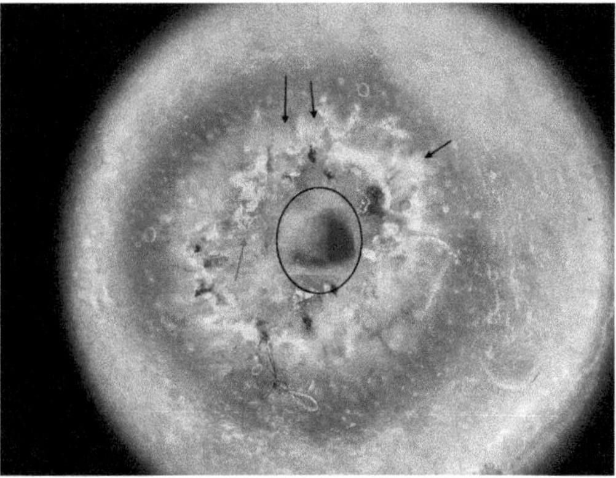

FIGURE 5.58 A moderately differentiated squamous cell carcinoma displaying white-yellow scales (red arrow), white structureless areas (black arrows), and peripheral hairpin vessels. A central ulceration is also observed (circle).

5.3 Basosquamous Carcinoma

Basosquamous carcinoma (BSC) is a rare skin tumor characterized by both basaloid and squamoid differentiation, in an apparent continuum between BCC and SCC. Although traditionally classified among BCC subtypes (metatypical BCC), it seems that the natural course of BSC is rather closer to SCC, and its biological nature remains to be further elucidated. The clinical recognition of BSC is almost impossible, with most BSCs diagnosed either as BCCs or as SCCs (Figure 5.59). Dermatoscopy mirrors the peculiar histopathology of BSC by revealing at least one BCC-related and one SCC-related dermatoscopic feature (Figure 5.60).

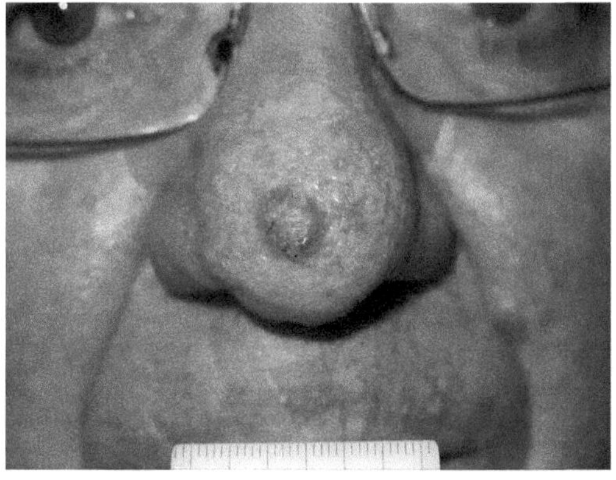

FIGURE 5.59 A nonpigmented nodule on the tip of the nose clinically diagnosed as basal cell carcinoma.

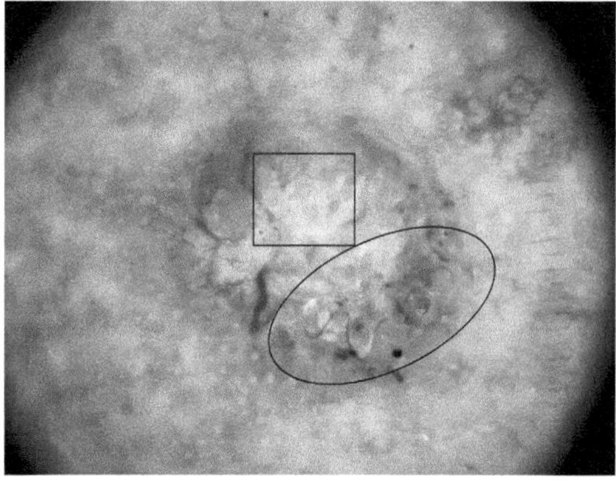

FIGURE 5.60 Dermatoscopy of the previous nodule reveals arborizing vessels and blue-gray globules (circle), which are features suggestive of basal cell carcinoma, but also white perifollicular circles (square), which is a feature suggestive of squamous cell carcinoma. This is a typical example of basosquamous carcinoma.

5.4 Merkel Cell Carcinoma

Merkel cell carcinoma (MCC) is a very aggressive neoplasm associated with a high risk of local, regional, and distant spread and poor prognosis. Clinically, MCC usually presents as a persistent, asymptomatic, red/pink nodular lesion rapidly increasing in size and might ulcerate or bleed (Figures 5.61 and 5.62). It is most commonly located on the head/neck and extremities, followed by trunk and oral and genital mucosa. The diagnosis is often delayed since more than 50% of MCCs are thought to be benign at the time of biopsy.

Dermatoscopically, MCC is typified by a milky-red background and a polymorphous vascular pattern, composed of dotted, arborizing, linear irregular and glomerular vessels (Figure 5.63). White shiny structures (streaks/blotches/strands) might also be seen (Figure 5.61). The aforementioned features are highly unspecific, since they can also be seen in poorly differentiated SCC, amelanotic melanoma, and other malignant tumors. However, dermatoscopy enhances the discrimination of MCC from benign tumors by revealing features indicative of malignancy.

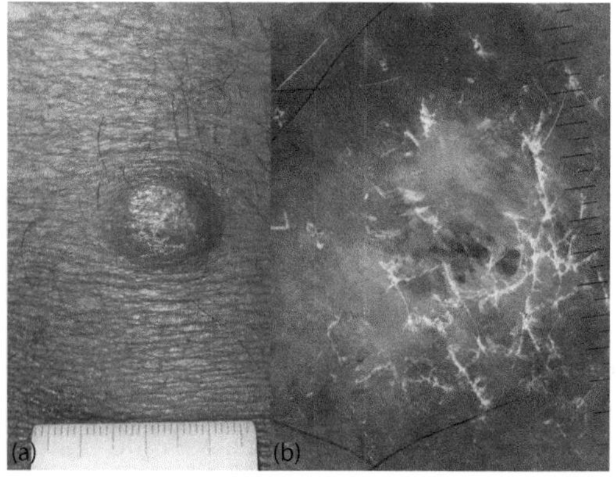

FIGURE 5.61 A Merkel cell carcinoma developing as a fast-growing red nodule (a). Dermatoscopy reveals a milky-red background and white shiny blotches and strands (b).

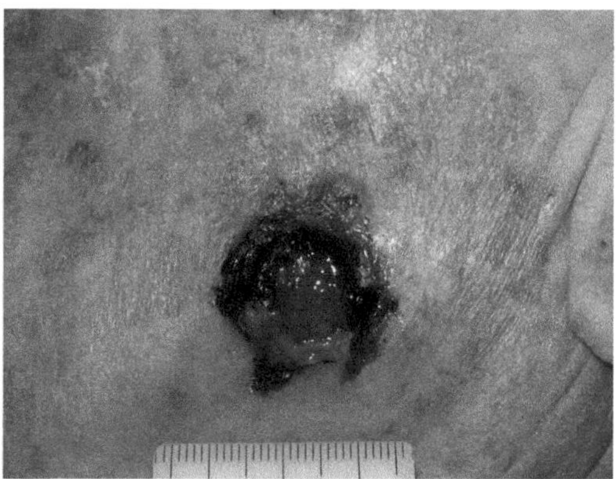

FIGURE 5.62 A Merkel cell carcinoma manifesting as an ulcerated, rapidly growing nodule.

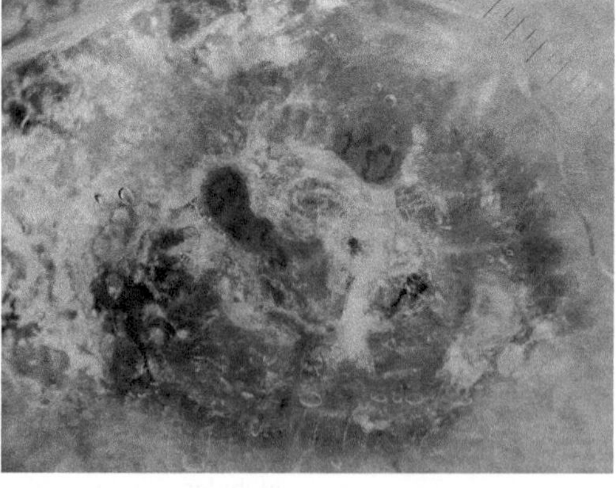

FIGURE 5.63 Dermatoscopy of the tumor of Figure 5.62 reveals a polymorphous vascular pattern, a milky-red background, and keratin masses.

Specifically, benign lesions rarely exhibit a polymorphous vascular pattern or milky-red areas (with the exception of pyogenic granuloma). Consequently, recognition of one or both of these criteria should warrant urgent surgical excision.

5.5 Atypical Fibroxanthoma and Malignant Fibrous Histiocytoma

Atypical fibroxanthoma (AFX) and malignant fibrous histiocytoma (MFH) are rare malignant tumors that share similar clinical and histopathologic characteristics. Biologically, AFX is characterized by a high tendency to locally recur but a low metastatic potential. In contrast, MFH is associated with poor survival.

Both tumors clinically develop as enlarging subcutaneous nodules located almost always on the head/neck area that rapidly increase in size and may ulcerate (Figure 5.64).

Dermatoscopically, AFX and MFH exhibit red and white structureless areas along with linear irregular vessels or a polymorphous vascular pattern consisting of linear, dotted, hairpin, and highly tortuous vessels, irregularly distributed within the lesion (Figure 5.65). Ulceration and keratin masses represent additional features. Although not specific, these dermatoscopic features are strongly suggestive of malignancy, warranting complete surgical excision.

5.6 Malignant Vascular Tumors

5.6.1 Kaposi Sarcoma

Kaposi sarcoma (KS) typically manifests with reddish, violaceous, or bluish-black macules and patches that coalesce to form nodules or plaques. The most common locations are the toes, soles, and legs.

Although lacking specific dermoscopic features, KS has been described to exhibit a "rainbow pattern," which is composed of structureless areas of confluent red, purple, blue, yellow, and green color (Figure 5.66).

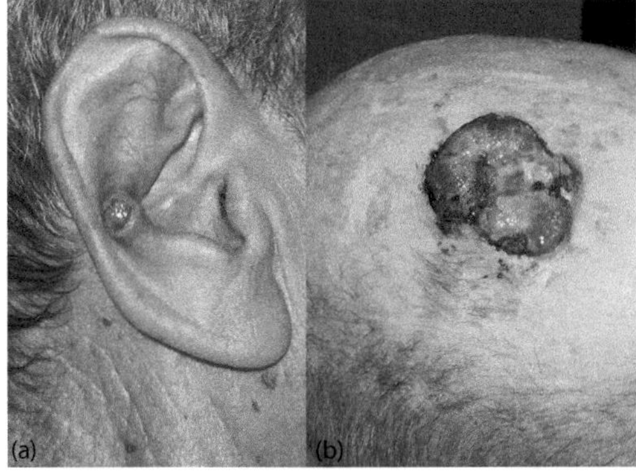

FIGURE 5.64 Atypical fibroxanthoma (a) and malignant fibrous histiocytoma (b) that clinically present as ulcerated nonpigmented nodules.

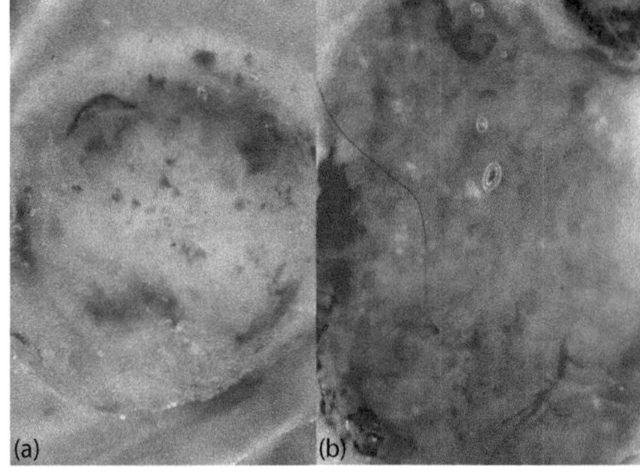

FIGURE 5.65 Dermatoscopy of both tumors reveals red and white areas, ulceration, and a polymorphous vascular pattern (a,b).

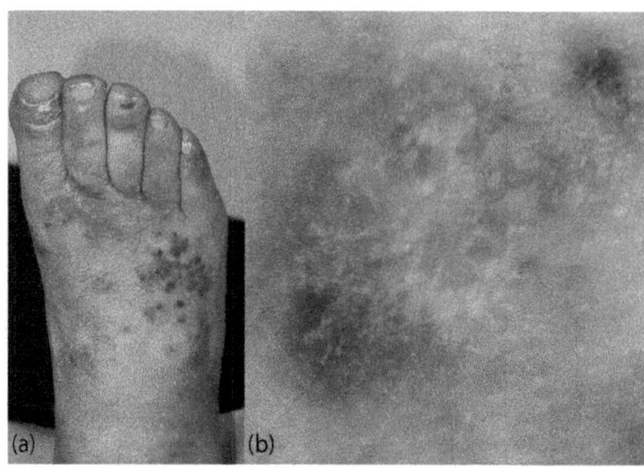

FIGURE 5.66 A typical example of Kaposi sarcoma clinically manifesting with confluent violaceous macules and patches (a). Dermatoscopy reveals structureless areas of red, purple, blue, and white colors (b).

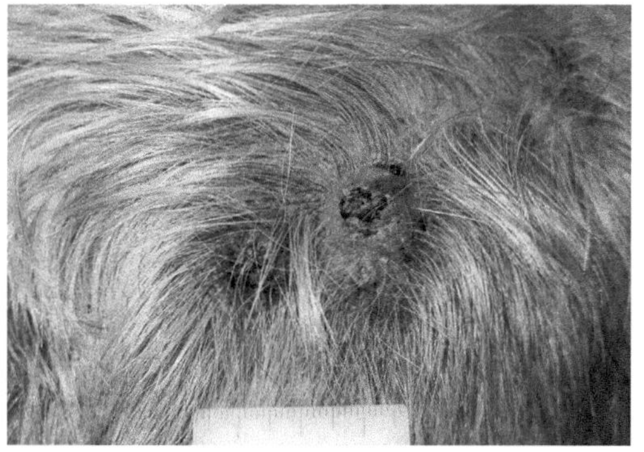

FIGURE 5.67 Typical clinical presentation of angiosarcoma of the head and scalp.

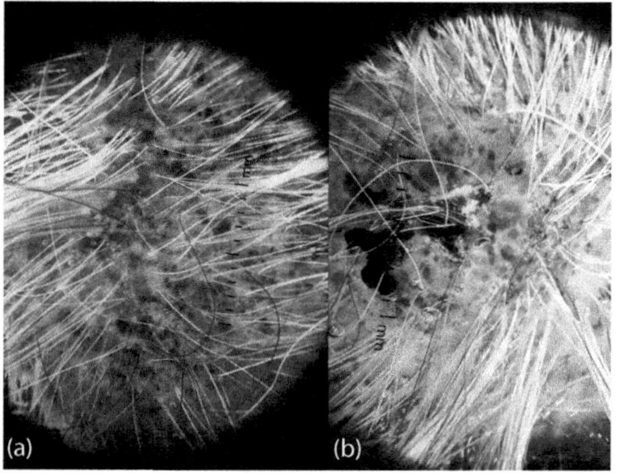

FIGURE 5.68 Dermatoscopy reveals red, purple, and blue colors and white lines (a,b).

5.6.2 Angiosarcoma

Cutaneous angiosarcoma is divided into three clinical variants: angiosarcoma of the head and scalp, lymphedema-associated angiosarcoma, and radiation-induced angiosarcoma. Clinically, angiosarcoma manifests with ill-defined violaceous to bluish areas with an indurated border that might become elevated, nodular, or occasionally ulcerated (Figure 5.67).

Dermatoscopically, angiosarcomas display the typical colors of vascular tumors, namely, red, purple, and blue, while white lines might also be present (Figure 5.68).

BIBLIOGRAPHY

Cameron A, Rosendahl C, Tschandl P et al. Dermatoscopy of pigmented Bowen's disease. *J Am Acad Dermatol.* 2010;62(4):597–604.

Dalle S, Parmentier L, Moscarella E et al. Dermoscopy of Merkel cell carcinoma. *Dermatology.* 2012;224:140–4.

Giacomel J, Lallas A, Argenziano G et al. Dermoscopy of basosquamous carcinoma. *Br J Dermatol.* 2013;169:358–64.

Giacomel J, Zalaudek I. Dermoscopy of superficial basal cell carcinoma. *Dermatol Surg.* 2005;31:1710–3.

Lallas A, Apalla Z, Argenziano G et al. The dermatoscopic universe of basal cell carcinoma. *Dermatol Pract Concept.* 2014;4(03):11–24.

Lallas A, Apalla Z, Ioannides D et al. Dermoscopy in the diagnosis and management of basal cell carcinoma. *Future Oncol.* 2015;11(22):2975–84.

Lallas A, Argenziano G, Zendri E et al. Update on non-melanoma skin cancer and the value of dermoscopy in its diagnosis and treatment monitoring. *Expert Rev Anticancer Ther.* 2013;13:541–58.

Lallas A, Moscarella E, Argenziano G et al. Dermoscopy of uncommon skin tumours. *Australas J Dermatol.* 2014;55(1):53–62.

Lallas A, Tzellos T, Kyrgidis A et al. Accuracy of dermoscopic criteria for discriminating superficial from other subtypes of basal cell carcinoma. *J Am Acad Dermatol.* 2014;70(2):303–11.

Longo C, Lallas A, Kyrgidis A et al. Classifying distinct basal cell carcinoma subtype by means of dermatoscopy and reflectance confocal microscopy. *J Am Acad Dermatol.* 2014;71(4):716–24.e1.

Menzies SW, Westerhoff K, Rabinovitz H et al. Surface microscopy of pigmented basal cell carcinoma. *Arch Dermatol.* 2000;136:1012–6.

Pan Y, Chamberlain AJ, Bailey M et al. Dermatoscopy aids in the diagnosis of the solitary red scaly patch or plaque—Features distinguishing superficial basal cell carcinoma, intraepidermal carcinoma, and psoriasis. *J Am Acad Dermatol.* 2008;59(2):268–74.

Papageorgiou C, Apalla Z, Variaah G et al. Accuracy of dermoscopic criteria for the differentiation between superficial basal cell carcinoma and Bowen's disease. *J Eur Acad Dermatol Venereol.* 2018;32:1914–9.

Rosendahl C, Cameron A, Argenziano G et al. Dermoscopy of squamous cell carcinoma and keratoacanthoma. *Arch Dermatol.* 2012;148(12):1386–92.

Zalaudek I, Argenziano G. Dermoscopy of actinic keratosis, intraepidermal carcinoma and squamous cell carcinoma. *Curr Probl Dermatol.* 2015;46:70–6.

Zalaudek I, Argenziano G, Leinweber B et al. Dermoscopy of Bowen's disease. *Br J Dermatol.* 2004;150:1112–6.

Zalaudek I, Di Stefani A, Argenziano G. The specific dermoscopic criteria of Bowen's disease. *J Eur Acad Dermatol Venereol.* 2006;20(3):361–2.

Zalaudek I, Giacomel J, Argenziano G et al. Dermoscopy of facial nonpigmented actinic keratosis. *Br J Dermatol.* 2006;155:951–6.

Zalaudek I, Giacomel J, Schmid K et al. Dermatoscopy of facial actinic keratosis, intraepidermal carcinoma, and invasive squamous cell carcinoma: A progression model. *J Am Acad Dermatol.* 2012;66:589–97.

6

Inflammatory Skin Diseases

General principles

The value of dermatoscopy in the diagnosis of pigmented and nonpigmented skin neoplasms has been well documented. Cumulative, recent data suggest usefulness of dermatoscopy also in inflammatory and infectious skin diseases. For many of us, our dermatoscope has become an irreplaceable diagnostic tool, used in every aspect of our daily practice, ranging from diagnosis to treatment monitoring. Along with patients' history and clinical examination, the dermatoscopic evaluation of structures and features invisible to the naked eye facilitates discrimination among different inflammatory and infectious diseases.

Five main parameters should be examined with the dermatoscope: (1) morphology and arrangement of vascular structures, (2) color and distribution of the scales, (3) follicular abnormalities, (4) color and shape of other structures, and (5) specific clues.

6.1 Psoriasis

Dermatoscopy in psoriasis is used in both diagnosis and treatment monitoring.

Dotted vessels (or red dots or red globules) in a regular distribution, as well as white scales, in a light red background represent the main dermatoscopic features of psoriasis (Figure 6.1). In higher magnification (×400), dotted vessels appear as dilated, convoluted loops corresponding to the spiral hypertrophic capillaries in the dermal papillae. Detection of any other type of vessels probably excludes the diagnosis of psoriasis. Although dotted vessels are present in every psoriatic plaque, they are not pathognomonic, since they may also be seen in various dermatoses, such as dermatitis and pityriasis rosea. However, their symmetric, regular, and homogeneous distribution all over the lesion is characteristic for psoriasis and rules out the diagnosis of other inflammatory diseases. Removal of thick superficial scales, when present, reveals the underlying vascular pattern, probably along with tiny red blood drops, which has been described as the dermatoscopic "Auspitz sign" (Figure 6.2). Other vascular patterns are rare in psoriasis exception for the "red globular rings" pattern consisting of vessels distributed as a network or in plexus. The latter, although not so frequent, is highly specific (Figure 6.3).

Scale color is also crucial for the differentiation of psoriasis from other erythematous scaly dermatoses. Specifically, while white scales are common, yellow scales are negatively associated with psoriasis and are indicative of dermatitis.

Concerning the dermatoscopic criteria of the other subtypes of the disease or specific anatomical sites, the vascular pattern (regularly distributed dotted vessels or red dots) remains unaltered, whereas the amount of superficial scales varies according to the anatomical location. For example, in psoriatic balanitis and inverse psoriasis that lack scaling, the vascular pattern is dermatoscopically evident (Figure 6.4). In contrast, in the hyperkeratotic scalp, or palmoplantar psoriasis, visualization of the typical vascular pattern is only feasible after removal of the scale (Figures 6.5 and 6.6). Scalp psoriasis displays additional features including ring vessels, red

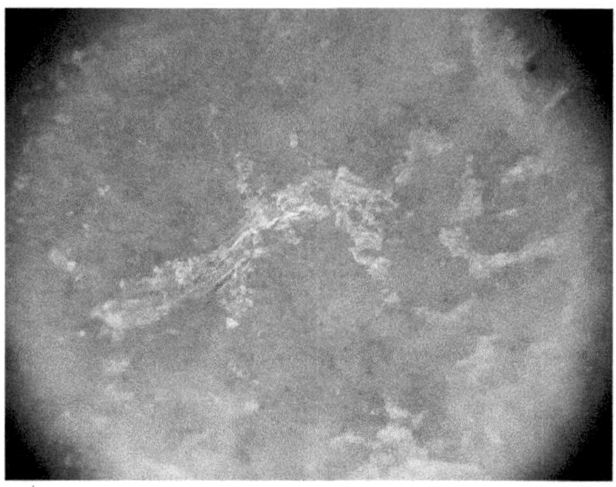

FIGURE 6.1 A psoriatic plaque dermatoscopically displaying dotted vessels, symmetrically and regularly distributed, along with white scales in a light red background.

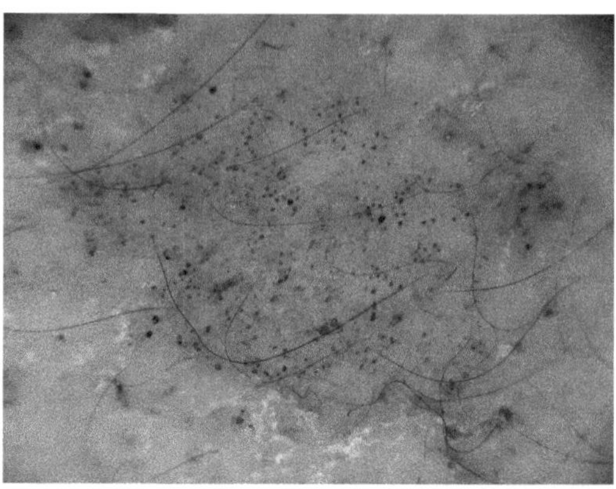

FIGURE 6.2 Red tiny blood drops (Auspitz sign) and dotted vessels following scale removal in a hyperkeratotic psoriatic lesion.

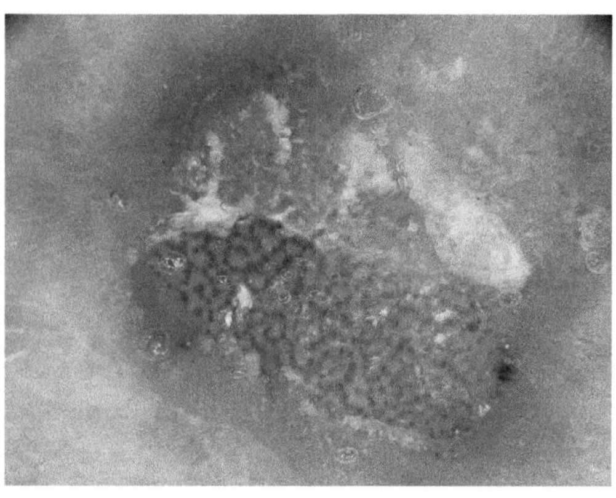

FIGURE 6.3 "Red globular rings" pattern in a psoriatic plaque.

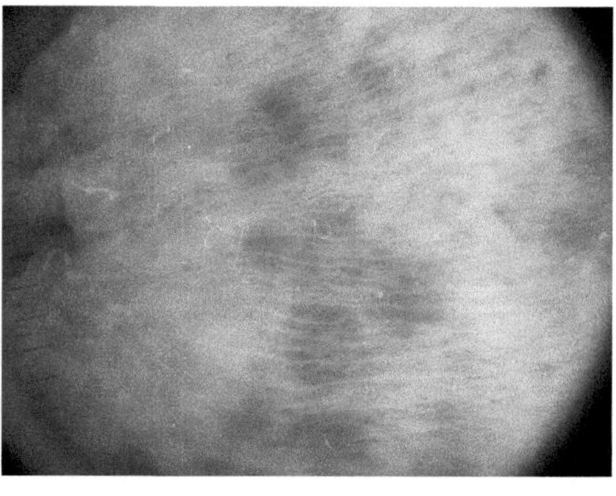

FIGURE 6.4 Psoriatic balanitis dermatoscopically displaying the typical vascular pattern of regularly arranged dotted vessels.

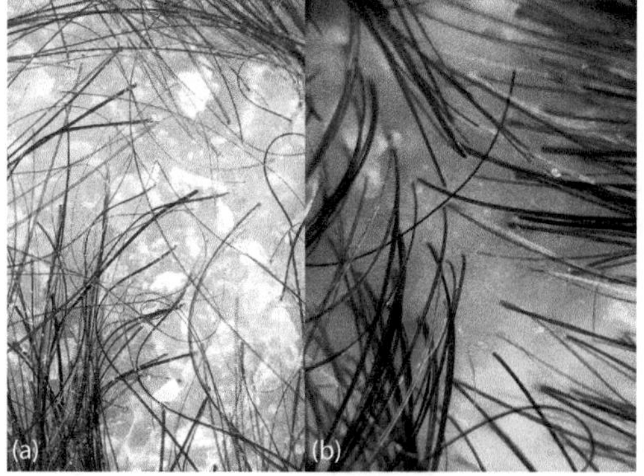

FIGURE 6.5 Thick white scales in a psoriatic lesion of the scalp (a), and visible dotted vessels symmetrically distributed after scaling removal (b).

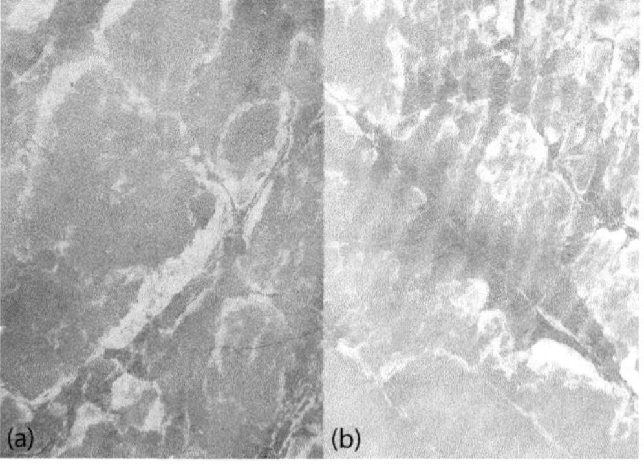

FIGURE 6.6 Thick white scales in palmoplantar psoriasis (a), and visible dotted vessels symmetrically arranged after the removal of scales (b).

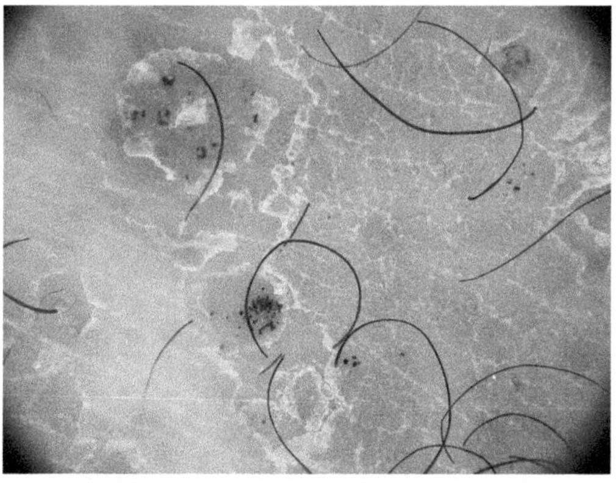

FIGURE 6.7 Psoriatic lesion in a patient under treatment with biologic agent. Dermatoscopy reveals the presence of hemorrhagic dots, suggestive of favorable response to treatment.

FIGURE 6.8 Detection of short, linear vessels, indicative of skin atrophy due to chronic use of corticosteroids.

loops, punctate hemorrhages, and perifollicular plugs, while palmoplantar pustulosis displays the typical yellow and brown pustules.

Beyond its role in the diagnosis, dermatoscopy is also useful for monitoring the treatment outcome (either with topical or systematic treatments). Specifically, the disappearance of dotted vessels along with the appearance of punctate red hemorrhagic dots suggest a favorable response to treatment (Figure 6.7). Opposed to that, the reappearance of dotted vessels indicates possible recurrence. Moreover, the early dermatoscopic detection of short linear vessels (before telangiectasias is clinically evident) suggests early steroid-induced skin atrophy (Figure 6.8).

6.2 Dermatitis

Dermatitis is a term used to include a wide spectrum of itchy inflammatory dermatoses, including contact dermatitis, seborrheic dermatitis, and nummular eczema. These entities may vary in etiology and clinical characteristics; however, they share similar histopathologic and dermatoscopic features. The dermatoscopic hallmark of dermatitis consists of dotted vessels in a patchy distribution and yellow scales/serocrusts, histologically corresponding to dermal spongiosis. The vessels' morphology is similar in psoriasis and dermatitis. However, contrary to psoriasis, vessels in dermatitis are asymmetrically distributed and tend to aggregate in clusters in some parts of a lesion or be unspecifically arranged (patchy vascular distribution) (Figures 6.9 through 6.11). Concerning the color of scales, it depends on the disease phase. Specifically, yellow scales and serocrusts are found in the acute phase, in which spongiosis is very prominent; a combination of yellow and white scales predominates in subacute lesions, while yellow scales in chronic lesions are usually absent. The term *yellow clod* sign has been used to describe the coalescent yellow scales seen in dermatitis.

6.3 Lichen Planus

The dermatoscopic hallmark of lichen planus (LP) is Wickham striae (WS) (Figures 6.12 and 6.13). WS consists of linear reticulated, or annular, white structures that may develop starburst projections. They are usually combined with dotted or linear vessels at the periphery

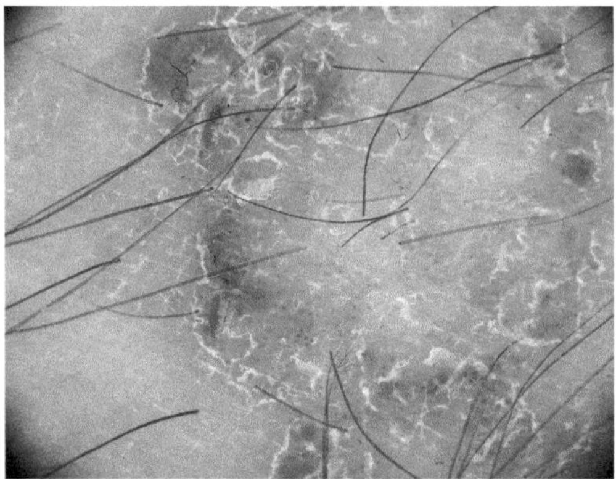

FIGURE 6.9 Dermatoscopic image of dermatitis exhibiting dotted vessels, asymmetrically and irregularly arranged (patchy distribution).

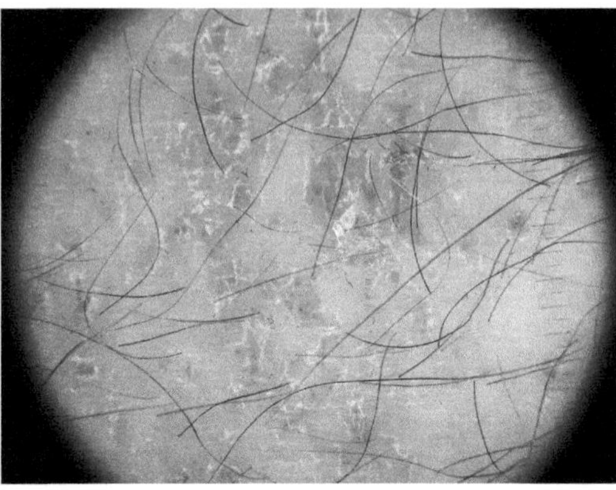

FIGURE 6.10 Diffuse, yellow, superficial scales in dermatitis.

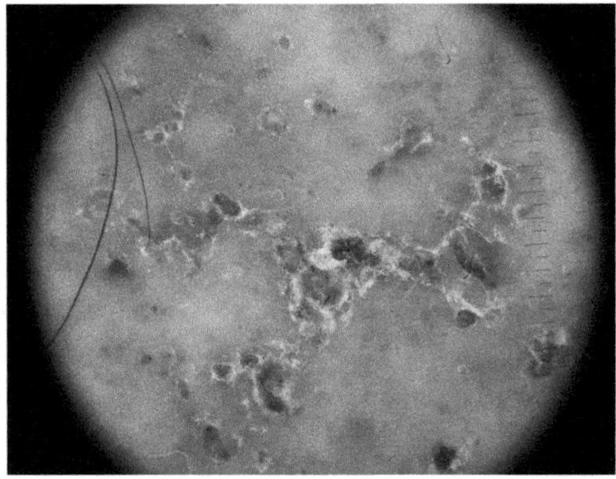

FIGURE 6.11 Yellow crusts and dotted vessels in a patchy distribution in eczema.

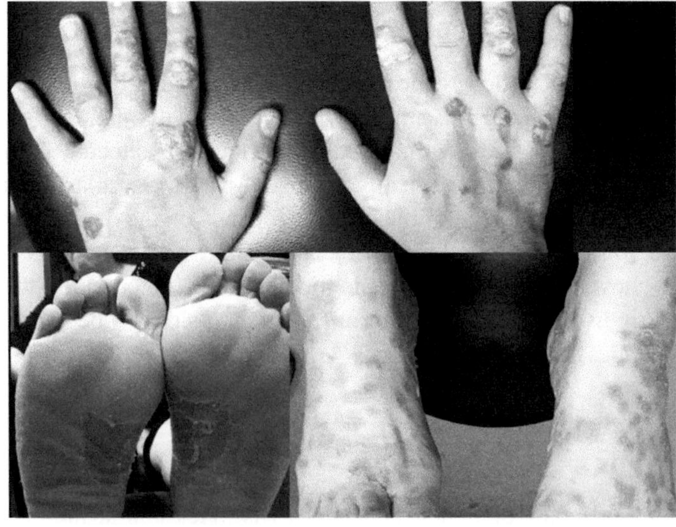

FIGURE 6.12 Clinical image of lichen planus located on palms and soles mimicking psoriasis.

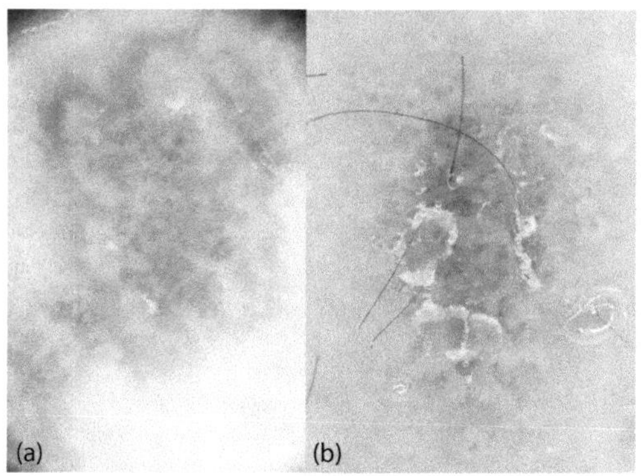

FIGURE 6.13 Dermatoscopy reveals the hallmark of lichen planus, namely, Wickham striae. Dotted or linear vessels are also seen at the periphery (a,b).

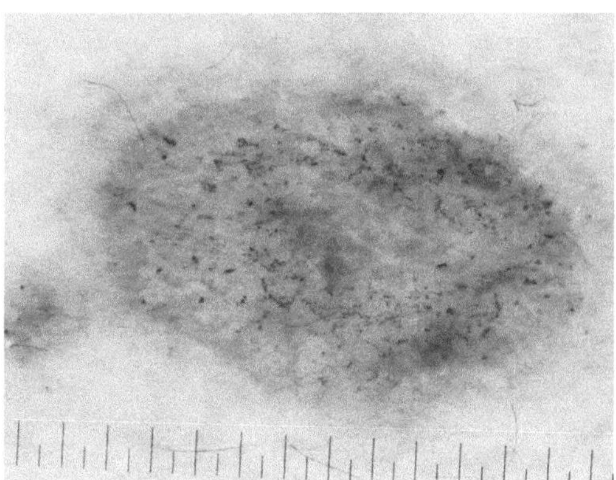

FIGURE 6.14 Blue-gray granules in a chronic lichen planus lesion.

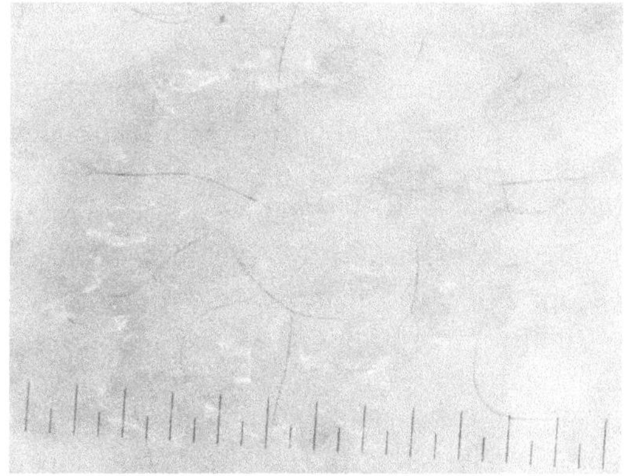

FIGURE 6.15 Dermatoscopic image of pityriasis rosea displaying peripheral white fine scales (collarette) and dotted vessels irregularly distributed.

(Figure 6.14). Histologically, WS correlates to hypergranulosis and acanthosis, mainly seen around the acrotrichia and acrosyringia. At chronic LP lesions, the presence of melanophages in the upper dermis is shown as blue-gray dots or granules, or as brown structureless areas. In late lesions, the vessels and the WS are less evident (Figure 6.15).

6.4 Pityriasis Rosea

The most common dermatoscopic feature of pityriasis rosea (PR) is the whitish fine scales at the periphery of the patches (collarette) (Figure 6.16). The vessels are dotted, but unlike psoriasis, they are usually irregularly distributed. Eczematous reaction is common in the background of PR. In this scenario, dermatoscopy reveals eczematoid features, namely, yellow serocrusts.

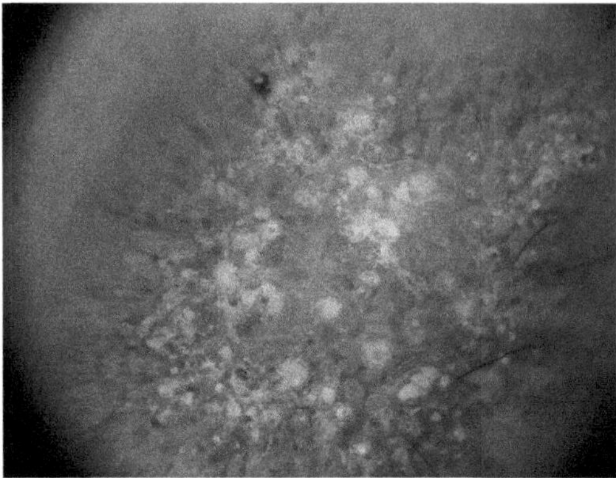

FIGURE 6.16 Dermatoscopy of early discoid lupus erythematosus revealing follicular plugs and perifollicular whitish halos as the predominant features.

6.5 Discoid Lupus Erythematosus

There are different dermatoscopic criteria for discoid lupus erythematosus (DLE) depending on the stage of the disease and the underlying histopathologic alterations. In early lesions, follicular criteria as follicular plugs, perifollicular whitish halos (correspond to perifollicular fibrosis), and white scales are the main dermatoscopic characteristics (Figure 6.17). As the disease evolves, atrophy-related structures, including erythema, hyperkeratosis, and telangiectasias become more evident. Furthermore, blue/gray pigmented granules, dots, or network-like white structures may appear as well. In long-standing lesions, white structureless areas, histologically corresponding to diffuse dermal fibrosis, represent the only dermatoscopic clue (Figures 6.18 and 6.19). Although DLE, sarcoidosis, and lupus vulgaris share similar clinical characteristics, the aforementioned dermatoscopic criteria of DLE, and the yellowish-orange structureless areas with linear or branching vessels seen in granulomatous diseases, facilitate differentiation between these entities. Differential diagnosis of DLE should also include actinic keratosis. Discrimination between the two entities is sometimes challenging. Actinic keratosis is typified by the "strawberry pattern" (i.e., erythema interrupted by white follicular openings).

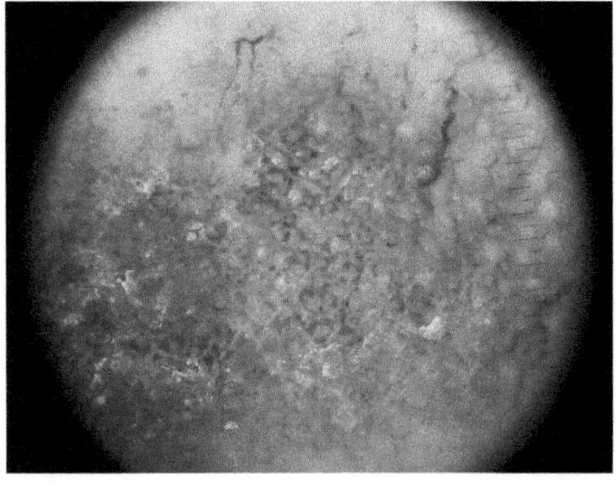

FIGURE 6.17 Early discoid lupus erythematosus dermatoscopically displaying follicular plugs, perifollicular whitish halos, white scales, and linear vessels.

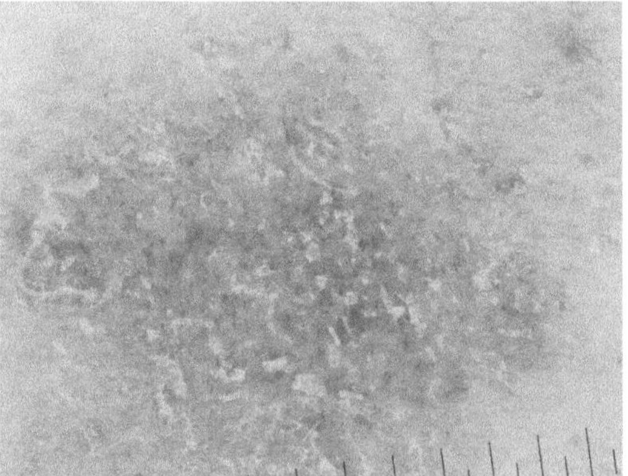

FIGURE 6.18 Discoid lupus erythematosus at a later stage: follicular plugs are less evident and telangiectatic vessels are more prominent.

FIGURE 6.19 White structureless areas and telangiectasia in a long-standing lesion of discoid lupus erythematosus.

6.6 Lichen Sclerosus and Morphea

Dermatoscopically, lichen sclerosus (LS) is characterized by the presence of white structureless areas. Dotted or short linear vessels usually typify genital LS, while yellowish keratotic plugs (or comedo-like openings) are commonly seen in extragenital LS (Figures 6.20 and 6.21). Lesions of extragenital LS may occasionally exhibit an erythematous halo at the periphery, which indicates disease activity.

The predominant dermatoscopic features of morphea are linear vessels on the lilac ring and fibrotic beams, which histopathologically correspond to dermal sclerosis.

6.7 Granulomatous Skin Diseases

Granulomatous skin diseases exhibit a repetitive dermatoscopic pattern, consisting of orange-yellow structureless areas and linear vessels. Orange-yellow areas originate from granulomas in the dermis.

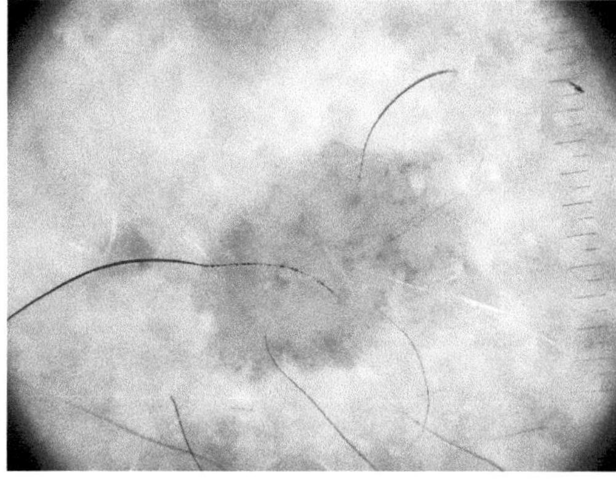

FIGURE 6.20 Dermatoscopy of genital lichen sclerosus revealing a central erythema with dotted and short linear vessels surrounded by white structureless areas.

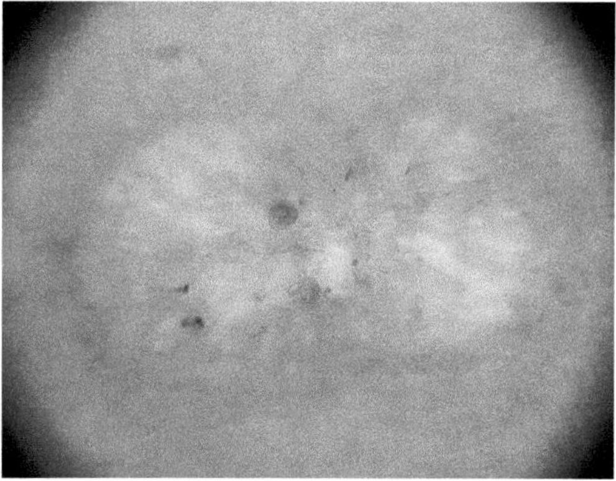

FIGURE 6.21 Dermatoscopic image of extragenital lichen sclerosus displaying white structureless areas, linear vessels, and the characteristic keratotic plugs.

6.7.1 Sarcoidosis and Lupus Vulgaris

In sarcoidosis and lupus vulgaris, the presence of yellow/orange, translucent, globular, or structureless areas (diffuse or focal), usually combined with linear branching vessels, typifies the diagnosis. Additional dermatoscopic features include pigmentation structures, follicular plugs, scales, dilated follicles, milia-like cysts, and crystalline structures (Figures 6.22 and 6.23).

Dermatoscopy is not sufficient to differentiate among granulomatous diseases. However, the presence of orange/yellow color and linear vessels favors the diagnosis of a granulomatous disease in general.

6.7.2 Necrobiosis Lipoidica and Granuloma Annulare

Necrobiosis lipoidica is dermatoscopically typified by the presence of diffuse or focal yellow/orange structureless areas combined with a highly specific vascular pattern. This pattern, which facilitates

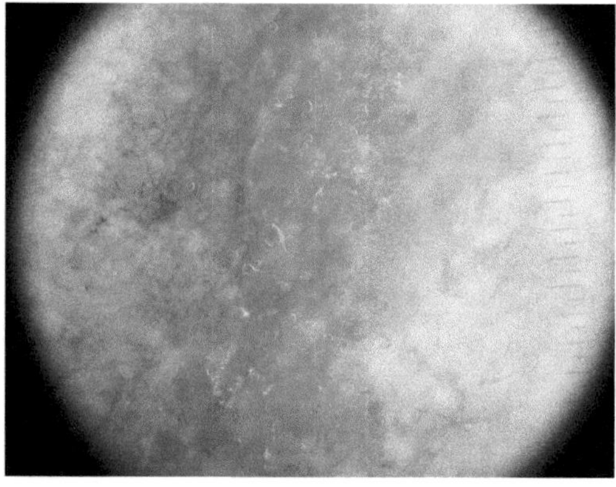

FIGURE 6.22 Cutaneous sarcoidosis, dermatoscopically characterized by translucent yellow/orange areas and short linear vessels.

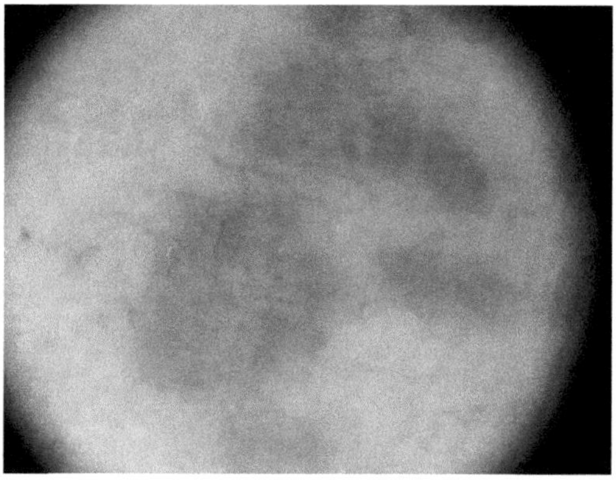

FIGURE 6.23 Cutaneous sarcoidosis, dermatoscopically typified by translucent yellow/orange areas and short linear vessels.

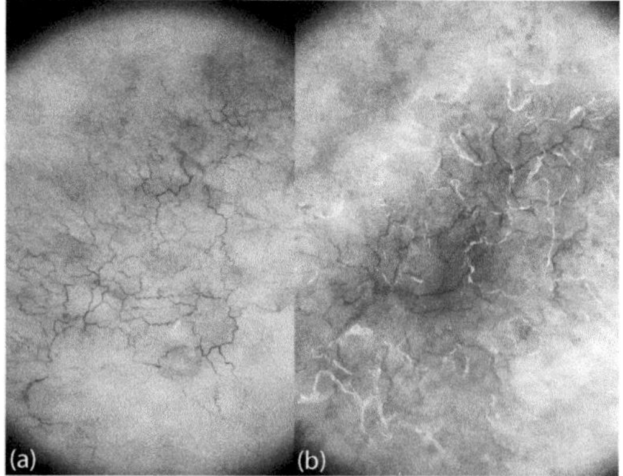

FIGURE 6.24 Dermatoscopic images of necrobiosis lipoidica displaying the characteristic prominent vascular pattern of fine, linear, branching, network-like vessels in a yellow background (a,b).

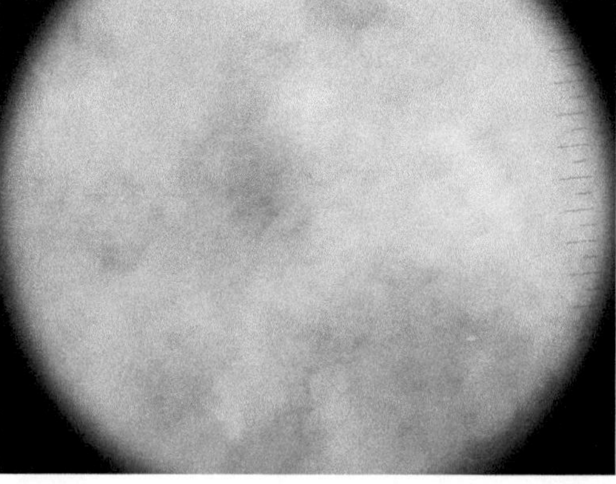

FIGURE 6.25 Dermatoscopic image of granuloma annulare showing linear vessels and a background erythema. No specific dermoscopic pattern is identified. Dotted or linear vessels in an erythematous background are observed.

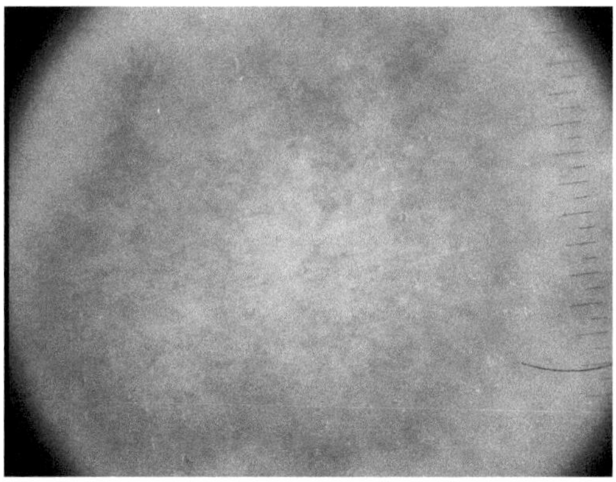

FIGURE 6.26 Granuloma annulare dermatoscopically displaying linear vessels over a whitish background.

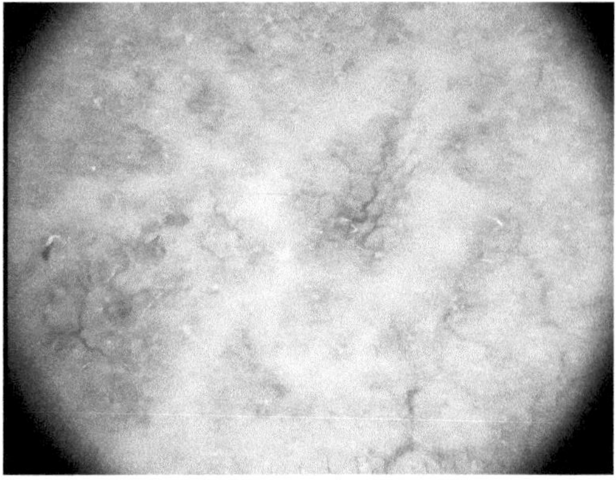

FIGURE 6.27 Granuloma annulare dermatoscopically displaying linear vessels over a rather whitish background and focal pigmented structures.

the discrimination of necrobiosis lipoidica from sarcoidosis and lupus vulgaris, consists of dotted, linear, or glomerular vessels in early stages, while linear branching vessels forming a prominent dense vascular network (often also seen macroscopically) in a yellow background are observed in late stages. Ulceration and yellow crusts are the most common additional features (Figure 6.24).

In comparison with other granulomatous diseases, granuloma annulare lacks the well-formed granulomas in histology and, subsequently, lacks the yellow/orange structureless areas in dermatoscopy. Vessels might be either dotted or linear in an erythematous, or whitish, or white and pink, or occasionally, white and yellow background (Figures 6.25 through 6.27). Furthermore, focal pigmented structures are not uncommon (Figure 6.27).

6.8 Rosacea

The dermatoscopic hallmark of erythematotelangiectatic rosacea and the main differential sign from other diseases is the large polygonal vessels (linear vessels forming polygons) (Figures 6.28 and 6.29). Although telangiectasias may also be observed in sun-damaged,

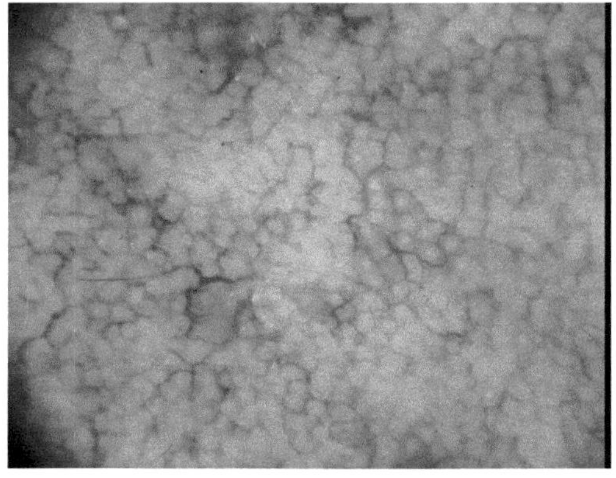

FIGURE 6.28 Rosacea is dermoscopically typified by a characteristic vascular pattern consisting of linear vessels forming polygons (polygonal vessels).

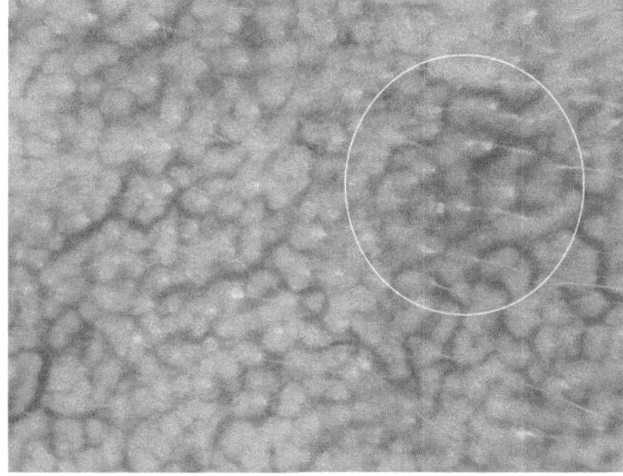

FIGURE 6.29 A case of rosacea-associated demodicosis. Dermoscopy reveals prominent polygonal vessels and white follicular spiny structures protruding from the follicular openings (circle).

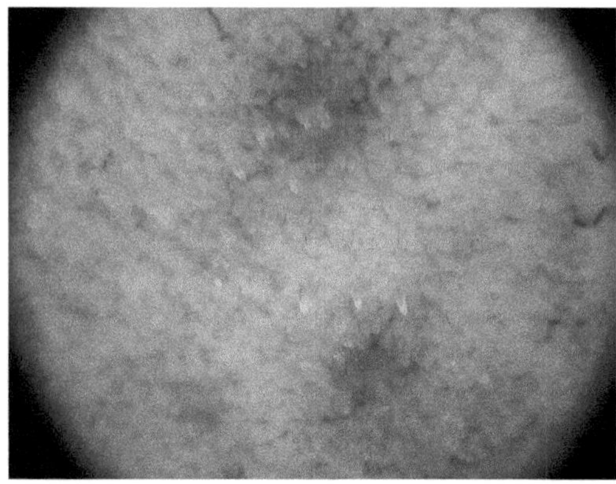

FIGURE 6.30 A case of demodicosis with dermatoscopically evident white follicular spiny structures protruding from the follicular openings (*Demodex* "tails").

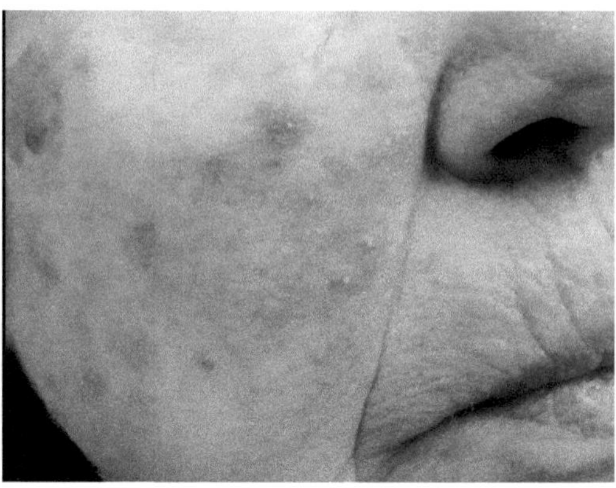

FIGURE 6.31 Clinical image of rosacea.

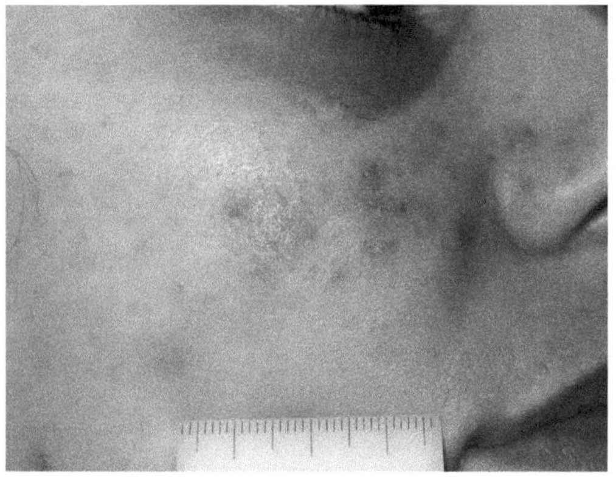

FIGURE 6.32 Clinical image of discoid lupus erythematosus.

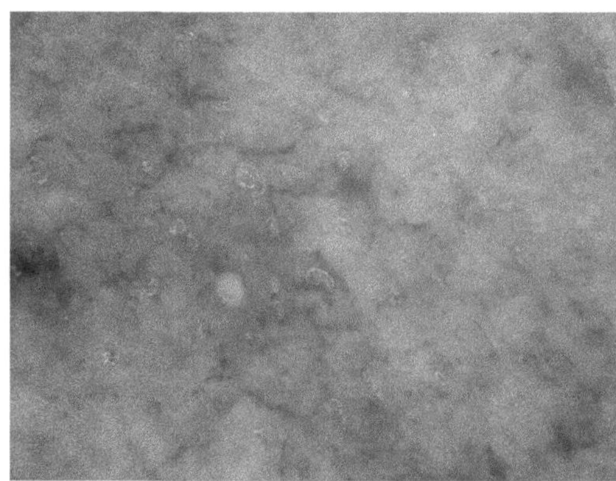

FIGURE 6.33 Dermatoscopy facilitates the discrimination of papulopustular rosacea from discoid lupus erythematosus by highlighting the pustules.

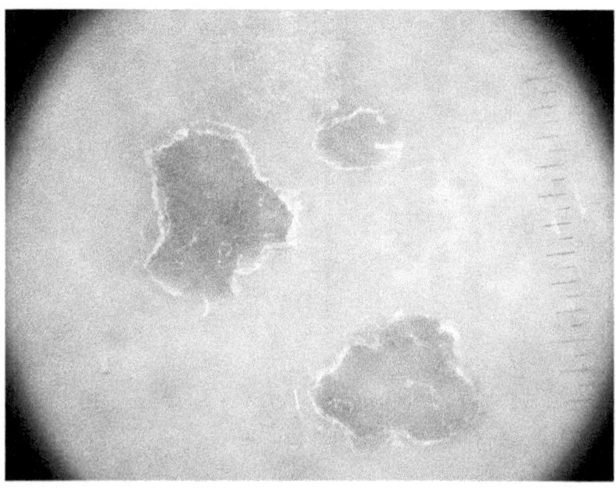

FIGURE 6.34 Dermatoscopic image of porokeratosis, which is typified by a well-defined, peripheral, white rim (cornoid lamella). Dotted and linear vessels are observed in the center of the lesion, due to atrophy.

atrophic facial skin, they usually lack the characteristic polygonal pattern. In cases of demodicidosis (an eruption caused by *Demodex folliculorum*), white spines protruding out of the follicular openings (*Demodex* "tails") combined with polygonal vessels are observed (Figures 6.29 and 6.30).

Depending on the clinical subtype of the disease, additional features may appear. For example, in papulopustular rosacea, the polygonal vessels are not so prominent, but dermatoscopy reveals pustules (sometimes not visible by naked-eye clinical examination), facilitating the discrimination from discoid lupus erythematosus (Figures 6.31 through 6.33). Glandular rosacea, including rhinophyma, may additionally exhibit follicular criteria, namely, dilated follicles filled with keratin plugs.

6.9 Porokeratosis

Porokeratosis displays a pathognomonic dermatoscopic pattern consisting of two parts: the peripheral rim (corresponding to the cornoid lamella) and the atrophic center. The rim is a thin, well-defined, white-yellowish scale, continuous or broken in some parts ("white track") (Figure 6.34). Occasionally, the peripheral rim is pigmented and slightly elevated, simulating the volcanic crater. The previously mentioned pattern allows a straightforward diagnosis of porokeratosis, even in clinically equivocal cases. In the central part of the lesion, the dermatoscopic criteria vary accordingly to the phase of evolution. In early active lesions, dotted and globular vessels prevail, while in the late stage, a central white color is present corresponding to dermal fibrosis/atrophy. Blue/gray dots or granules indicate resolving lesions.

6.10 Urticaria and Urticarial Vasculitis

Urticaria dermatoscopically displays a network of linear vessels. Alternations between vascular and avascular areas due to dermal edema are an additional clue (Figure 6.35). The detection of purpuric dots or globules in urticariform lesions is highly indicative of urticarial vasculitis (Figure 6.36).

FIGURE 6.35 Avascular areas, due to edema, in urticaria.

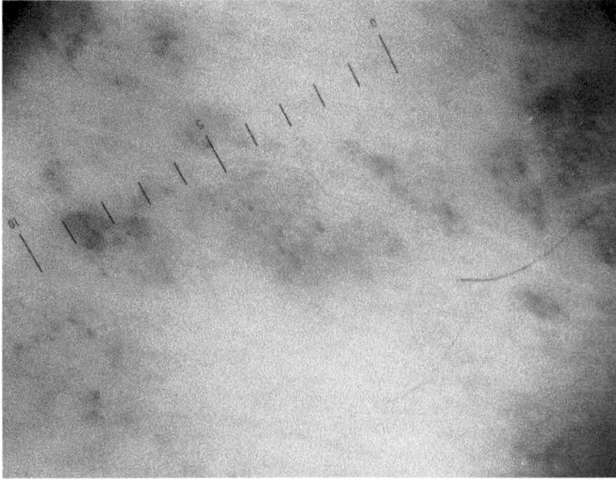

FIGURE 6.36 Purpuric dots and globules in urticarial vasculitis.

6.11 Mastocytosis

Multiple dermatoscopic features have been described in mastocytosis, depending on the clinical subtype of the disease. As a result, overlapping criteria are frequent among the several subtypes. Specifically, a light-brown blot and a uniform pigment network typify maculopapular mastocytosis, while a reticular vascular pattern on an erythematous/brownish background characterizes telangiectasia macularis eruptiva perstans. Dotted or thin linear vessels may be present in both types. Solitary mastocytoma displays diffuse orange-yellow color or multifocal yellow-orange areas (Figures 6.37 and 6.38). The reticular vascular pattern has been related with more severe symptoms and indicates an increased risk for continuous medication.

6.12 Pigmented Purpuric Dermatoses

Pigmented purpuric dermatoses represent a group of disorders that includes Schamberg disease, Majocchi purpura, eczematoid purpura of Doucas and Kapetanakis, lichen aureus, and pigmented purpuric lichenoid dermatitis of Gougerot-Blum. Round to oval, red, purpuric dots and/or globules, developing in an orange-brownish to reddish background are the dermatoscopic result of the extravasated erythrocytes and dermal deposits of hemosiderin, respectively (Figure 6.39). Linear or dotted vessels, white scales, and pigmented structures (pigmented dots/globules, network) represent frequent additional features. Similar dermatoscopic features have been described, also, in mycosis fungoides. Consequently, such lesions should be thoroughly evaluated to facilitate early diagnosis and adequate treatment.

6.13 Pityriasis Rubra Pilaris

The most frequent dermatoscopic pattern of classic pityriasis rubra pilaris consists of round/oval yellowish areas surrounded by linear and dotted vessels (Figure 6.40). Central keratin plugs may also be present. Dermatoscopy contributes in the diagnosis of keratoderma occurring in pityriasis rubra pilaris with the recognition of homogenous, patchily distributed orange areas and white scales. Erythrodermic pityriasis rubra pilaris displays a distinct

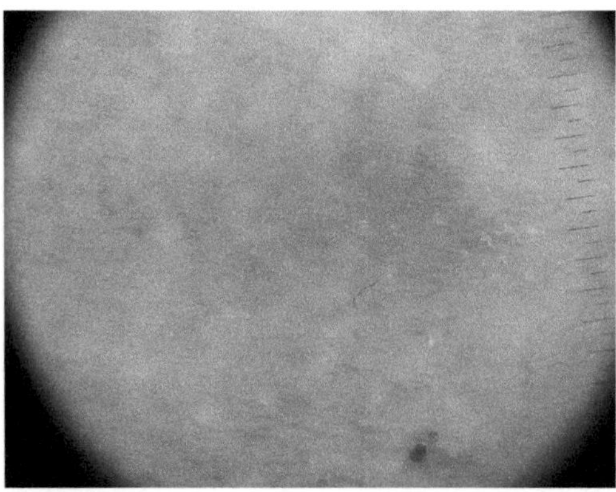

FIGURE 6.37 A dermatoscopic yellow-orange blot in a solitary mastocytoma.

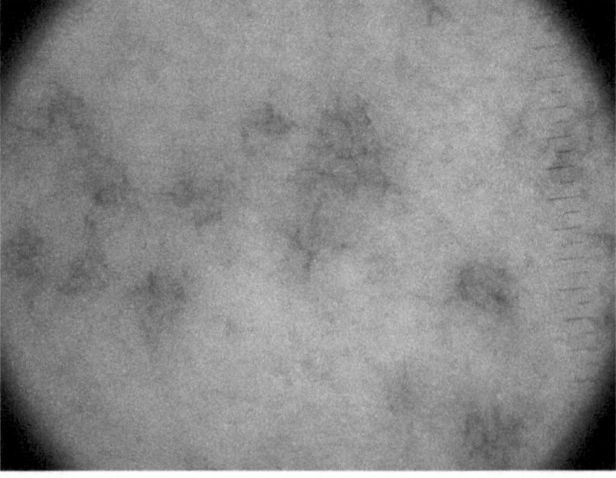

FIGURE 6.38 Telangiectasia macularis eruptiva perstansis, dermatoscopically characterized by reticular vessels on an erythematous background.

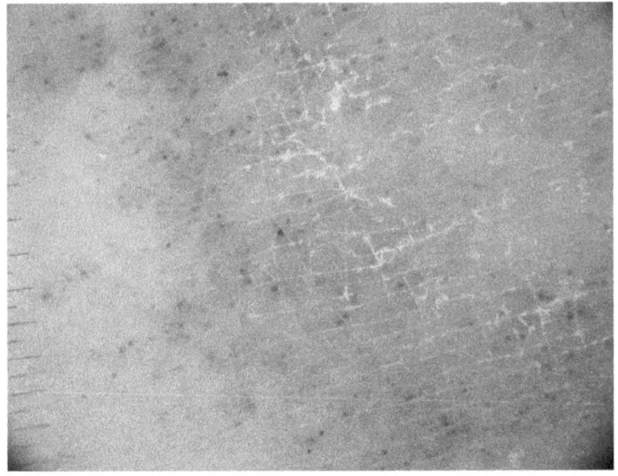

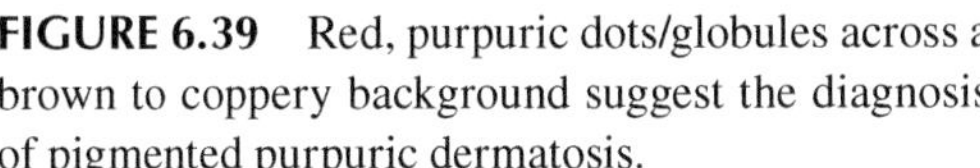

FIGURE 6.39 Red, purpuric dots/globules across a brown to coppery background suggest the diagnosis of pigmented purpuric dermatosis.

FIGURE 6.40 Round/oval yellowish areas surrounded by linear and dotted vessels in pityriasis rubra pilaris.

dermatoscopic feature, consisting of orange blotches and islands of nonerythematous (spared) skin with reticular vessels.

6.14 Pityriasis Lichenoides et Varioliformis Acuta

Although both pityriasis lichenoides et varioliformis acuta (PLEVA) and pityriasis lichenoides chronica (PLC) belong to the same clinical spectrum, they differ in dermatoscopy. Concerning PLEVA, the dermatoscopic features vary according to the disease stage. In early lesions, purpuric dots or diffuse hemorrhagic areas, typically in the canter of the lesion, are seen and histologically correspond to epidermal necrosis, ulceration, and microhemorrhages. As the disease progresses, lesions exhibit whitish-structureless areas and central white crust within a whitish-structureless rim. Scale, focal bluish-grayish areas or centrifugal strands irregularly distributed at the periphery of the lesion are additional findings.

Opposed to PLEVA, the histological alterations in PLC result in a totally different dermatoscopic pattern. Orange-yellow structureless areas corresponding to extravasated erythrocytes (and consequent hemosiderin deposition) are the main dermatoscopic findings in PLC. Moreover, focal mainly dotted vessels, due to dilatation of superficial dermal vessels without significant and constant papillomatosis, represent the major vascular component. The main differential diagnosis for PLC is guttate psoriasis. However, dermatoscopy is a very helpful diagnostic tool for the discrimination between them. Focusing on vascular criteria, diffuse regularly distributed dotted vessels displayed in guttate psoriasis (corresponding to tortuous and dilated blood vessels within elongated dermal papillae) facilitate differentiation from PLC, in which dotted vessels are focally arranged.

6.15 Prurigo Nodularis

In both hyperkeratotic and excoriated lesions of prurigo nodularis, the predominant dermatoscopic pattern is the "white starburst pattern," which consists of either radially arranged whitish lines or a peripheral whitish halo with a few centrifugal coarse projections (Figure 6.41). Additional features include brown or red/brown or yellow crust(s), erosion(s) and/or hyperkeratosis and scales in a brown-pinkish background.

6.16 Acquired Perforating Dermatoses

The term *perforating dermatoses* describes a group of skin disorders characterized by "perforation," and/or elimination, of degraded dermal connective tissue through the epidermis. There are four main, primary perforating dermatoses based on clinical features, types of epidermal disruption, and nature of eliminated material: reactive perforating collagenosis, elastosis perforans serpiginosa, perforating folliculitis, and acquired perforating dermatosis (Kyrle disease). These entities are often associated with either chronic renal failure or diabetes mellitus.

The different histological subtypes of acquired perforating dermatoses correspond to different dermatoscopic features. The "trizonal concentric" pattern is a common feature (Figure 6.42). It consists of a central, brown-green/yellowish-brown structureless area surrounded by a white keratotic collarette and an outer erythematous halo, with or without dotted vessels. A peripheral, brown, delicate pigmentation has also been described, especially in Kyrle disease.

6.17 Grover's Disease and Darier Disease

The dermatoscopic hallmark of Darier disease is the peculiar giant pseudocomedones, seen as centrally located polygonal brownish areas, surrounded by a whitish halo and linear vessels.

Grover disease is typified by "stellate erosion," which is a central yellow or brown area with radial (star-like) projections, in an erythematous background (Figure 6.43). Peripheral dotted or linear vessels may also be present. Sometimes, the central tan-brown area may be relatively large and round or ovoid in shape, reminiscent of the pseudocomedones of Darier disease.

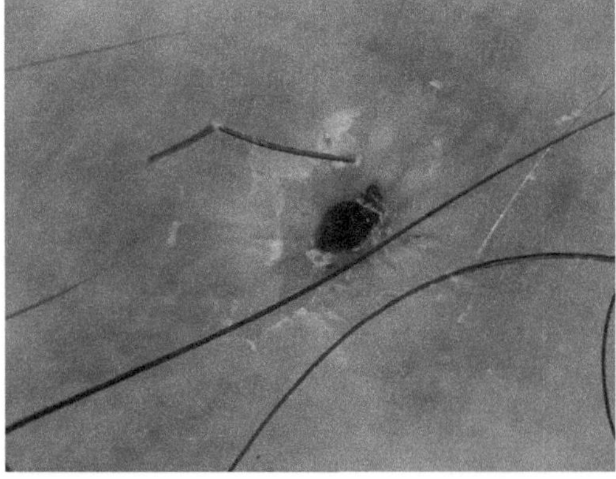

FIGURE 6.41 Dermatoscopic white starburst pattern (radially arranged whitish lines) of prurigo nodularis combined with a central erosion.

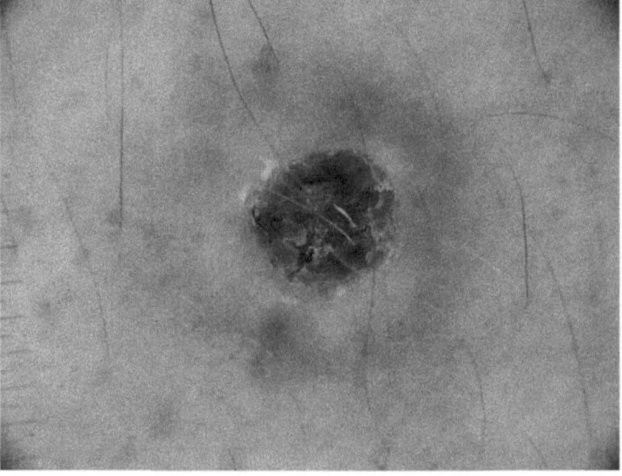

FIGURE 6.42 The "trizonal concentric pattern" is common in perforating dermatoses.

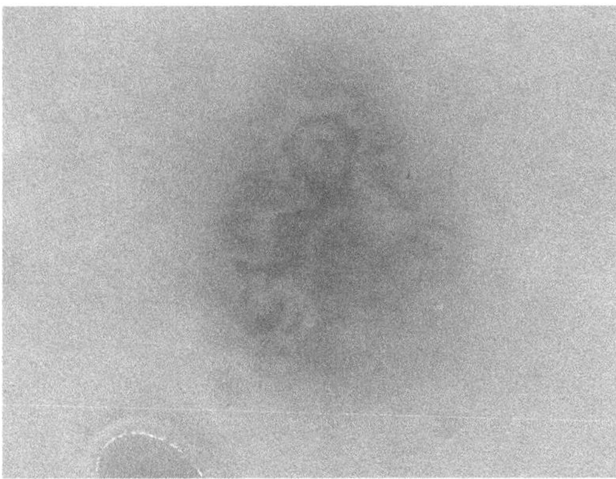

FIGURE 6.43 The "stellate erosion" of Grover disease: a central yellow or brownish eroded area with radial projections.

6.18 Mycosis Fungoides

Dermatoscopy of mycosis fungoides (MF) displays several features that offer insight into the underlying histopathology. Fine, short linear vessels and orange-yellow patchy areas predominate in patch-stage MF and correspond to dilated dermal vessels and deposits of hemosiderin in the dermis, respectively (Figure 6.44). A peculiar vascular pattern ("spermatozoon-like structure") consisting of short linear vessels starting from a red dot has also been described in a certain proportion of MF cases (Figure 6.45).

The vascular structures may vary according to disease subtype. In the poikilodermic variant of the disease, short linear vessels are much more prominent; in the erythrodermic variant, the number of vessels is significantly decreased, and sparse whitish scales along with widespread dotted vessels are commonly seen. Dermatoscopic evaluation of the vascular pattern allows the discrimination of MF from chronic dermatitis, which is the main differential diagnosis. Specifically, short linear vessels, spermatozoon-like structures, and orange-yellow areas favor the diagnosis of MF, while dotted vessels and yellow scales favor the diagnosis of dermatitis.

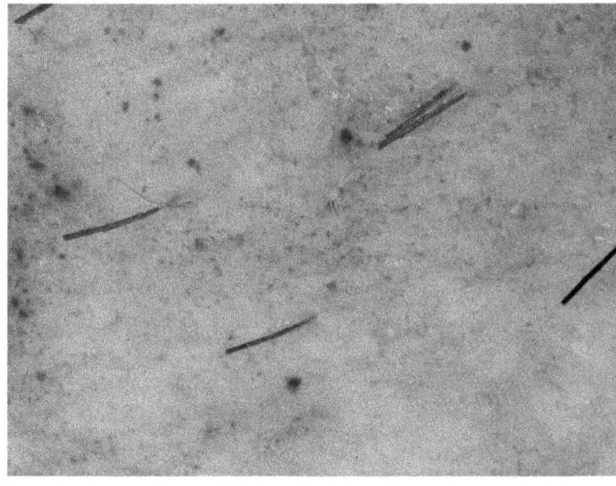

FIGURE 6.44 Patch-stage mycosis fungoides, dermoscopically displaying short linear vessels.

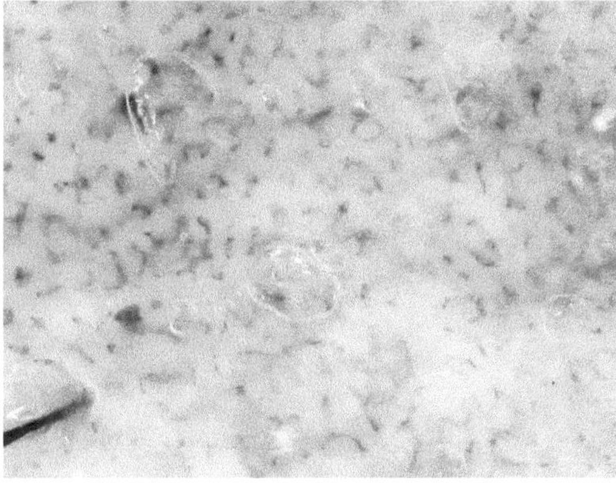

FIGURE 6.45 The "spermatozoon-like structures," consisting of a short curved linear vessel originating from a dotted vessel, in mycosis fungoides.

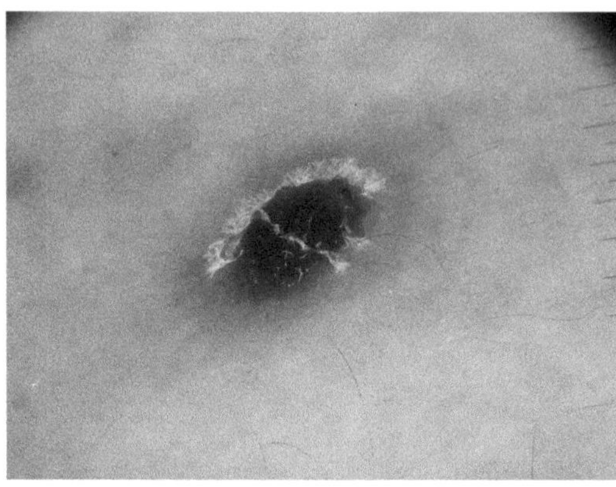

FIGURE 6.46 Dermatoscopy of a necrotic lesion of lymphomatoid papulosis displaying central brown-yellowish crust and peripheral vessels.

6.19 Lymphomatoid Papulosis

Several dermatoscopic patterns for lymphomatoid papulosis (LyP) have been described depending on the stage of evolution of each lesion. In early lesions, the vascular pattern is predominant and consists of dotted or tortuous/irregular vessels over an erythematous background. Purpuric spots are common at this stage. Progressively, scales become more prominent, and the vessels are limited at the periphery. In hyperkeratotic lesions, white or yellow scales cover the central part of the papules, while in a necrotic lesion, the main dermatoscopic feature is the central brownish-yellow crusts (Figure 6.46). Finally, postinflammatory pigmentation, seen as brown structureless areas, typifies healing lesions.

BIBLIOGRAPHY

Akay BN, Kittler H, Sanli H, Harmankaya K, Anadolu R. Dermatoscopic findings of cutaneous mastocytosis. *Dermatology.* 2009;218:226–30.

Ankad BS, Beergouder SL. Pityriasis lichenoides et varioliformis acuta in skin of color: New observations by dermoscopy. *Dermatol Pract Concept.* 2017;7:27–34.

Apalla Z, Lallas A. Photoletter to the editor: Dermoscopy of atypical lichen sclerosus involving the tongue. *J Dermatol Case Rep.* 2012;6:57–8.

Arpaia N, Cassano N, Vena GA. Lessons on dermoscopy: Pigment network in nonmelanocytic lesions. *Dermatol Surg.* 2004;30:929–30.

Bakos RM, Cartell A, Bakos L. Dermatoscopy of early-onset necrobiosis lipoidica. *J Am Acad Dermatol.* 2012;66:e143–4.

Brasiello M, Zalaudek I, Ferrara G et al. Lupus vulgaris: A new look at an old symptom – The lupoma observed with dermoscopy. *Dermatology.* 2009;218(2):172–4.

Chuh AA. Collarette scaling in pityriasis rosea demonstrated by digital epiluminescence dermatoscopy. *Australas J Dermatol.* 2001;42:288–90.

Chuh AA. The use of digital epiluminescence dermatoscopy to identify peripheral scaling in pityriasis rosea. *Comput Med Imaging Graph.* 2002;26:129–34.

Coelho de Sousa V, Oliveira A. Inflammoscopy in the diagnosis of hypertrophic lichen planus. *J Am Acad Dermatol.* 2015;73:e171–3.

Conde-Montero E, Aviles-Izquierdo JA, Mendoza-Cembranos MD, Parra-Blanco V. Dermoscopy of necrobiosis lipoidica. *Actas Dermosifiliogr.* 2013;104:534–7.

Errichetti E, Lacarrubba F, Micali G, Piccirillo A, Stinco G. Differentiation of pityriasis lichenoides chronica from guttate psoriasis by dermoscopy. *Clin Exp Dermatol.* 2015;40:804–6.

Errichetti E, Piccirillo A, Stinco G. Dermoscopy of prurigo nodularis. *J Dermatol.* 2015;42:632–4.

Errichetti E, Piccirillo A, Stinco G. Dermoscopy as an auxiliary tool in the differentiation of the main types of erythroderma due to dermatological disorders. *Int J Dermatol.* 2016;55:e616–8.

Errichetti E, Stinco G. The practical usefulness of dermoscopy in general dermatology. *G Ital Dermatol Venereol.* 2015;150:533–46.

Errichetti E, Stinco G. Dermoscopy in differential diagnosis of palmar psoriasis and chronic hand eczema. *J Dermatol.* 2016;43:423–5.

Friedman P, Sabban EC, Marcucci C, Peralta R, Cabo H. Dermoscopic findings in different clinical variants of lichen planus. Is dermoscopy useful? *Dermatol Pract Concept.* 2015;5:51–5.

Garrido-Rios AA, Alvarez-Garrido H, Sanz-Munoz C, Aragoneses-Fraile H, Manchado-Lopez P, Miranda-Romero A. Dermoscopy of extragenital lichen sclerosus. *Arch Dermatol.* 2009;145:1468.

Giacomel J, Zalaudek I, Argenziano G. Dermatoscopy of Grover's disease and solitary acantholytic dyskeratoma shows a brown, star-like pattern. *Australas J Dermatol.* 2012;53:315–6.

Giacomel J, Zalaudek I, Argenziano G, Lallas A. Dermoscopy of hypertrophic lupus erythematosus and differentiation from squamous cell carcinoma. *J Am Acad Dermatol.* 2015;72(1 Suppl):S33–6.

Inui S, Itami S, Murakami M, Nishimoto N. Dermoscopy of discoid lupus erythematosus: Report of two cases. *J Dermatol.* 2014;41:756–7.

Kibar M, Aktan S, Bilgin M. Dermoscopic findings in scalp psoriasis and seborrheic dermatitis; two new signs; signet ring vessel and hidden hair. *Indian J Dermatol.* 2015;60:41–5.

Kittisak P, Tanaka M. Dermoscopic findings in a case of reactive perforating collagenosis. *Dermatol Pract Concept.* 2015;5:75–7.

Lacarrubba F, Micali G. Dermoscopy of pityriasis lichenoides et varioliformis acuta. *Arch Dermatol.* 2010;146:1322.

Lallas A, Apalla Z, Argenziano G, Moscarella E, Longo C, Zalaudek I. Clues for differentiating discoid lupus erythematosus from actinic keratosis. *J Am Acad Dermatol.* 2013;69:e5–6.

Lallas A, Apalla Z, Karteridou A, Lefaki I. Photoletter to the editor: Dermoscopy for discriminating between pityriasis rubra pilaris and psoriasis. *J Dermatol Case Rep.* 2013;7:20–2.

Lallas A, Apalla Z, Lefaki I et al. Dermoscopy of discoid lupus erythematosus. *Br J Dermatol.* 2013;168:284–8.

Lallas A, Apalla Z, Lefaki I et al. Dermoscopy of early stage mycosis fungoides. *J Eur Acad Dermatol Venereol.* 2013;27:617–21.

Lallas A, Apalla Z, Tzellos T, Lefaki I. Photoletter to the editor: Dermoscopy in clinically atypical psoriasis. *J Dermatol Case Rep.* 2012;6:61–2.

Lallas A, Argenziano G, Apalla Z et al. Dermoscopic patterns of common facial inflammatory skin diseases. *J Eur Acad Dermatol Venereol.* 2014;28:609–14.

Lallas A, Argenziano G, Longo C et al. Polygonal vessels of rosacea are highlighted by dermoscopy. *Int J Dermatol.* 2014;53:e325–7.

Lallas A, Giacomel J, Argenziano G et al. Dermoscopy in general dermatology: Practical tips for the clinician. *Br J Dermatol.* 2014;170:514–26.

Lallas A, Kyrgidis A, Tzellos TG et al. Accuracy of dermoscopic criteria for the diagnosis of psoriasis, dermatitis, lichen planus and pityriasis rosea. *Br J Dermato.* 2012;166:1198–205.

Lallas A, Zaballos P, Zalaudek I et al. Dermoscopic patterns of granuloma annulare and necrobiosis lipoidica. *Clin Exp Dermatol.* 2013;38:425–7.

Larre Borges A, Tiodorovic-Zivkovic D, Lallas A et al. Clinical, dermoscopic and histopathologic features of genital and extragenital lichen sclerosus. *J Eur Acad Dermatol Venereol.* 2013;27:1433–9.

Lopez-Tintos BO, Garcia-Hidalgo L, Orozco-Topete R. Dermoscopy in active discoid lupus. *Arch Dermatol.* 2009;145:358.

Moura FN, Thomas L, Balme B, Dalle S. Dermoscopy of lymphomatoid papulosis. *Arch Dermatol.* 2009;145:966–7.

Navarini AA, Feldmeyer L, Tondury B et al. The yellow clod sign. *Arch Dermatol.* 2011;147:1350.

Oiso N, Kawada A. Dermoscopic features in disseminated superficial actinic porokeratosis. *Eur J Dermatol.* 2011;21:439–40.

Panasiti V, Rossi M, Curzio M, Bruni F, Calvieri S. Disseminated superficial actinic porokeratosis diagnosed by dermoscopy. *Int J Dermatol.* 2008;47:308–10.

Pellicano R, Caldarola G, Filabozzi P, Zalaudek I. Dermoscopy of necrobiosis lipoidica and granuloma annulare. *Dermatology.* 2013;226:319–23.

Pellicano R, Tiodorovic-Zivkovic D, Gourhant JY et al. Dermoscopy of cutaneous sarcoidosis. *Dermatology.* 2010;221:51–4.

Pizzichetta MA, Canzonieri V, Massone C, Soyer HP. Clinical and dermoscopic features of porokeratosis of Mibelli. *Arch Dermatol.* 2009;145:91–2.

Ramirez-Fort MK, Khan F, Rosendahl CO, Mercer SE, Shim-Chang H, Levitt JO. Acquired perforating dermatosis: A clinical and dermatoscopic correlation. *Dermatol Online J.* 2013;19:18958.

Rubegni P, Tataranno DR, Nami N, Fimiani M. Rosettes: Optical effects and not dermoscopic patterns related to skin neoplasms. *Australas J Dermatol.* 2013;54:271–2.

Segal R, Mimouni D, Feuerman H, Pagovitz O, David M. Dermoscopy as a diagnostic tool in demodicidosis. *Int J Dermatol.* 2010;49:1018–23.

Shim WH, Jwa SW, Song M et al. Diagnostic usefulness of dermatoscopy in differentiating lichen sclerous et atrophicus from morphea. *J Am Acad Dermatol.* 2012;66:690–1.

Stinco G, Buligan C, Errichetti E, Valent F, Patrone P. Clinical and capillaroscopic modifications of the psoriatic plaque during therapy: Observations with oral acitretin. *Dermatol Res Pract.* 2013;2013:781942.

Stinco G, Buligan C, Maione V, Valent F, Patrone P. Videocapillaroscopic findings in the microcirculation of the psoriatic plaque during etanercept therapy. *Clin Exp Dermatol.* 2013;38:633–7.

Stinco G, Lautieri S, Valent F, Patrone P. Cutaneous vascular alterations in psoriatic patients treated with cyclosporine. *Acta Derm Venereol.* 2007;87:152–4.

Uhara H, Kamijo F, Okuyama R, Saida T. Open pores with plugs in porokeratosis clearly visualized with the dermoscopic furrow ink test: Report of 3 cases. *Arch Dermatol.* 2011;147:866–8.

Vano-Galvan S, Alvarez-Twose I, De las Heras E et al. Dermoscopic features of skin lesions in patients with mastocytosis. *Arch Dermatol.* 2011;147:932–40.

Vazquez-Lopez F, Fueyo A, Sanchez-Martin J, Perez-Oliva N. Dermoscopy for the screening of common urticaria and urticaria vasculitis. *Arch Dermatol.* 2008;144:568.

Vazquez-Lopez F, Lopez-Escobar M, Maldonado-Seral C, Perez-Oliva N, Marghoob AA. The handheld dermoscope improves the recognition of giant pseudocomedones in Darier's disease. *J Am Acad Dermatol.* 2004;50:454–5.

Vazquez-Lopez F, Maldonado-Seral C, Soler-Sanchez T, Perez-Oliva N, Marghoob AA. Surface microscopy for discriminating between common urticaria and urticarial vasculitis. *Rheumatology.* 2003;42:1079–82.

Vazquez-Lopez F, Marghoob AA. Dermoscopic assessment of long-term topical therapies with potent steroids in chronic psoriasis. *J Am Acad Dermatol.* 2004;51:811–3.

Vazquez-Lopez F, Vidal AM, Zalaudek I. Dermoscopic subpatterns of ashy dermatosis related to lichen planus. *Arch Dermatol.* 2010;146:110.

Vazquez-Lopez F, Zaballos P, Fueyo-Casado A, Sanchez-Martin J. A dermoscopy subpattern of plaque-type psoriasis: Red globular rings. *Arch Dermatol.* 2007;143:1612.

Zaballos P, Puig S, Malvehy J. Dermoscopy of pigmented purpuric dermatoses (lichen aureus): A useful tool for clinical diagnosis. *Arch Dermatol.* 2004;140:1290–1.

Zaballos P, Puig S, Malvehy J. Dermoscopy of disseminated superficial actinic porokeratosis. *Arch Dermatol.* 2004;140:1410.

Zalaudek I, Ferrara G, Brongo S, Giorgio CM, Argenziano G. Atypical clinical presentation of pigmented purpuric dermatosis. *J Dtsch Dermatol Ges.* 2006;4:138–40.

7

Infectious Skin Diseases

7.1 Parasitoses

7.1.1 Scabies

Scabies is a skin infestation caused by the parasite *Sarcoptes scabiei* var. *hominis.* It is an infectious disease, and, although not life threatening, it impairs patients' quality of life due to intense pruritus. The incubation time after the initial infection ranges from 2 to 6 weeks, while in the case of reinfection, itching may start within the first 24 hours.

The adult female of *Sarcoptes scabiei,* after fertilization, burrows into the stratum corneum, creating a tunnel in which it incubates and deposits its eggs. In a healthy adult, the overall number of mites is less than 10. Sites of predilection include the interdigital clefts, the wrists, the trunk, the gluteus area, the axillae, the nipple and areola complex in females, and the shaft of the penis in males. Primary lesions clinically develop as itchy papules, often eroded, and are either solitary or gathered in groups at the aforementioned body sites. Burrows are often shaped as "Z," "S," or "L." However, during clinical examination with the naked eye, they are barely seen.

Clinical diagnosis of scabies may be challenging due to similarities with other inflammatory skin disorders, including dermatitis and folliculitis (Figure 7.1). The definite diagnosis is usually established by microscopy with the detection of the parasite or its eggs in a skin sample collected by scraping the lesions. However, this process requires collaboration with a laboratory and/or the use of a microscope. Literature data suggest that dermatoscopy facilitates scabies diagnosis with thorough examination of all the lesions and allows for the *in vivo* recognition of the parasite and its eggs within the burrows and furrows. The dermatoscopic hallmark of scabies is the "jet with contrail" pattern. Specifically, it consists of small black/brown triangular structures (jet) located at the end of whitish structureless lines (curved or wavy) (contrail), which correspond to the pigmented part of the mite and the burrow, respectively (Figure 7.2). Within the burrow, the parasites' eggs may be dermatoscopically detected as white, tiny, oval-shaped structures in a linear distribution (Figure 7.3). The most useful diagnostic clue to distinguish the burrow from white erosions or scales observed in several dermatoses is the tubular or cylindrical shape of the burrow. In case of excessive scratching, the upper part of the burrow along with the mite might be removed. In this scenario, the morphology of the lesions is altered, making clinical diagnosis extremely challenging. Dermatoscopy might prove useful since angular or tortuous furrows without the mite may be observed, together with erosions and erythematosquamous papules.

7.1.2 Pediculosis

Pediculosis is one of the most common contagious infestations worldwide. It is divided into phthiriasis of the scalp, caused by the pediculus humanus capitis, and phthiriasis of the body and pubis, caused by pediculus humanus corporis and pediculus humanus pubis, respectively.

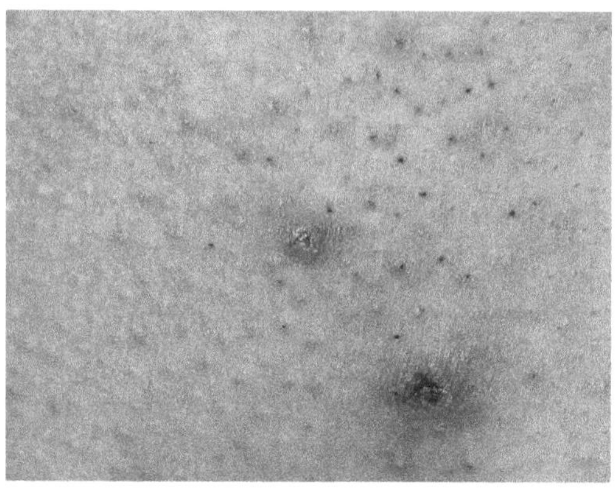

FIGURE 7.1 Clinical aspect of scabies mimicking folliculitis of the axillae.

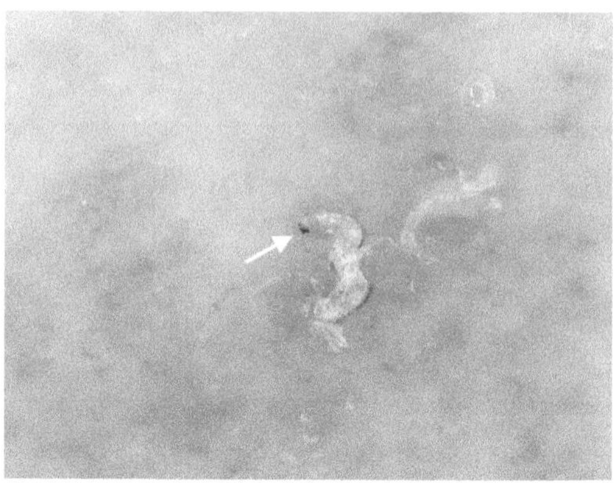

FIGURE 7.2 "Jet with contrail" pattern. The parasite appears as a small black/brown triangular structure (arrow) located at the end of a whitish wavy line (burrow).

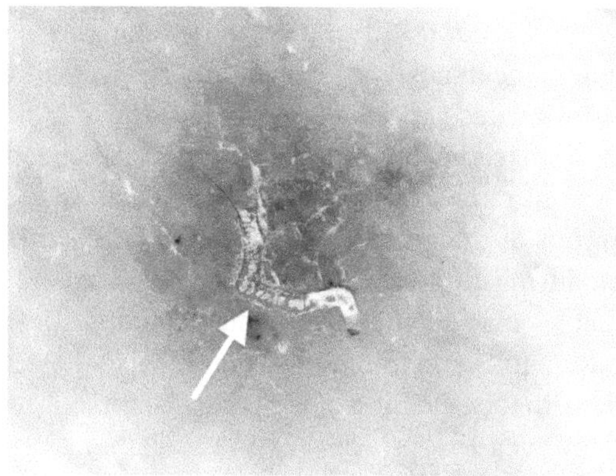

FIGURE 7.3 Tiny, white, oval structures in a linear arrangement along the burrow correspond to the parasite's eggs (arrow).

Phthiriasis of The Scalp

The female lice, 1–2 days after fertilization, deliver eggs (nits), which fix to the hair shafts, near the proximal end, within 1–2 mm of the scalp. At this site, the increased temperature is optimal for incubation. Sites of predilection are the temporal and occipital area of the scalp. Each mature louse lays about 7–10 eggs (nits) per day. After 6–10 days, nymphs (immature lice) hatch from the nits, and after 9–12 days, they become mature and live as adults for about 1–3 months. The parasite is white to gray in color, 1–3 mm in length, and has three pairs of clawed legs. As an ectoparasite, whose only hosts are humans, the adult louse survives only 24–48 hours away from the human body.

The clinical diagnosis of phthiriasis of the scalp is usually easy. However, in case of "pseudonits," the discrimination may be challenging. Pseudonits (also called "hair casts") represent cylindrical white scales that encircle the hair shaft and closely simulate nits. They usually result from the debris of hair spray or gel. Distinguishing between the two entities may be almost impossible with a naked-eye clinical examination. However, dermatoscopy allows

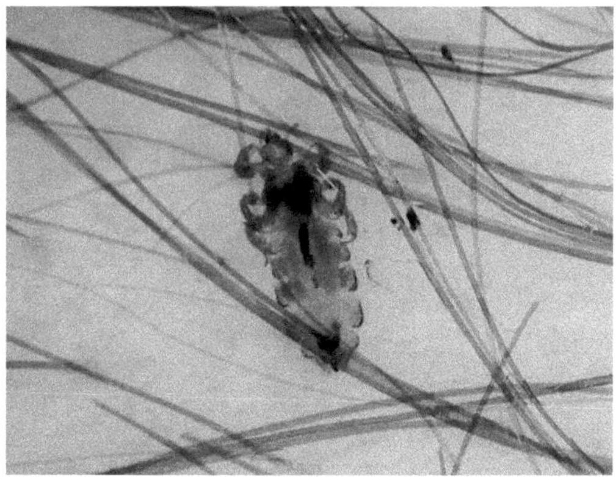

FIGURE 7.4 Dermatoscopic aspect of the pediculus humanus capitis.

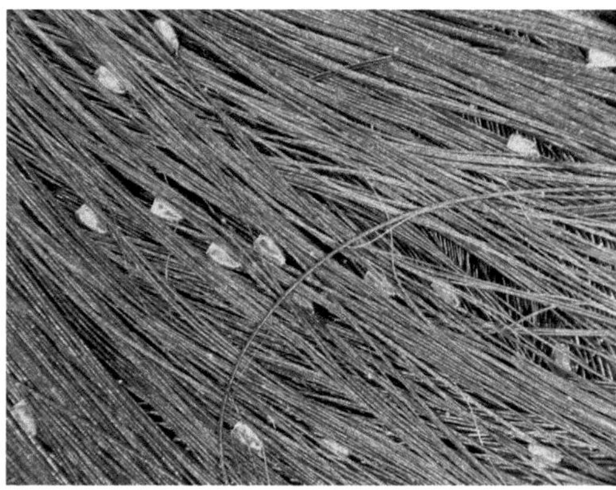

FIGURE 7.5 Dermatoscopy of nits that are fixed to the hair shaft.

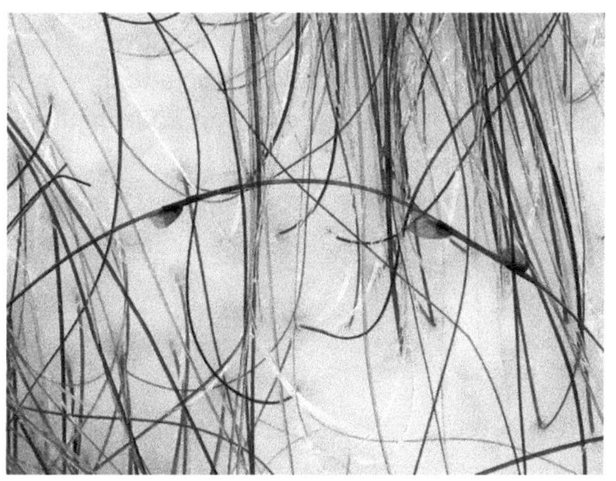

FIGURE 7.6 Empty nits are seen as semitranslucent, white/gray, ovoid structures attached on the hair shafts.

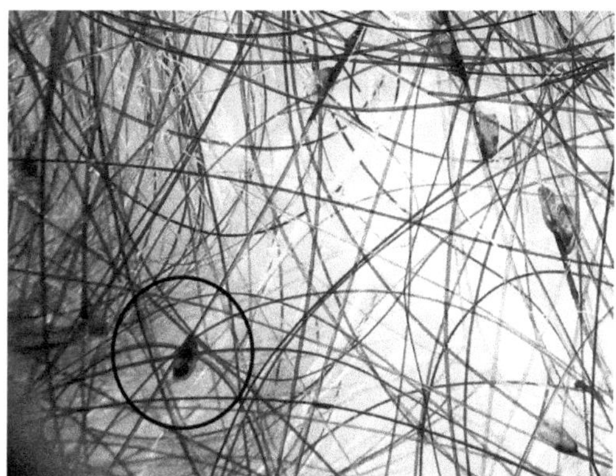

FIGURE 7.7 Live nits are dark brown in color.

a rapid and straightforward diagnosis since it enables visualization of both parasite and nits (Figure 7.4). Nits are dermatoscopically seen as brown to white ovoid structures that are firmly attached to the hair shaft (Figure 7.5). Apart from the diagnosis, dermatoscopy is very useful for monitoring the treatment outcome. Specifically, dermatoscopy allows for the discrimination between the empty (dead) nits from those containing vital nymphs (alive) and running the incubation phase. The latter suggests continuation or modification of treatment. The empty nits appear whitish in color, are semitranslucent, and typically show a plane and fissured free ending (Figure 7.6). Live nits dermatoscopically exhibit ovoid dark brown structures in smooth tense shells (Figure 7.7).

Phthiriasis of the Body (Phthiriasis Corporis)

Phthiriasis of the body is rare in the Western world. Overcrowded living conditions or camps and poor personal hygiene are risk factors associated with small epidemics of phthiriasis corporis. The parasite is larger in size compared to the *Pediculus humanus capitis*, but it also feeds on

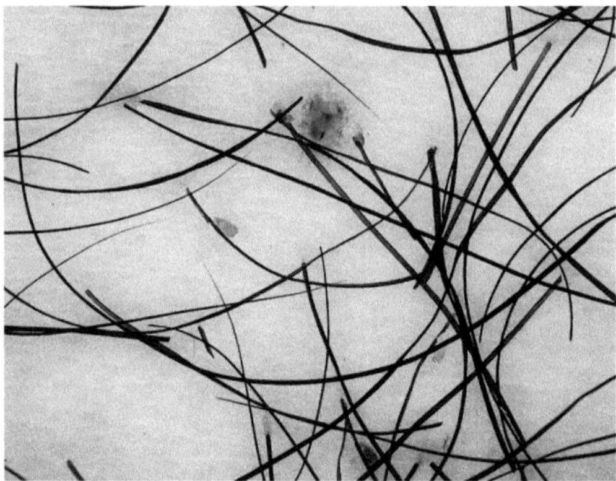

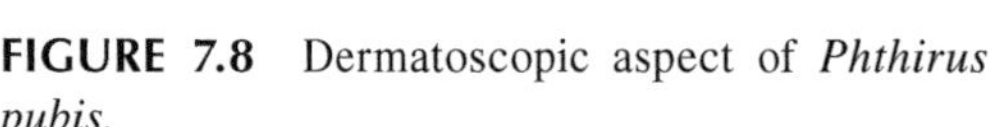

FIGURE 7.8 Dermatoscopic aspect of *Phthirus pubis.*

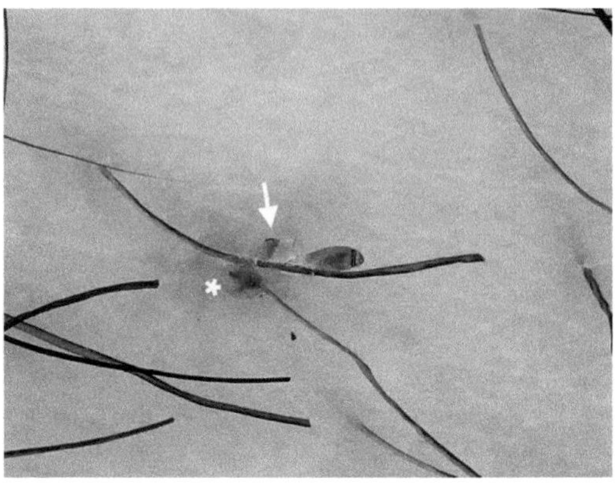

FIGURE 7.9 Live nit (brown colored) and empty translucent shell (arrow) on the same hair shaft, out of which there is a young, newly born parasite (asterisk).

human blood. The lice are usually found on clothes and linen, mainly along the fabric seams, where they reproduce and lay their eggs. Common clinical sites of involvement include the lower back, the axillae, and the groin area. Transmission occurs via infected clothing and linen and direct contact with infected individuals, as well.

Literature data reporting dermatoscopic findings of phthiriasis corporis are very limited. However, dermatoscopy seems to be substantially helpful as it enables the visualization of both the parasite and its nits.

Phthiriasis Pubis

Even though phthiriasis pubis mainly affects the pubic hairs in the groin, it can also involve the eyebrows, eyelashes, trunk, thighs, axillary areas, and occasionally, the scalp. The pubic louse (*Phthirus pubis*, also called "crab" due to its short, broad body and its large front claws) is an ectoparasite whose host is human, and it feeds exclusively on blood. Morphologically, it differs from all the other *Phthirus* species. Specifically, an adult louse is about 1.3–2 mm long, and its body is oval shaped. Moreover, its hind two pairs of legs are thicker than the front legs and have large claws for better traction. Its eggs are gray in color and are grouped in small piles at the base of hair fibers. The pubic lice are transmitted via close body contact (usually sexual) and less commonly through clothing, linen, and towels used by an infested individual. Clinical examination and history of itching are usually sufficient to establish the diagnosis. In case of diagnostic doubts, dermatoscopy may prove helpful, since it can easily point out the parasite and the nits (Figure 7.8). Similar to phthiriasis capitis, dermatoscopy facilitates the evaluation and monitoring of the therapeutic outcome, by identifying live and dead nits (Figure 7.9).

7.2 Viral Infections

7.2.1 Molluscum Contagiosum

Molluscum contagiosum (MC) is a viral infection of the skin caused by the MC virus (MC types I–IV), which belongs to the Poxviridae family. The virus is transmitted by direct body contact, as well as via clothes or towels used by an infested individual. MC virus causes characteristic skin lesions, either solitary or, most commonly, multiple that present in small groups of shiny, flesh-colored, nontender, round-shaped papules (Figures 7.10 and 7.11). The papules are characterized by an umbilicated center, which is filled with white-yellow material that contains molluscum bodies. In the case of giant MC, the size of the lesions varies from a few millimeters to 1.5 centimeters. The infection is mostly seen in young ages; the most common sites of involvement include face, trunk, extremities, thighs, perineum, and pubic area. Although a rare event, the virus may also infect mucosa. Immunosuppression and inflammatory dermatoses of childhood (e.g., atopic dermatitis) represent risk factors of widespread and resistant-to-treatment MC infections.

The differential diagnosis of MC includes human papillomavirus infection, sebaceous hyperplasia, keratoacanthoma, and in more widespread cases, lichen planus.

Dermatoscopy enhances the diagnosis of MC as a result of the almost pathognomonic dermatoscopic pattern of the disease. The dermatoscopic hallmark of MC is the combination of a central pore or umbilication combined with white-yellowish, multilobular, amorphous structures with fine, linear, often branching vessels at the periphery (crown vessels). The vessels are characteristically restricted at the periphery and never cross the center of the lesion (Figures 7.12 and 7.13).

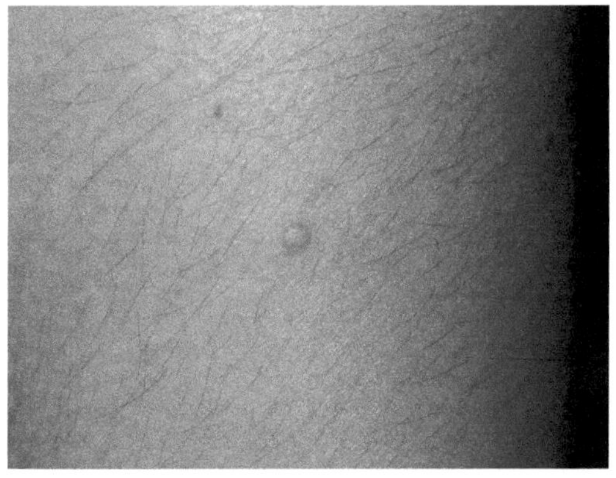

FIGURE 7.10 Clinical aspect of a typical molluscum contagiosum.

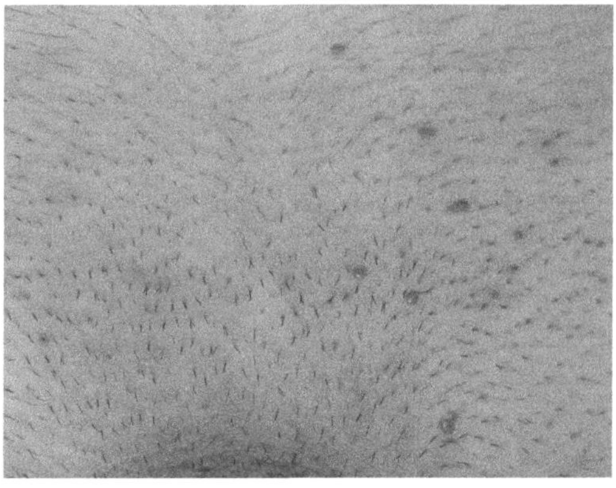

FIGURE 7.11 Clinical aspect of multiple typical molluscum contagiosum lesions located on the groin.

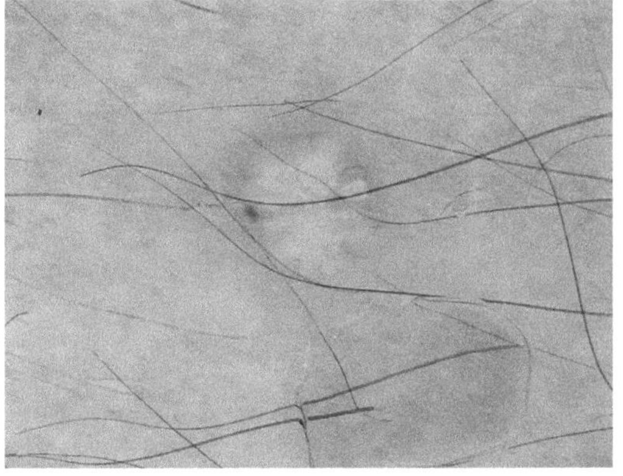

FIGURE 7.12 Dermatoscopy of molluscum contagiosum displaying a multilobular, white-yellowish center and "crown vessels" at the periphery.

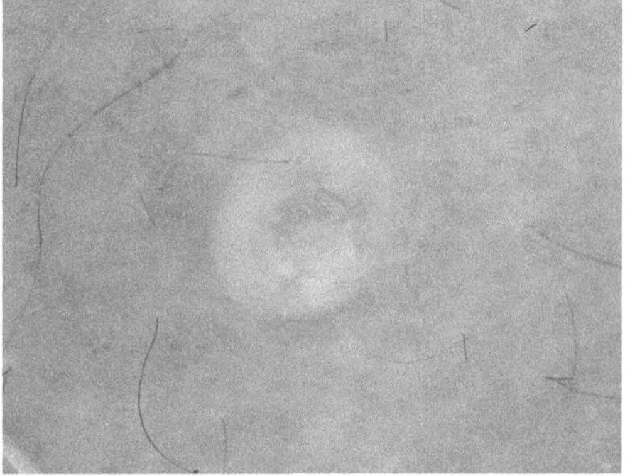

FIGURE 7.13 Dermatoscopic aspect of molluscum contagiosum exhibiting a white-yellowish center and peripheral, linear vessels that do not cross the center of the lesion.

In adult patients who present with tiny papules involving the pubic area, dermatoscopy is very helpful in discriminating between MC and anogenital warts, since the dermatoscopic patterns of MC and warts have major differences, as explained in the following sections.

7.2.2 Human Papillomavirus Infections

Anogenital Warts (Condyloma Acuminatum)

Anogenital warts are the clinical manifestation of infection by certain types of human papillomavirus (HPV). Specifically, types 6 and 11 are responsible for more than 90% of anogenital warts. The virus enters the body through insignificant traumas or erosions of the skin, and after the incubation period that ranges from 3 weeks to 9 months, the patient develops clinically visible lesions. Condyloma acuminatum manifests as one or multiple papules with a cauliflower or plaque-like appearance and can be smooth, verrucous, or lobulated. The color may vary from flesh-colored to brownish (Figure 7.14). In moist areas, such as the glans penis, when left untreated and due to constant maceration, the warts may appear white in color (Figure 7.15). Occasionally, HPV lesions coalesce into large, verrucous plaques mimicking seborrheic keratoses (Figure 7.16).

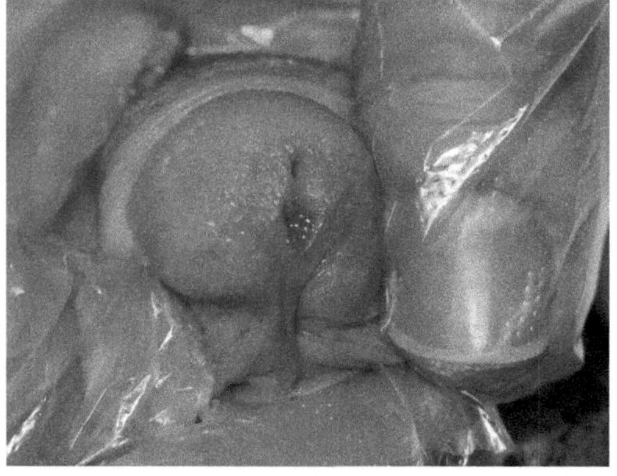

FIGURE 7.14 Clinical aspect of a genital wart, involving the urethral opening. Due to the size of the lesion and the site of involvement, a certain diagnosis cannot be safely established.

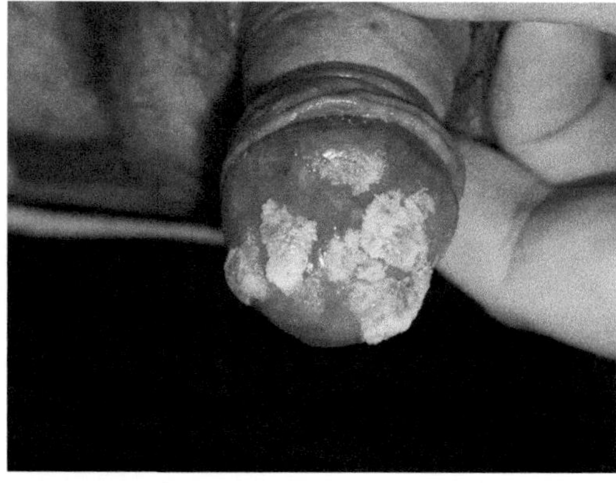

FIGURE 7.15 Multiple white-colored warts located on the glans penis.

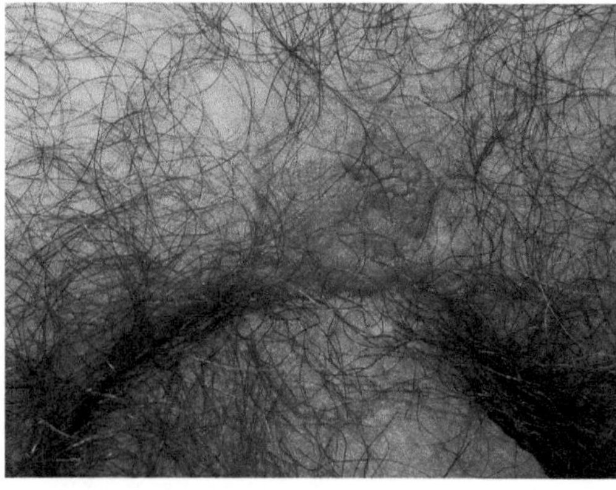

FIGURE 7.16 Genital wart presenting as a plaque with verrucous surface and resembling seborrheic keratosis.

The diagnosis of anogenital warts does not usually pose significant difficulties and can be easily established from a clinical point of view. However, sometimes, the diagnosis may be confusing due to normal anatomical structures of the genital area, such as the pearly penile papules and Fordyce papules. Moreover, the differential diagnosis should include other dermatoses that affect the area and are morphologically similar to anogenital warts, such as lichen planus and MC. In such cases, dermatoscopy highlights the cauliflower appearance of the anogenital warts, as well as the characteristic white halos surrounding dotted and/or hairpin vessels, facilitating their diagnosis (Figures 7.17 through 7.19).

Common, Plane, and Palmoplantar Warts

Common, plane, and palmoplantar warts are caused by certain types of HPV that inoculate, via small erosions or traumas, in our skin, during direct or indirect contact with the virus. After a long incubation period that ranges from a few weeks to several months, the patient develops the first clinically visible lesions. Autoinoculation is also frequent, causing local spread of lesions.

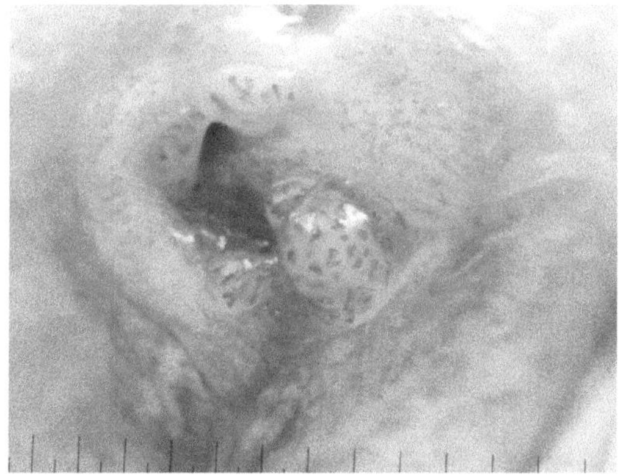

FIGURE 7.17 Dermatoscopic aspect of the lesion clinically presented in Figure 7.14. Lack of thick keratin in the mucosal area enables visualization of the glomerular and hairpin vessels surrounded by white halo in a white-reddish background.

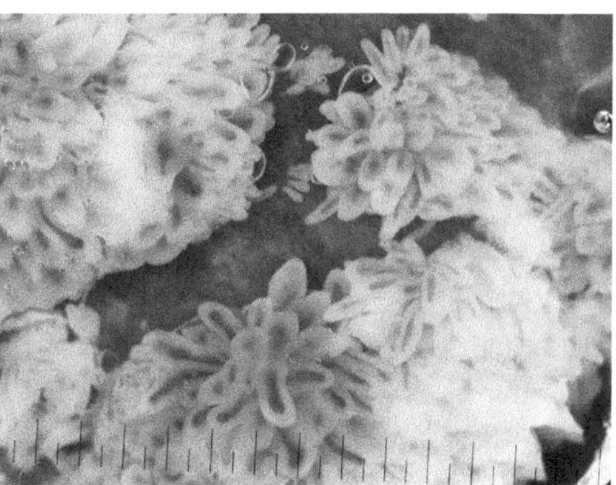

FIGURE 7.18 Characteristic dermatoscopic pattern of white halo surrounding a vessel (1).

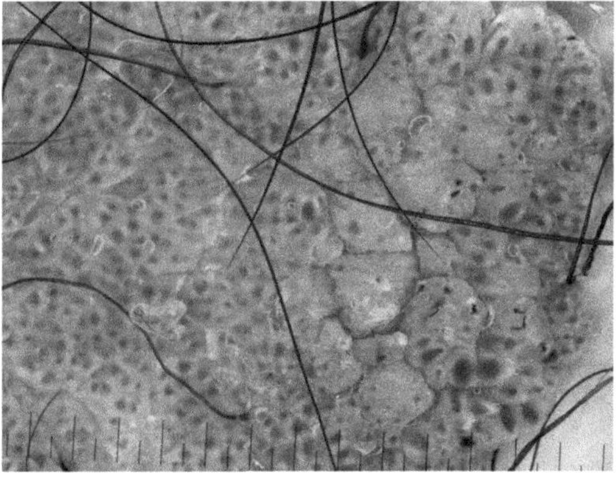

FIGURE 7.19 Characteristic dermatoscopic pattern of white halo surrounding a vessel (2).

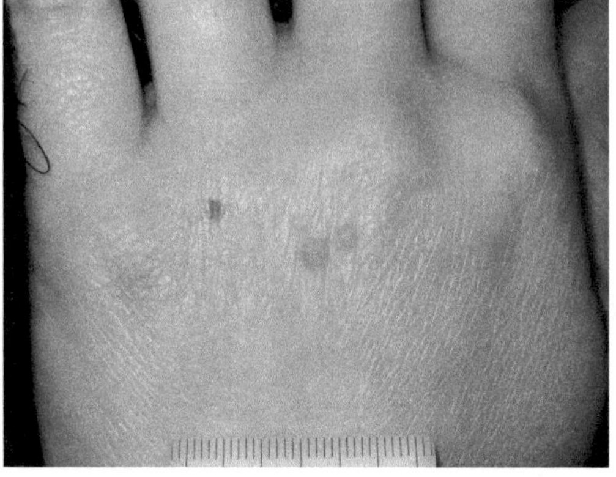

FIGURE 7.20 Clinical aspect of a typical common wart.

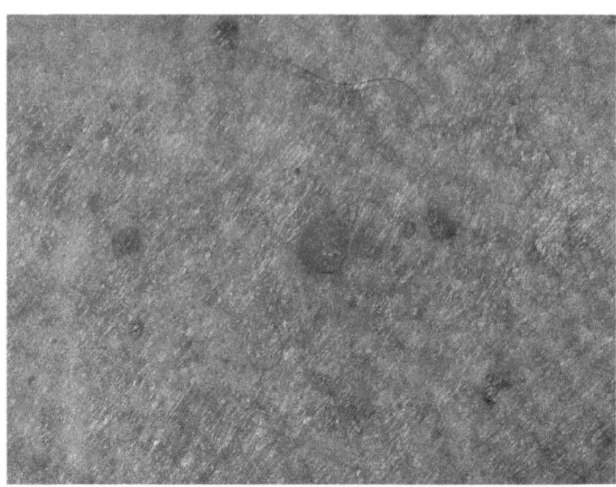

FIGURE 7.21 Clinical aspect of a typical common wart with cauliflower appearance.

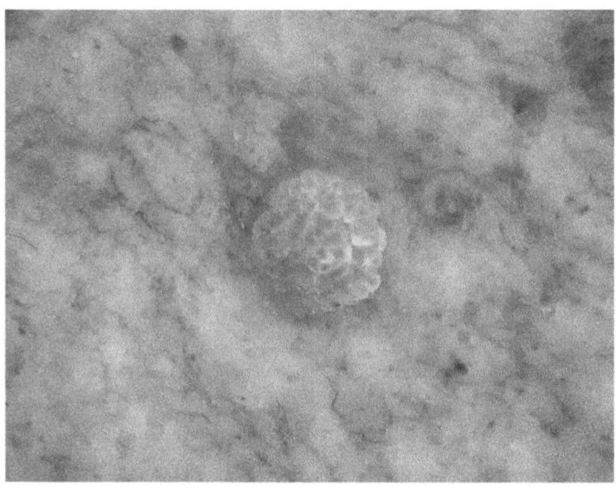

FIGURE 7.22 Dermatoscopic image of common wart exhibiting multiple papillae with red dots surrounded by white halos that correspond to perpendicularly oriented vessels within the papillary dermis.

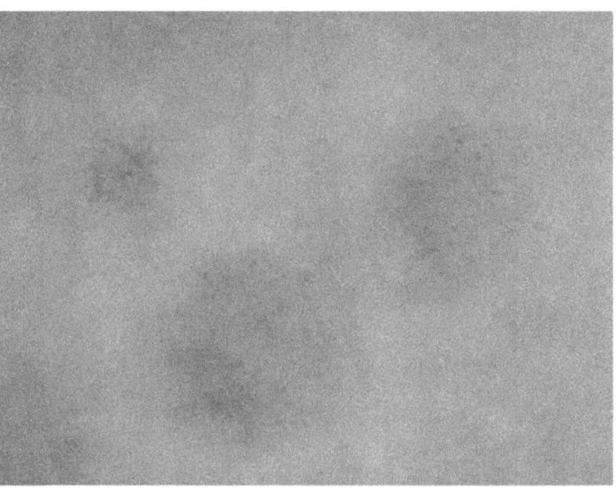

FIGURE 7.23 The most common dermatoscopic pattern of common warts consists of dotted vessels surrounded by white color.

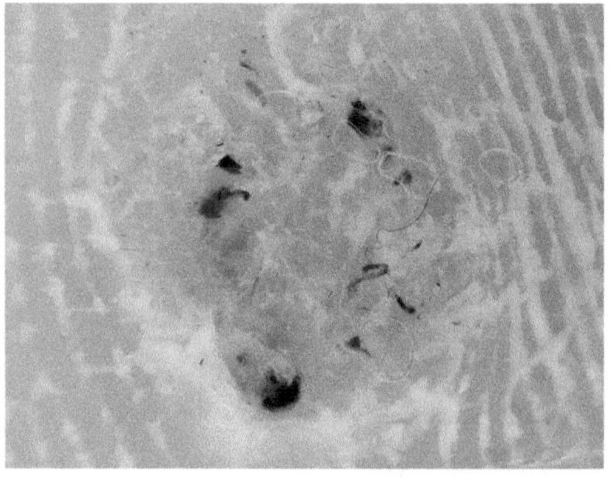

FIGURE 7.24 Hemorrhages and red spots in a plantar wart.

FIGURE 7.25 Multiple tiny red dots dermatoscopically typify plane warts.

About 65% of the warts may spontaneously resolve without any treatment, within the first 2 years of infection, without scarring.

Common warts develop as hard in palpation, asymptomatic, flesh-colored to grayish papules, with a rough, verrucous surface (Figures 7.20 and 7.21).

Dermatoscopic examination reveals multiple densely packed papillae containing red dots surrounded by white halo corresponding to perpendicularly oriented, often thrombosed, vessels within the elongated dermal papillae (Figures 7.22 and 7.23). This finding is more prominent in plantar warts in which the increased pressure results in vascular thrombosis, dermatoscopically seen as red to brown/black hemorrhages and blood spots (Figure 7.24). The latter is very useful for the discrimination of plantar warts from calluses, which lack the aforementioned features. In addition to this, dermatoscopy reveals the well-defined yellowish papilliform surface of a plantar wart in which the normal skin lines are interrupted following HPV infection.

Concerning plane warts, they dermatoscopically display regularly arranged, tiny red dots on a light brown to yellow background allowing for their discrimination from acne or folliculitis lesions, which exhibit a central white to yellow pore (Figure 7.25).

7.3 Other Infections

7.3.1 Tick Bites

Ixodes ricinus (commonly known as tick) is a parasite that causes several infectious diseases such as borreliosis and ehrlichiosis. The site of the tick bite clinically appears as a black dot of about 1 mm in diameter and in many cases can be misdiagnosed as a small melanocytic nevus. The diagnosis of a tick bite is straightforward with the use of dermatoscopy. Specifically, dermatoscopy allows for the recognition of the posterior part of the body and the posterior pair of the legs of the parasite that remain out of the human body at the site of the bite; in contrast, the head of the parasite is dipped into the skin (Figure 7.26). Beyond the diagnosis, dermatoscopy is also helpful for the evaluation of whether the attempt to remove the parasite was successful.

7.3.2 Demodicosis

Demodicosis is a common parasitic infestation that clinically manifests as erythema and papulopustules, combined with pruritus and a burning sensation. The most common site

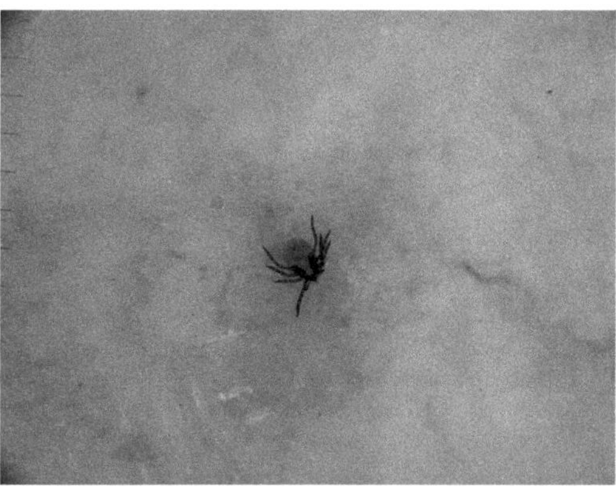

FIGURE 7.26 The posterior part of the tick body and its posterior pairs of legs as seen in dermatoscopy; the head of the parasite is dipped into the skin.

of involvement is the face (Figure 7.27). The responsible parasite is *Demodex folliculorum*. *Demodex folliculorum* is normally present on the human skin and remains nonpathogenic in many individuals. However, under certain circumstances, excessive proliferation of the parasite may result in demodicosis. The disease may clinically mimic periocular and perioral dermatitis, seborrheic dermatitis, acne vulgaris, and discoid lupus erythematosus from which it should be differentiated.

Dermatoscopy reveals cylindrical, whitish, scaly structures within the openings of the hair follicles. This feature corresponds to the "tail" of the *Demodex* (Figure 7.28). Dermatoscopy is also useful for monitoring and evaluation of the treatment outcome.

7.3.3 Leishmaniasis

In cutaneous leishmaniasis, generalized erythema, white clods that correspond to follicular plugs and have also been described as "yellow tears," hyperkeratosis, central erosion/ulceration, and vascular structures (such as linear, dotted, comma, hairpin vessels) are the most frequent

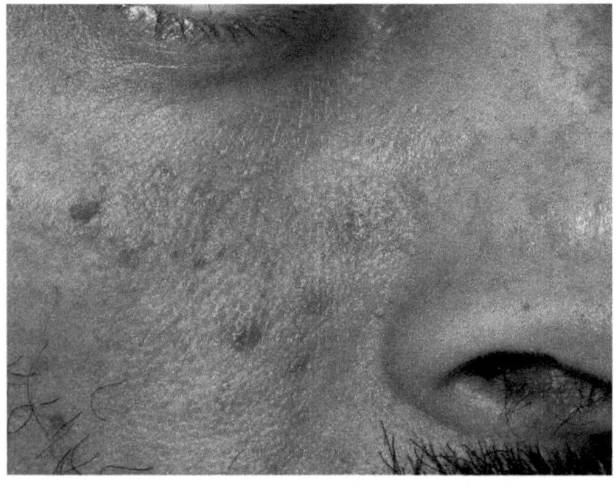

FIGURE 7.27 Clinical aspect of demodicosis manifesting as an erythematous papulopustular eruption on the face.

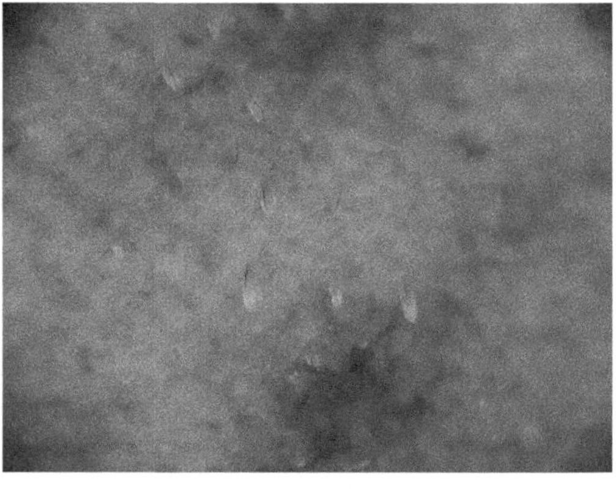

FIGURE 7.28 Whitish squamoid projections ("*Demodex* tails"), protruding out of the follicular openings are indicative of demodicosis.

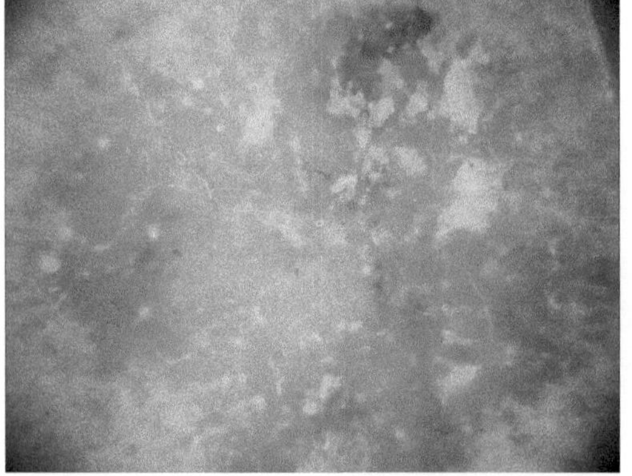

FIGURE 7.29 Dermatoscopic aspect of leishmaniasis consisting of diffuse orange-yellow areas, white scales, linear vessels, and white clods (follicular plugs).

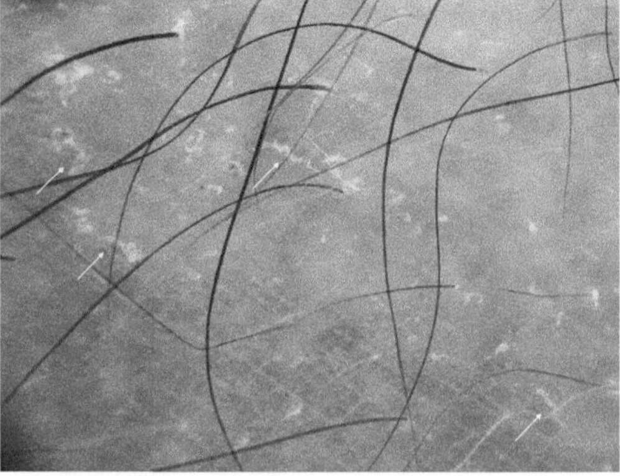

FIGURE 7.30 The dermatoscopic hallmark of tinea corporis is the inward-to-outward direction of the peripheral scales (arrows).

dermatoscopic findings (Figure 7.29). Moreover, translucent yellow/orange areas may sometimes be observed.

7.3.4 Tinea Corporis

The dermatoscopic hallmark of tinea corporis is peripherally distributed white scales. A peculiar characteristic of tinea scales is that the desquamation process progresses in an inward-to-outward direction (Figure 7.30). The outer border of the scales is typically intact and sharply demarcated and might acquire a "moth-eaten appearance." Multiple circular peripheral scales often coalesce to form larger multicyclic lesions. The vascular pattern is usually monomorphic, consisting of dotted vessels with unspecific distribution.

BIBLIOGRAPHY

Bae JM, Kang H, Kim HO, Park YM. Differential diagnosis of plantar wart from corn, callus and healed wart with the aid of dermoscopy. *Br J Dermatol.* 2009;160:220–2.

Bakos RM, Bakos L. Dermoscopy for diagnosis of pediculosis capitis. *J Am Acad Dermatol.* 2007;57(4):727–8.

Chuh A, Lee A, Wong W, Ooi C, Zawar V. Diagnosis of *Pediculosis pubis*: A novel application of digital epiluminescence dermatoscopy. *J Eur Acad Dermatol Venereol.* 2007;21(6):837–8.

Di Stefani A, Hofmann-Wellenhof R, Zalaudek I. Dermoscopy for diagnosis and treatment monitoring of *Pediculosis capitis. J Am Acad Dermatol.* 2006;54(5):909–11.

Dong H, Shu D, Campbell TM, Frühauf J, Soyer HP, Hofmann-Wellenhof R. Dermatoscopy of genital warts. *J Am Acad Dermatol.* 2011;64:859–64.

Dupuy A, Dehen L, Bourrat E, Lacroix C, Benderdouche M, Dubertret L, Morel P, Feuilhade de Chauvin M, Petit A. Accuracy of standard dermoscopy for diagnosing scabies. *J Am Acad Dermatol.* 2007;56(1):53–62.

Friedman P, Sabban EC, Cabo H. Usefulness of dermoscopy in the diagnosis and monitoring treatment of demodicidosis. *Dermatol Pract Concept.* 2017;7:35–8.

Kim SH, Seo SH, Ko HC, Kwon KS, Kim MB. The use of dermatoscopy to differentiate vestibular papillae, a normal variant of the female external genitalia, from condyloma acuminata. *J Am Acad Dermatol.* 2009;60:353–5.

Ku SH, Cho EB, Park EJ, Kim KH, Kim KJ. Dermoscopic features of molluscum contagiosum based on white structures and their correlation with histopathological findings. *Clin Exp Dermatol.* 2015;40:208–10.

Lallas A, Apalla Z, Lazaridou E, Sotiriou E, Vakirlis E, Ioannides D. Scabies escaping detection until dermoscopy was applied. *Dermatol Pract Concep.* 2017;7(1):49–50.

Lee DY, Park JH, Lee JH, Yang JM, Lee ES. The use of dermoscopy for the diagnosis of plantar wart. *J Eur Acad Dermatol Venereol.* 2009;23:726–7.

Marin-Cabanas I, Pascual JC. Image gallery: Dermoscopy of *Phthiriasis pubis*: A handy and useful tool. *Br J Dermatol.* 2016;175(1):e94.

Martins LG, Bernardes Filho F, Quaresma MV, Bellott TR, Botelho LN, Prata AC. Dermoscopy applied to pediculosis corporis diagnosis. *An Bras Dermatol.* 2014;89(3):513–4.

Segal R, Mimouni D, Feuerman H. Dermoscopy as a diagnostic tool in demodicidosis. *Int J Dermatol.* 2010;49:1018–23.

Walter B, Heukelbach J, Fengler G, Worth C, Hengge U, Feldmeier H. Comparison of dermoscopy, skin scraping, and the adhesive tape test for the diagnosis of scabies in a resource-poor setting. *Arch Dermatol.* 2011;147(4):468–73.

Watanabe T, Yoshida Y, Yamamoto O. Differential diagnosis of pearly penile papules and penile condyloma acuminatum by dermoscopy. *Eur J Dermatol.* 2010;20:414–5.
Zaballos P, Ara M, Puig S, Malvehy J. Dermoscopy of molluscum contagiosum: A useful tool for clinical diagnosis in adulthood. *J Eur Acad Dermatol Venereol.* 2006;20:482–3.
Zalaudek I, Giacomel J, Cabo H, Di Stefani A, Ferrara G, Hofmann-Wellenhof R, Malvehy J, Puig S, Stolz W, Argenziano G. Entodermoscopy: A new tool for diagnosing skin infections and infestations. *Dermatology.* 2008;216:14–23.

8

Trichoscopy

Dermatoscopy of the hair and scalp, also known as trichoscopy, has been successfully incorporated in our diagnostic armamentarium during the last decades. Today it is extensively used in our daily practice for diagnosing hair loss. Trichoscopy allows a detailed visualization of the skin of the scalp, including follicular openings and interfollicular epidermis (scales, coloration, vascularity), while it provides the opportunity to observe the morphology of the hair shafts (hair thickness, hair shaft anomalies, and different types of hairs).

Normal hair shaft

Each normal terminal hair is characterized by homogeneity in terms of color and thickness along the hair shaft. In an adult individual, hairs of different color and thickness may be present, while in the elderly, white and gray colored hairs may coexist. The presence of white hair during childhood, puberty, or in very young adults is a pathologic condition, indicative of a disease (e.g., vitiligo). A hair shaft is classified as thick, moderately thick, and thin based on hair shaft diameter. The diameter of a normal, thick, terminal hair usually ranges from 0.05 to 0.06 mm ($\approx$55 μm). A moderately thick hair is about 0.03–0.05 mm, while a thin hair is no more than 0.03 mm. Calculation of the hair shaft thickness is not feasible with the use of handheld dermatoscopes; however, it allows a rough classification of them into thick, moderately thick, and thin hairs. Thick hairs predominate in the scalp, but depending on the scalp site, all three types may coexist. Analytically, thin hairs at a rate up to 10% are present in frontal, occipital, and temporal areas; moderately thick hairs account for up to 30% in the frontal area and up to 40% in the occipital and temporal areas of the scalp. All the other anatomical sites of the scalp are covered by thick hairs at a very high rate greater than 50% (Figure 8.1).

Vellus hairs of about 10% are a normal finding in adult individuals. Unlike terminal hairs, vellus hairs are thin, pale, and short (less than 3 mm in length), and typically lack the medulla (Figure 8.2). The presence of vellus hairs in a higher than expected rate for the anatomical area may indicate alopecia, mostly androgenetic, or persistent alopecia areata. Taking into consideration that calculation of the rate of vellus hairs is tough, an easier way to go in our daily practice is to measure their absolute number per optical field during trichoscopy (×20 magnification). In this scenario, recognition of two to three vellus hairs per optical field in the frontal area is an indication of androgenetic alopecia. Vellus hairs should be differentiated from short, normal, regrowing hairs. The latter are usually 3–5 mm in length and 0.05 mm in thickness. They are pigmented and arranged in an upright position, with a sharp distal end, which significantly differs from the dull distal end of vellus hairs (Figure 8.3).

In the end, hair medulla may be complete, occupying continuously the central part of the hair shaft, fragmented, or absent. In the former occasion, it develops as a longitudinal, hypopigmented band along the center of the hair shaft, covering less than 50% of the hair thickness (continuous medulla). The fragmented medulla appears as an interrupted, usually whitish, longitudinal band, occupying less than 50% of the hair shaft thickness (interrupted medulla). The presence, or thickness of the hair medulla is not of significant clinical importance.

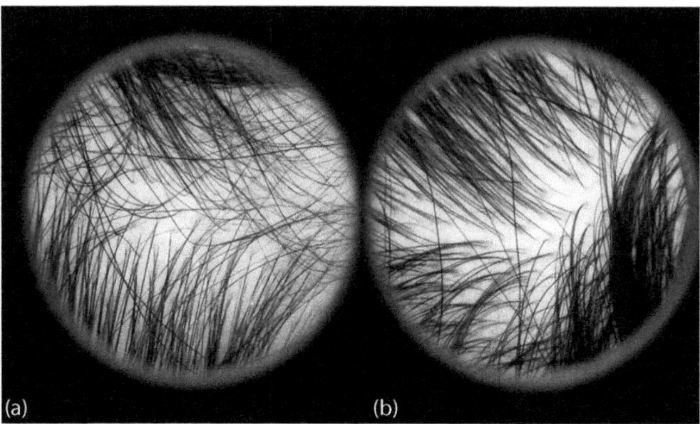

FIGURE 8.1 Trichoscopic findings in the temporal (a) and the occipital (b) areas of the scalp, in which we normally observe thin hairs at lower rates compared to moderately thick hairs. Thick terminal hairs predominate at these sites of the scalp.

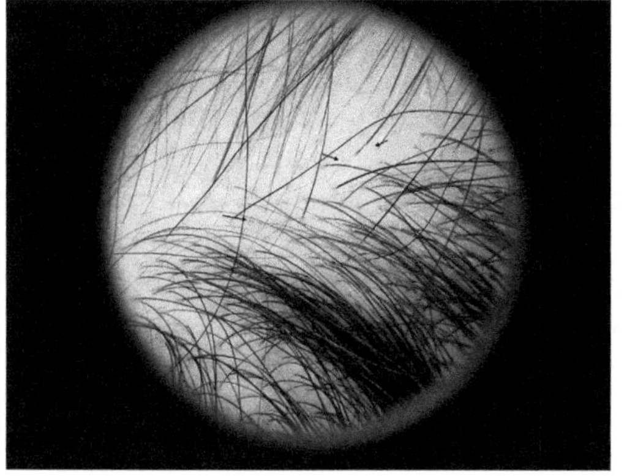

FIGURE 8.2 Vellus hair is a normal finding in the frontal area (arrows).

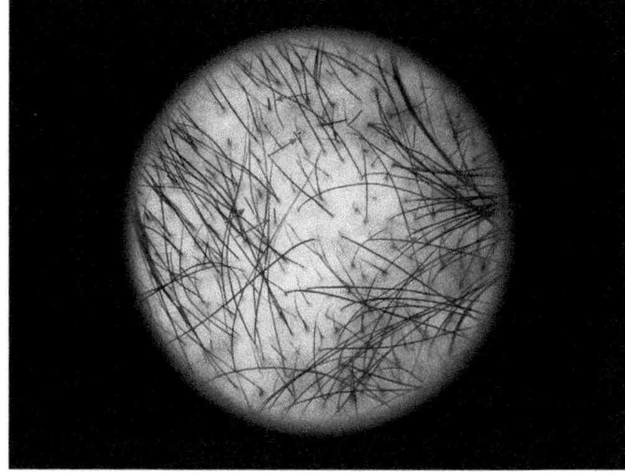

FIGURE 8.3 New, regrowing hairs in upright position and sharp distal end (arrows).

Alopecia

The term *alopecia* refers to hair loss independent of the causal factor, site, or extent of involvement. There are two distinct clinical groups of alopecia, namely, noncicatricial and cicatricial alopecia. In this chapter, we describe the more important diseases of each group, and we analyze their typical trichoscopic features.

8.1 Noncicatricial Alopecias

8.1.1 Androgenetic Alopecia (Male and Female Pattern Hair Loss)

Androgenetic alopecia (AGA) represents the most common type of hair loss. The terms *male* (MPHL) and *female pattern hair loss* (FPHL) are used for AGA in males and females, respectively. The precise pathogenesis of AGA has not been fully elucidated. Current data suggest a multifactorial process, with genetic predisposition in a central role. The course of the disease includes gradual miniaturization of the hair follicles, gradual shortening of the anagen phase, and prolongation of the post-exogen part of the telogen phase (latent phase, or kenogen phase). The process is driven by dihydrotestosterone that locally interferes with the hair follicle, while the level of circulating androgens is usually in normal range.

Clinical Presentation

On the clinical basis, AGA is characterized by distinct patterns of hair loss in females versus males. However, one of the features in common is that the central scalp is the most severely involved area.

MPHL (Hamilton-Norwood type), which is the most predominant pattern in men, involves recession of the frontal hair line in conjunction with vertex thinning (Figure 8.4).

In FPHL (Ludwig type), we observe maintenance of the frontal hairline and diffuse thinning of the centroparietal area. The latter is mostly seen in females (Figure 8.5); however, it has been occasionally observed in males, too. The Christmas tree pattern is similar to the Ludwig type, with diffuse centroparietal thinning, in combination with breached frontal hairline (Figure 8.6).

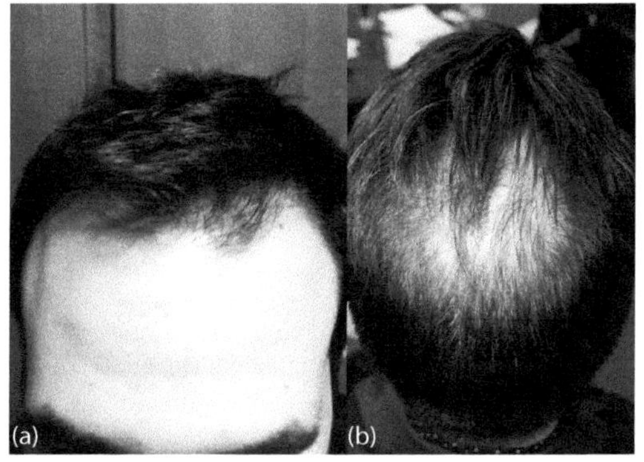

FIGURE 8.4 Clinical examples of androgenetic alopecia in a male patient: (a) recession of the frontal hairline, mainly at the temporal area and (b) thinning of hair in the parietal area.

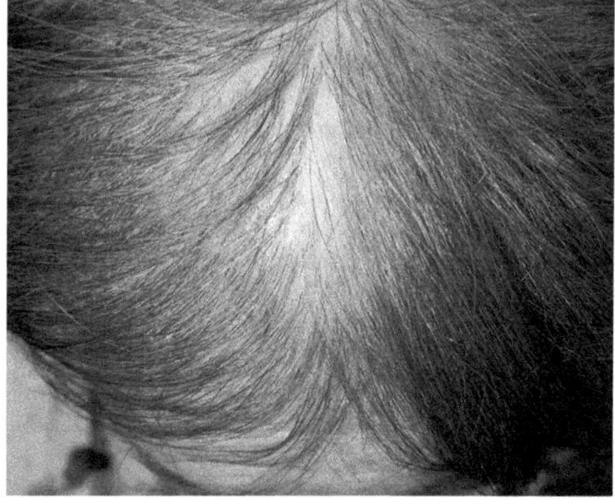

FIGURE 8.5 Clinical example of androgenetic alopecia in a female patient.

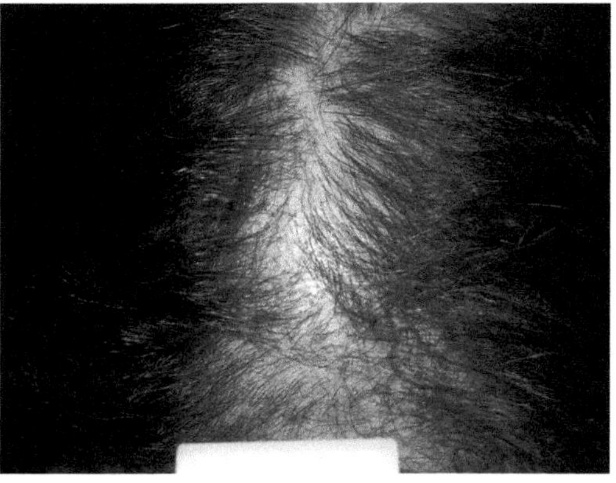

FIGURE 8.6 Christmas tree alopecia pattern in a woman.

Trichoscopy

In trichoscopy, there is hair shaft thickness heterogeneity (hair shafts of different thickness), with more than 20% of them being thinner compared to the normal terminal hairs. The latter represents a trichoscopic sign of progressive miniaturization. In addition, there are short hypopigmented vellus hairs in a higher than 10% rate. Yellow dots, corresponding to empty follicular openings filled with sebum and keratin, are associated to follicles in the kenogen phase. An additional clue for AGA is the predominance of follicular units with one or two hairs, versus the follicular units with three or more hairs. In the end, the peripilar sign (also called perifollicular hyperpigmentation) is related to the perifollicular microinflammation observed in histopathology (Figures 8.7 through 8.10).

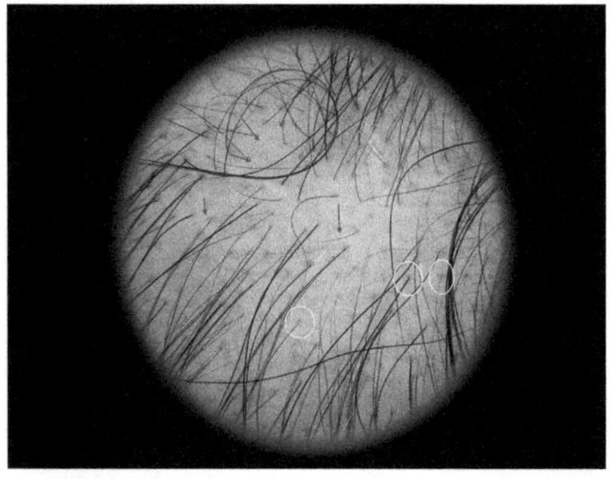

FIGURE 8.7 Androgenetic alopecia with miniaturization, perifollicular hyperpigmentation (yellow circles), and the presence of vellus hair (red arrows).

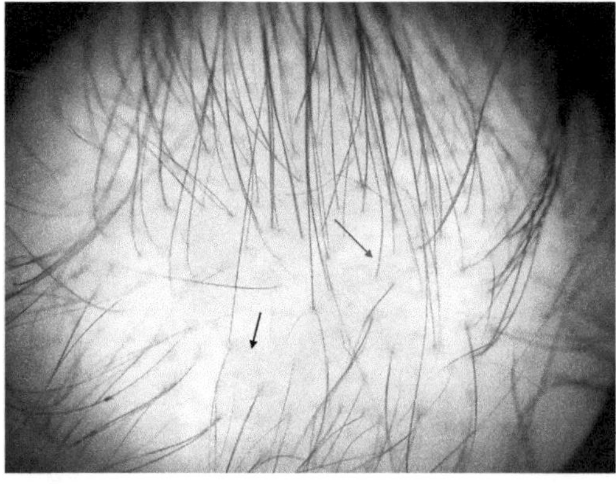

FIGURE 8.8 Androgenetic alopecia (AGA) trichoscopically typified by miniaturization, yellow dots (black arrow), follicles with one or two hair shafts (red arrow), and numerous vellus hairs in AGA.

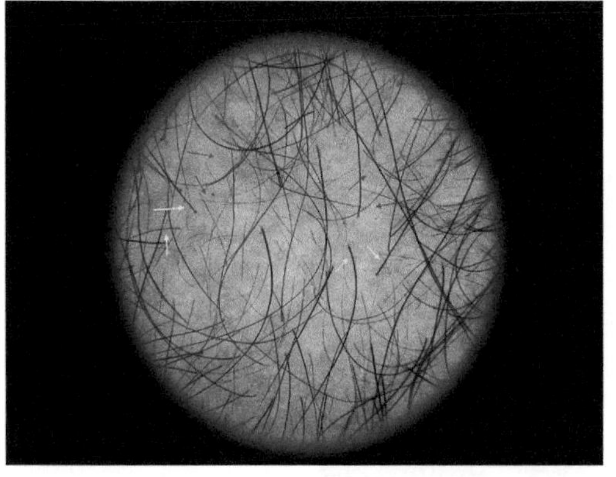

FIGURE 8.9 Trichoscopy of androgenetic alopecia revealing yellow dots (red arrows), follicles with one or two hair shafts (yellow arrows), and numerous vellus hairs (center).

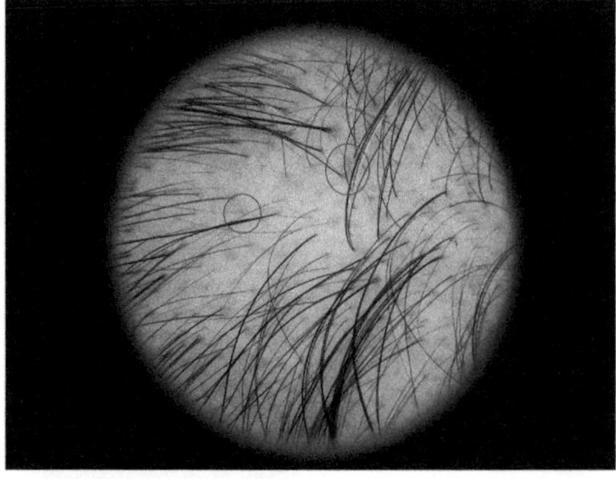

FIGURE 8.10 Trichoscopy of androgenetic alopecia revealing yellow dots, follicles with one or two hair shafts, vellus hairs, and perifollicular hyperpigmentation (circles).

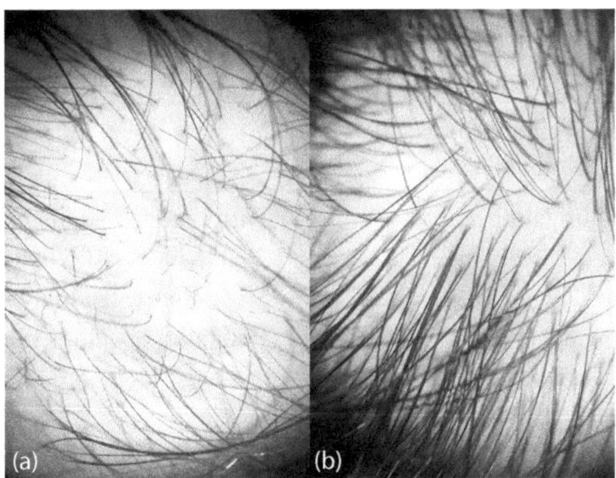

FIGURE 8.11 Comparison of trichoscopic images of the frontal (a) and occipital (b) areas in androgenetic alopecia.

A useful tip for the diagnosis of AGA is the comparison of trichoscopic images captured from frontal and occipital areas. The latter area is typically not affected in AGA (Figure 8.11).

The main trichoscopic criteria of AGA are listed in Table 8.1.

In the differential diagnosis, we should consider telogen effluvium (hair shafts of the same thickness, short, regrowing hairs in an upright orientation, and a similar trichoscopic profile between frontal and occipital areas) and diffuse alopecia areata (yellow dots and scattered exclamation mark hairs). Occasionally, fibrosing alopecia may appear in a patterned distribution. In the latter case, there is loss of follicular units resulting in empty areas among the normal hair follicles, follicular units with a single hair, lack of follicular miniaturization, and predominance of normal terminal hair shafts. In patients with frontal fibrosing alopecia who develop clinical features of AGA, trichoscopy is extremely useful, since it reveals features of cicatricial alopecia that do not conform to the clinical manifestation.

Beyond diagnosis, trichoscopy facilitates treatment monitoring in patients with AGA. Alterations in terms of hair shaft thickness, number of yellow dots, and rate of follicular units with three or more hairs indicate disease improvement, stability, or progress. Figure 8.12 illustrates a patient experiencing disease improvement based on multiple follicles with more than two hair shafts. With the use of trichoscopy, we can appreciate the outcome earlier, compared to the naked-eye clinical examination (6 versus 12 months of treatment).

8.1.2 Alopecia Areata

Alopecia areata (AA) belongs to the group of nonscarring alopecias, and it is a lymphocyte-driven autoimmune hair disorder.

Clinical Presentation

AA is clinically classified as patchy, totalis (entire loss of scalp hairs), and universalis (total body hair loss). Depending on the different patterns of hair loss, we recognize the patchy, ophiasis (band-like hair loss in the parieto-temporo-occipital area), ophiasis inversus (band-like hair loss in the fronto-parieto-temporal area), reticulate, and diffuse AA (Figures 8.13 through 8.16).

TABLE 8.1

Basic Trichoscopic Characteristics of the Most Common Nonscarring Alopecias

Disease	Trichoscopic Characteristics	Description
Androgenetic alopecia	Miniaturization	Different hair shafts in terms of thickness and diameter (>20%/optical field, ×20)
	Vellus hair	Hypopigmented thin hair >10%
	Yellow dots	Follicular openings filled with sebum and keratin
	Follicles with one to two hairs	
	Perifollicular hyperpigmentation	Brown color around the follicle
Alopecia areata	"Exclamation mark" hairs	Thin proximal and thick and darker distal end
	Broken hairs	Rapture of the shaft
	Pseudomonilethrix	Irregular (in terms of distance) beads along the shaft
	Circle hair	Hair shaft in circular arrangement
	"Pigtail" hair	Short coiled hair with thin distal end
	Black dots	Black spots
	Vellus hair	Hypopigmented thin hair >10%
Trichotillomania	Trichoptilosis	Splitting of the distal end of the hair shaft
	Coiled hairs	Short spiral hairs
	"Hook" hairs	Partially coiled short hairs
	"Flame" hairs	Semitransparent, wavy, cone-shaped hairs
	"Tulip hairs"	Short hairs with darker, tulip-shaped end
	"V" sign	Two or more short hairs in one follicular unit, broken at the same level
Tinea capitis	"Comma" hairs	Curved short hair homogenous in thickness and pigmentation
	"Corkscrew" hairs	Intensively bended hair
	"Zig-zag" hairs	Sharply bent hair in different sites
	"Morse-code" hair	Short hair with vertically oriented white band along the shaft
	i-hair	Short hair with darkened distal end
	Black dots	Black spots

Trichoscopic Findings

The clues for trichoscopic diagnosis of AA include "exclamation mark" hairs, tapered hairs, Pohl-Pinkus constrictions of the hair shafts, broken hairs, vellus hairs, and circle hairs (Figures 8.17 through 8.19). Black dots and yellow dots correspond to empty follicular openings (Figures 8.20 and 8.21).

"Exclamation mark" hairs represent an almost pathognomonic trichoscopic feature of AA. They are fractured hairs with thick hyperpigmented distal ends and thin, hypopigmented proximal ends, which are responsible for the characteristic morphology. They are more common in the border of the alopecia patch and represent an indication of disease activity.

Tapered hairs are longer compared to the "exclamation mark" hairs, but they have the same morphology, namely, a thinner proximal end. Recent data suggest that tapered hairs are an early dermoscopic feature of AA, preceding emergence of black dots and exclamation mark hairs.

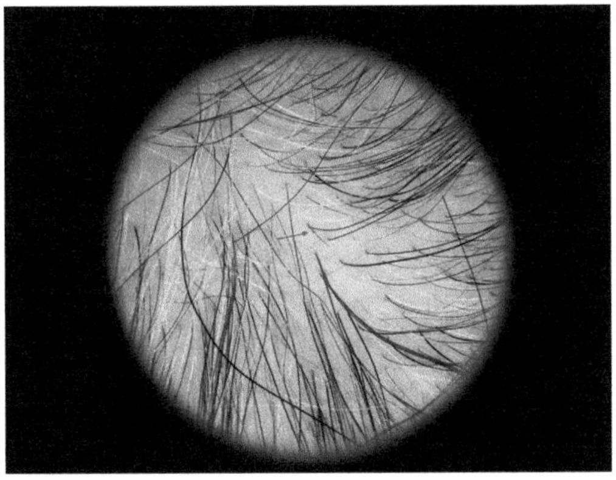

FIGURE 8.12 Trichoscopy of androgenetic alopecia after 6 months of treatment, in which there is visible decrease of the number of yellow dots and corresponding increase of the number of follicles with many hairs.

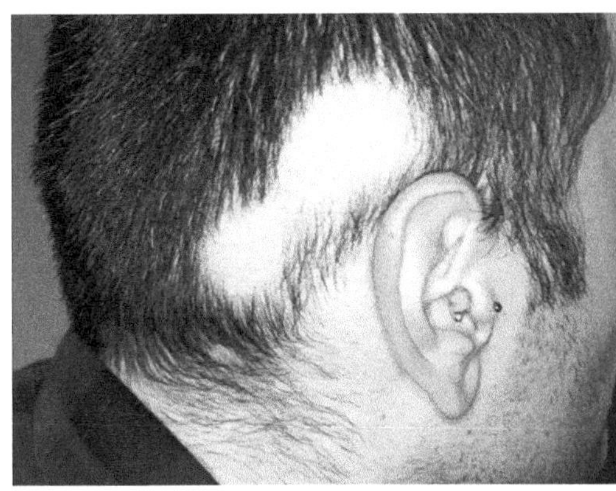

FIGURE 8.13 Clinical presentation of patch-type alopecia areata affecting the scalp.

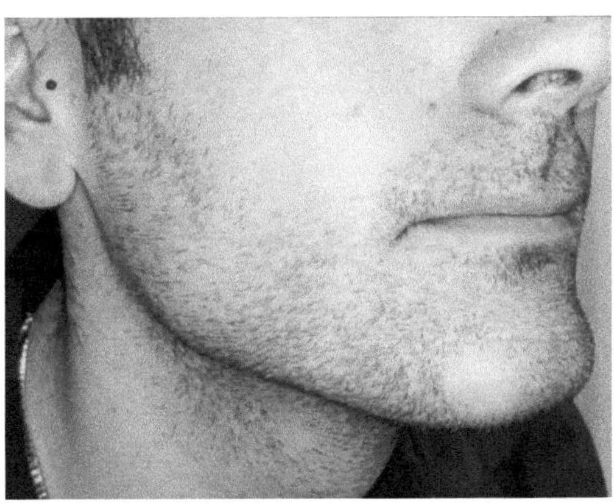

FIGURE 8.14 Clinical presentation of patch-type alopecia areata affecting the beard.

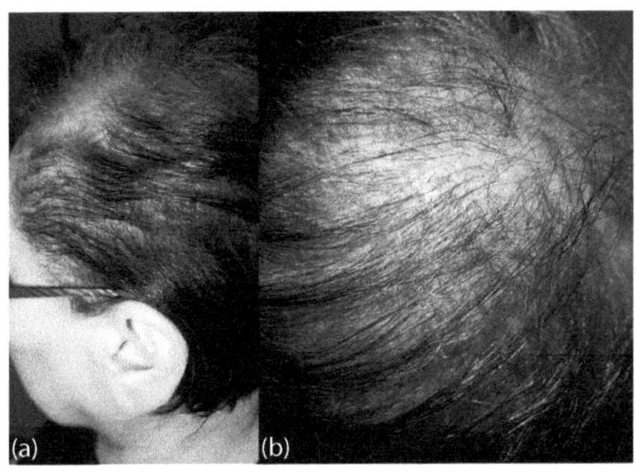

FIGURE 8.15 Clinical presentation of diffuse alopecia areata of the scalp (a,b).

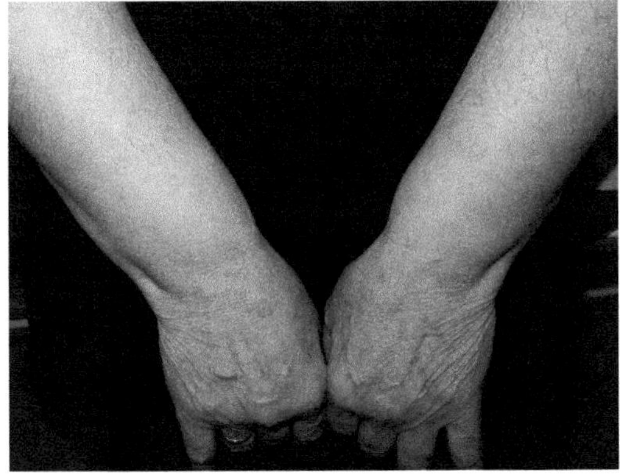

FIGURE 8.16 In the patient in Figure 8.15, the upper extremities were also affected by the diffuse alopecia areata.

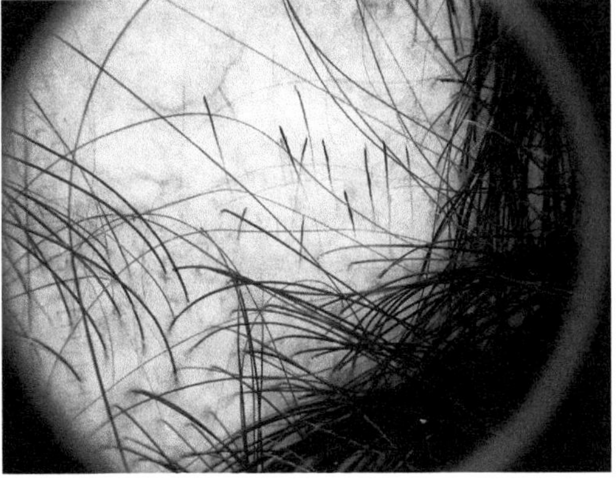

FIGURE 8.17 Exclamation mark hairs in alopecia areata.

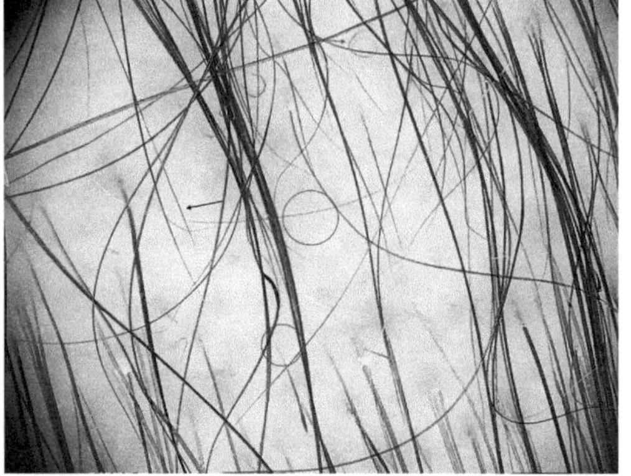

FIGURE 8.18 Exclamation mark hairs (yellow star) and tapered hairs (black arrow) in alopecia areata. Furthermore, there are yellow dots (red circles) and pigtail hairs (red arrow).

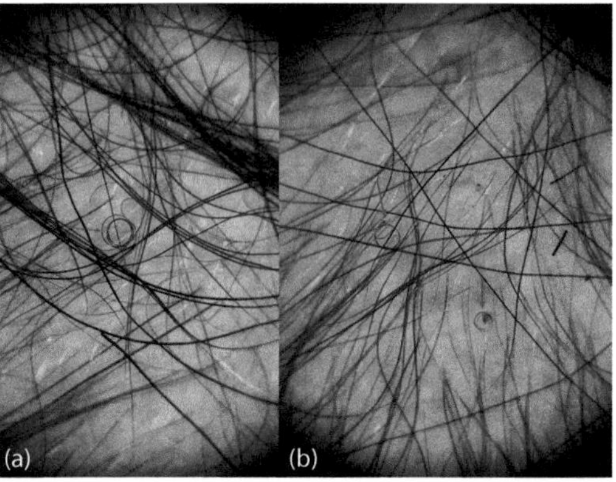

FIGURE 8.19 Circle hairs in alopecia areata (a,b—red arrows).

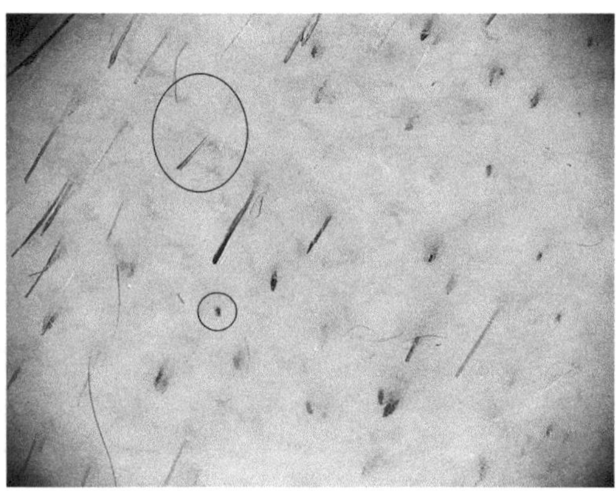

FIGURE 8.20 Broken hairs and black dots (black circles) in alopecia areata.

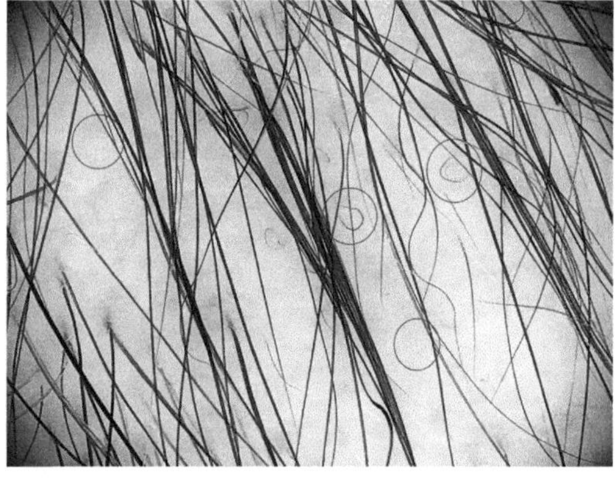

FIGURE 8.21 Pigtail hairs and yellow dots in alopecia areata.

Transverse fracture of a terminal hair shaft as a result of inflammation results in the broken hairs sign. Broken hairs may also result by rapid regrowth of dystrophic hairs that were previously seen as black dots. The fractures in AA are usually at the same level. Opposed to AA, in trichotillomania there are broken hair shafts at different levels as a result of retraction. Other hair disorders that display broken hairs in trichoscopy include tinea capitis, traction/traumatic alopecia, and primary cicatricial alopecia.

Pigtail hairs are short, coiled hairs with tapered ends, and they represent regrowing hairs that became thick, terminal hairs after a few months. They are more common in children.

Another characteristic feature is the Pohl-Pinkus constrictions, seen as zones of decreased hair thickness along the hair shaft. They are related to instant but repetitive interruptions of the metabolic and mitotic activity in the follicle, and they are most commonly observed in active disease.

AA displays yellow dots (Figures 8.18 and 8.21), which are practically present in all variants of the disease. As already mentioned, they correspond to the openings of the empty hair follicle filled with sebum and/or keratotic material. Yellow dots are not pathognomic of AA, since they can be found in various hair disorders, namely, loose anagen hair syndrome, dissecting cellulitis, telogen effluvium, and discoid lupus erythematosus. If they are numerous, they are regularly distributed within the alopecia field. As expected due to the immature sebaceous glands, they are less common during childhood.

Black dots (Figure 8.20) are seen during disease exacerbations, and they probably represent the end phase of exclamation marks, broken, or tapered hairs. Black hairs can also be observed in trichotillomania, tinea capitis, lichen planopilaris, discoid lupus erythematous, dissecting cellulitis, chemotherapy-associated alopecia, traction/traumatic alopecia, and subsequent to laser depilation, or after a trichogram.

Useful Tips

1. Exclamation mark hairs is an indication of disease activity.
2. Tapered hairs is an early trichoscopic feature.
3. In AA the rapture of the broken hairs is in the same length.
4. Pseudomonilethrix is an early finding of active disease.
5. Yellow dots are found in groups of three or more and are rarely present in children.
6. Black dots are remnants of broken, destroyed, or exclamation mark hairs and indicate disease activity.

8.1.3 Trichotillomania

Trichotillomania, also known as hair pulling disorder, is a mental disorder characterized by an irresistible conscious or unconscious pulling out of one's own hair. Hair pulling from the scalp often leaves patchy bald areas, or areas of thinned, or cut at different levels, hairs (Figure 8.22). Noticeable hair loss of other sites of the body may also be observed (e.g., sparse or missing eyelashes or eyebrows).

In trichotillomania, the hair shafts are ruptured at different lengths (Figures 8.23 through 8.30). They also differ in terms of shape. Ruptured hairs immediately after exiting the follicular opening appear as black dots in dermatoscopy. Longitudinal splitting of hair shafts (trichoptilosis); short hairs with coiled distal end; partially coiled short hairs ("hook" hairs); semitransparent, wavy, cone-shaped hairs ("flame" hairs); and "tulip" hairs (short hairs with darker, tulip-shaped

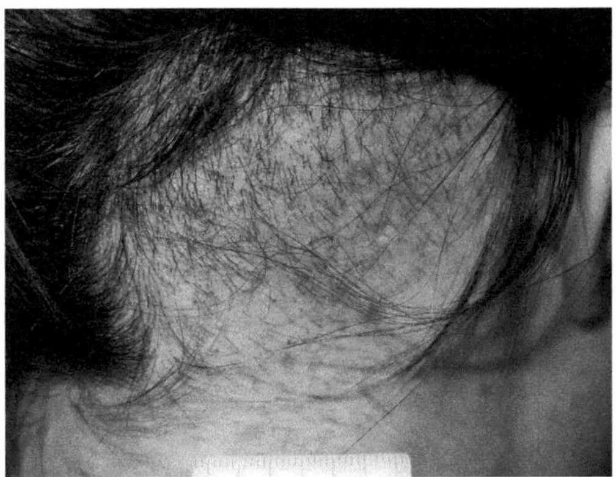

FIGURE 8.22 Clinical presentation of trichotillomania.

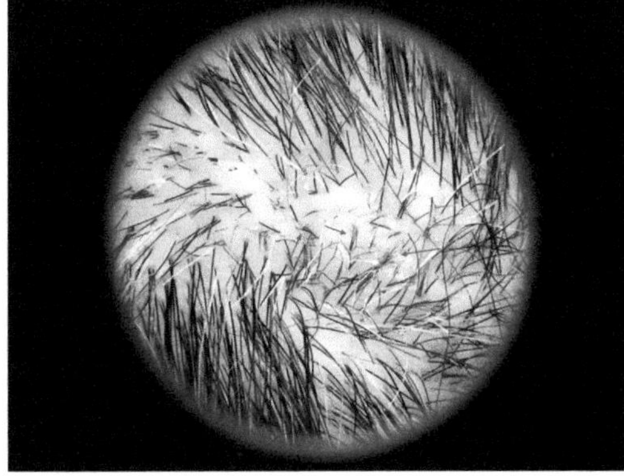

FIGURE 8.23 Trichoptilosis in trichotillomania.

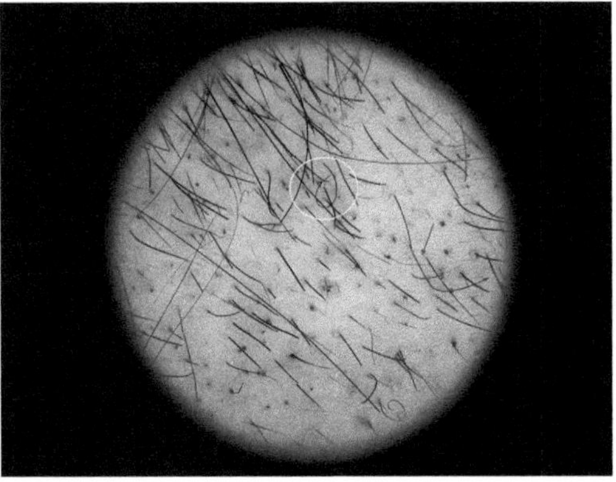

FIGURE 8.24 Coiled hairs (yellow circle) and "hook" hairs (red arrow) in trichotillomania.

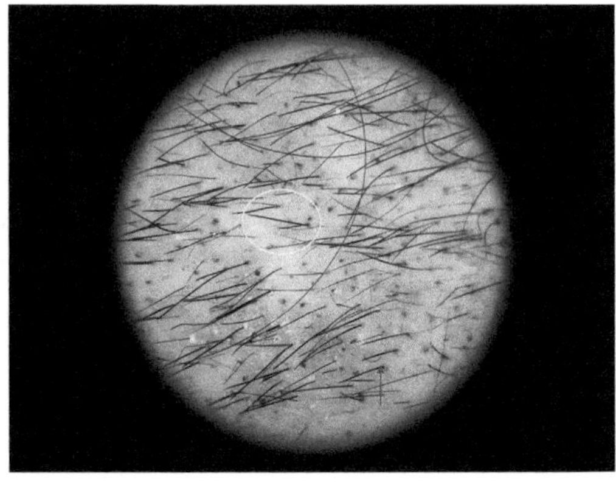

FIGURE 8.25 "Hook" hair (red arrow) and V sign (yellow circle) in trichotillomania.

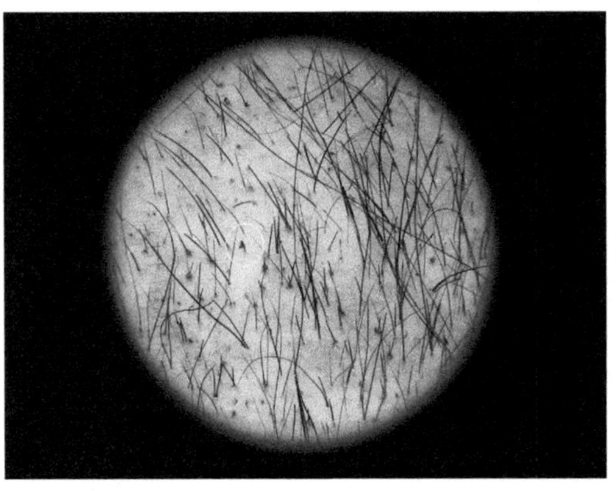

FIGURE 8.26 Flame hair in trichotillomania.

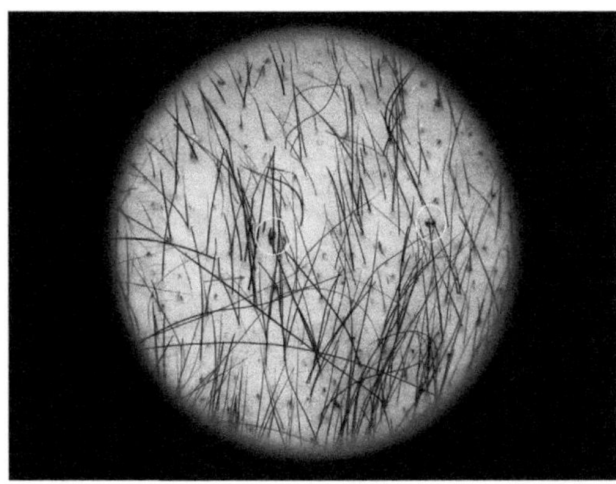

FIGURE 8.27 Tulip hair (red arrows) and flame hairs (yellow circles) in trichotillomania.

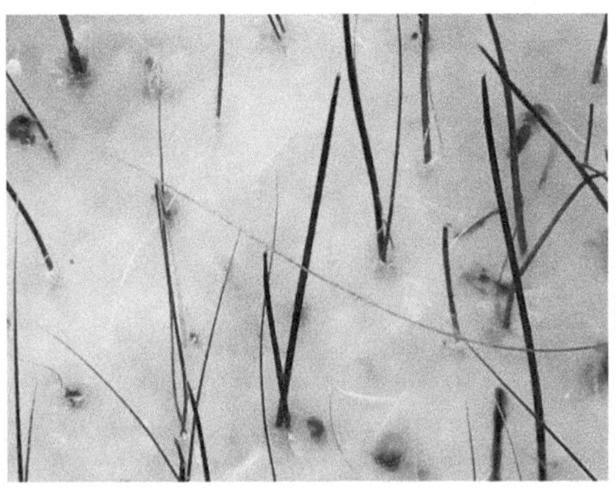

FIGURE 8.28 V sign in trichotillomania.

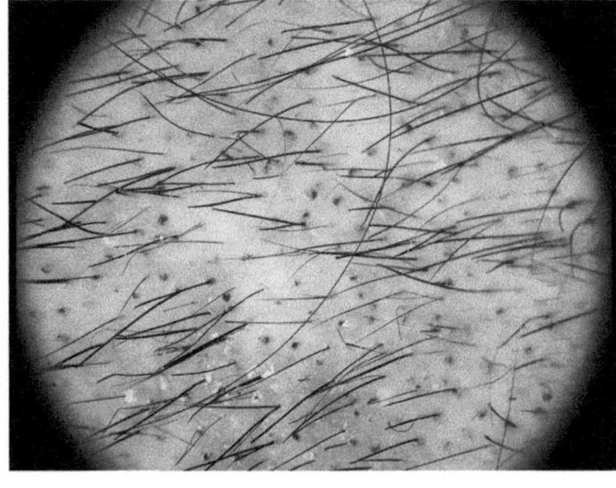

FIGURE 8.29 Black dots forming "hair dust" in trichotillomania.

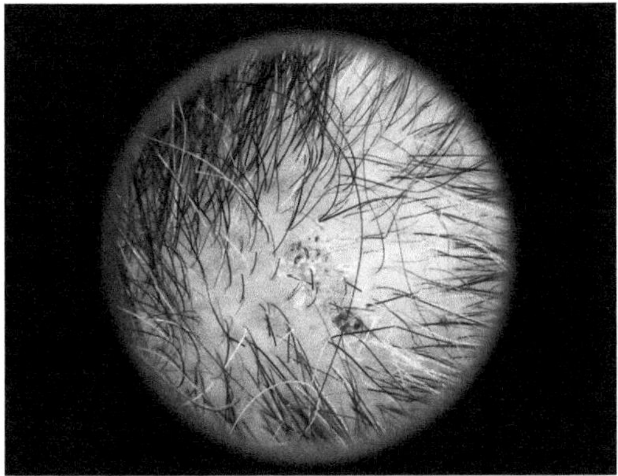

FIGURE 8.30 Focal hemorrhage as a result of trauma in trichotillomania.

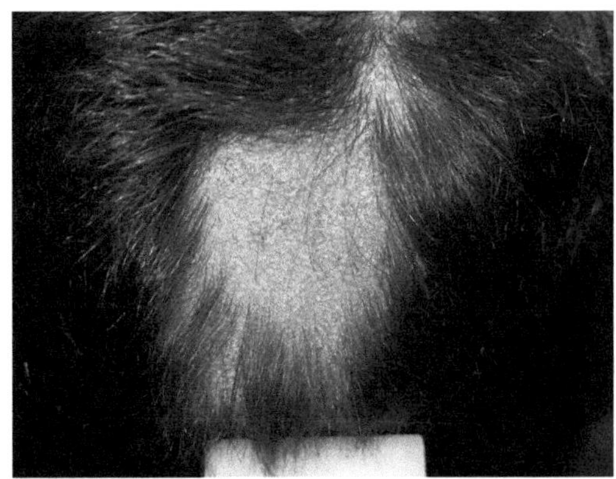

FIGURE 8.31 Clinical presentation of tinea capitis.

end that looks empty) represent classical trichoscopic clues for trichotillomania (Figures 8.23 through 8.27). A typical feature of trichotillomania is the V sign (Figures 8.25 and 8.28), resulting from two or more short hairs in one follicular unit, broken at the same level. In the end, the term *hair powder* is used to describe sprinkled hair residue, observed when the shafts are severely damaged by intense, repetitive trauma (Figure 8.29). Foci of hemorrhagic crusts are not uncommon (Figure 8.30).

8.1.4 Tinea Capitis

Tinea capitis is a fungal infection of the scalp, mostly seen during childhood. Adult cases are sporadically reported. Recognition of the characteristic trichoscopic pattern of tinea capitis may prove extremely useful in early diagnosis, which is ultimately confirmed by the microscopic examination and mycologic culture of the infected material. Tinea capitis results in scaly, focal alopecia (Figure 8.31).

The main trichoscopic features of tinea capitis include zig-zag hairs (hair shafts that are sharply bent in different directions), comma hairs (short hairs resembling commas), corkscrew or coiled hairs, and Morse code–like hairs (hair shafts transversely interrupted by vertical white bands, regularly distributed along the hair shaft). Figures 8.32 through 8.37 illustrate typical

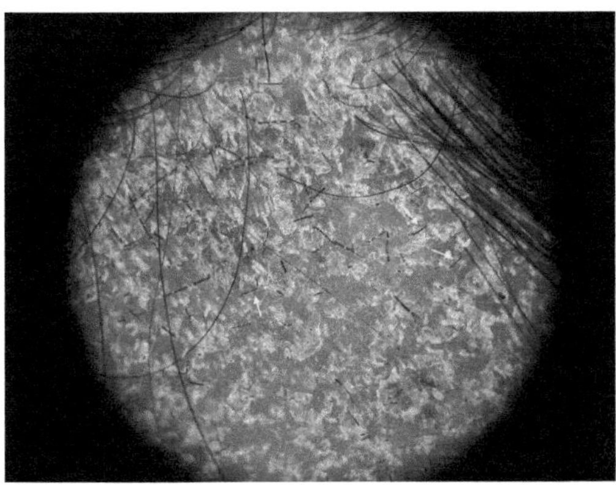

FIGURE 8.32 Coma hairs in tinea capitis (yellow arrows).

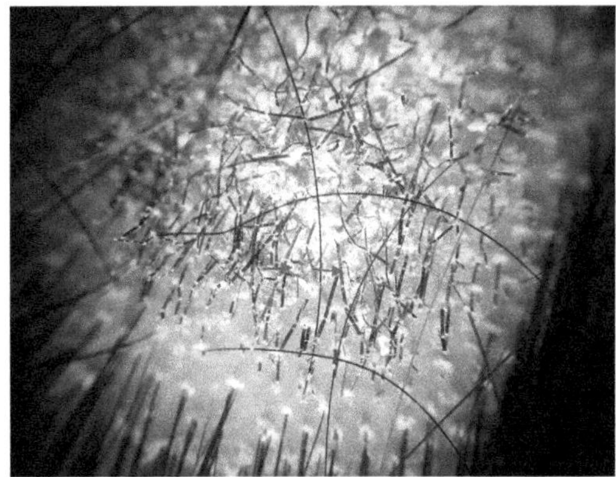

FIGURE 8.33 Corkscrew hairs in tinea capitis (red arrows).

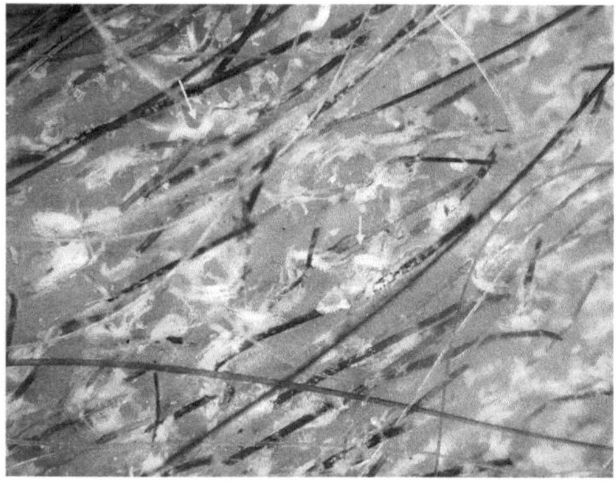

FIGURE 8.34 Higher magnification of the previous image, highlighting the abundant scales surrounding corkscrew hairs (yellow arrows).

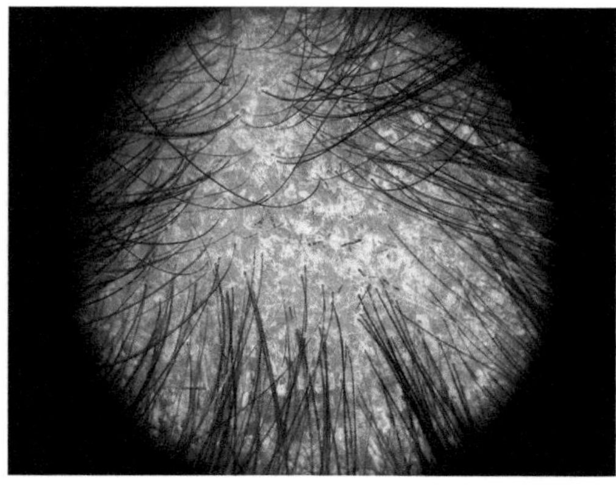

FIGURE 8.35 "Zig-zag" hairs in tinea capitis (red arrows).

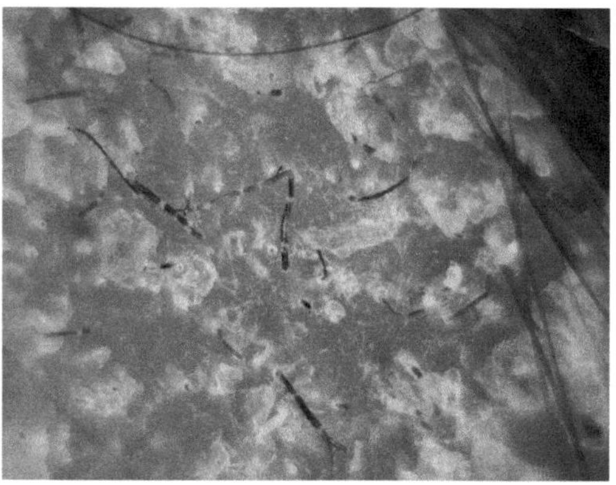

FIGURE 8.36 Higher magnification of the previous image highlighting the "zig-zag" hairs.

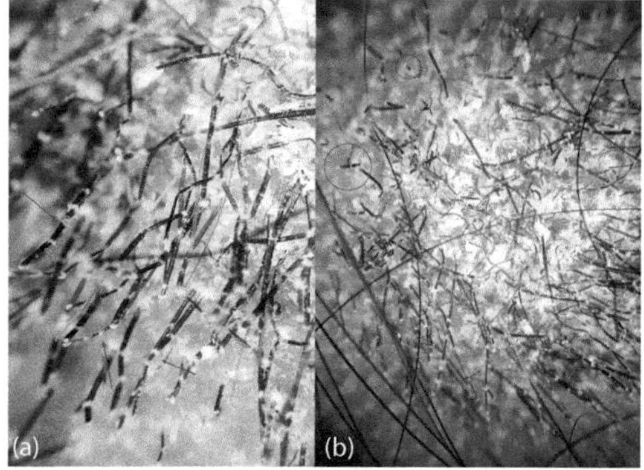

FIGURE 8.37 (a,b) Dermatoscopy of tinea capitis revealing Morse-code hairs and "i-hairs" (circles).

examples of the trichoscopic features in tinea capitis. Additional features are black dots and i-hairs (short hair with accentuated distal ends) (Figures 8.37 and 8.38).

8.2 Primary Cicatricial Alopecias

8.2.1 Lichen Planopilaris

Lichen planopilaris (LPP) is a rare variant of lichen planus that affects the hair follicles. LPP is the most common cause of primary cicatricial alopecia. The clinical spectrum of LPP includes the classic LPP, frontal fibrosing alopecia (FFA), fibrosing alopecia in a patterned distribution, and Graham-Little-Piccardi-Lassueur syndrome. The classic variant develops with patches of cicatricial alopecia, typically seen in the vertex area (Figure 8.39). FFA develops with progressive recession of the frontotemporal hairline, while fibrosing alopecia in a patterned distribution is characterized by numerous small areas of scarring alopecia in the androgen-dependent sites of the scalp (Figure 8.40). Graham-Little-Piccardi-Lassueur syndrome is a rare

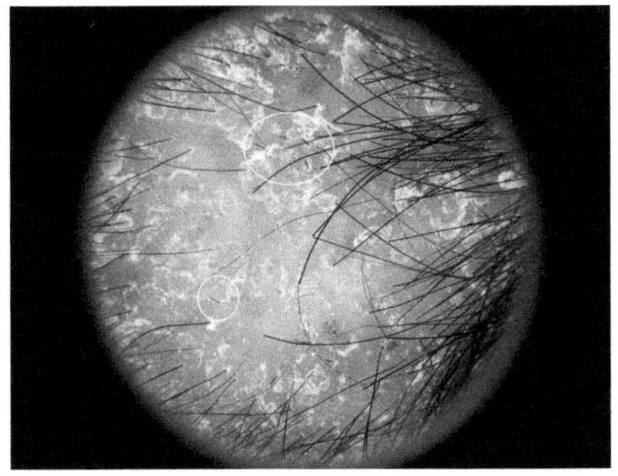

FIGURE 8.38 "i-Hairs" in tinea capitis.

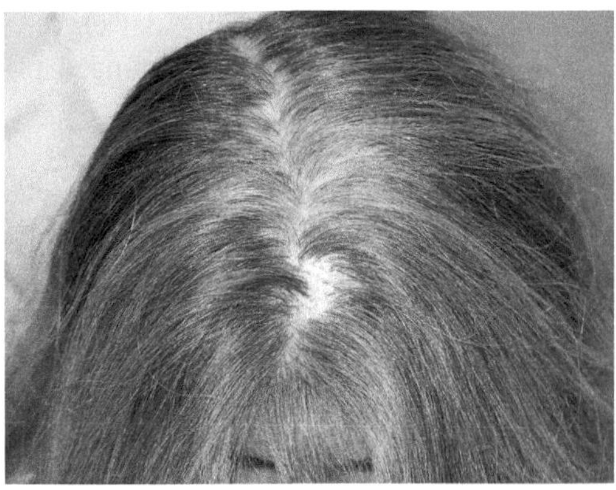

FIGURE 8.39 Classic clinical presentation of lichen planopilaris.

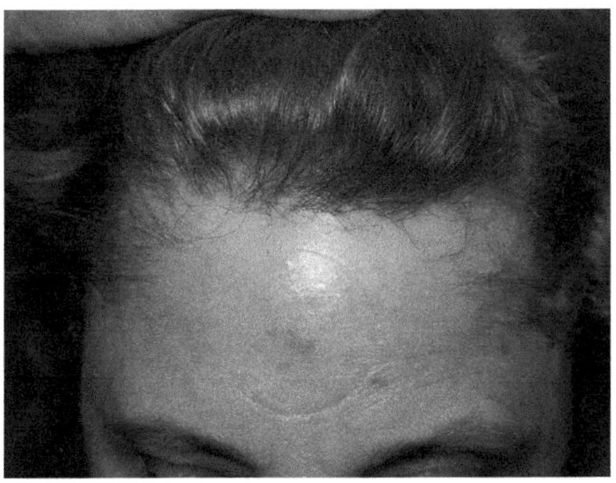

FIGURE 8.40 Clinical presentation of frontal fibrosing alopecia.

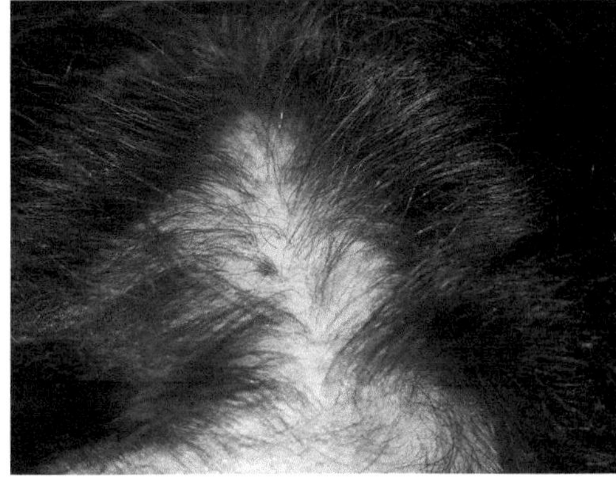

FIGURE 8.41 Graham-Little-Piccardi-Lassueur syndrome. The clinical presentation at the scalp is identical to lichen planopilaris.

entity that combines cicatricial alopecia of the scalp, noncicatricial hair loss in the axillary and pubic areas, as well as lichenoid pilar eruption (Figure 8.41).

Trichoscopic Features

In the early phase of the disease, trichoscopy reveals white dots corresponding to the fibrotic process in the dermis. Progressively, they coalesce into larger whitish areas that lack follicular openings and hair shafts (Figure 8.42).

The most typical trichoscopic feature in LPP is the perifollicular tubular silver-white scale (also known as peripilar casts) at the base of the hair shaft (Figures 8.42 and 8.43). It is mostly seen at the periphery of the alopecia patch. It is histopathologically correlated to perifollicular hyperkeratosis and vacuolar changes of the basal cell layer, as well as with apoptotic keratinocytes in the epidermis of the outer root sheath of the follicle. The same trichoscopic feature appears also in FFA; however, it is subtle and focal (Figure 8.44). The use of immersion fluid during trichoscopy highlights perifollicular erythema. Higher magnification facilitates visibility of elongated vessels concentrically arranged around the follicular units (Figure 8.45).

Blue-gray dots around the follicular structures ("target" pattern) correlate to melanophages in papillary dermis as a result of pigment incontinence.

Isolated hair shafts, separated from the frontal hairline, are typical, though not pathognomonic, of FFA. They are usually located in the upper part of the forehead, in the area of the original hairline (Figure 8.46). Furthermore, in FFA we lack the normally present vellus hair in the recessed hairline.

8.2.2 Discoid Lupus Erythematosus

Discoid lupus erythematosus (DLE) is the second most common cause of primary cicatricial alopecia. Typically, it appears as a hairless erythematous plaque with follicular plugging and

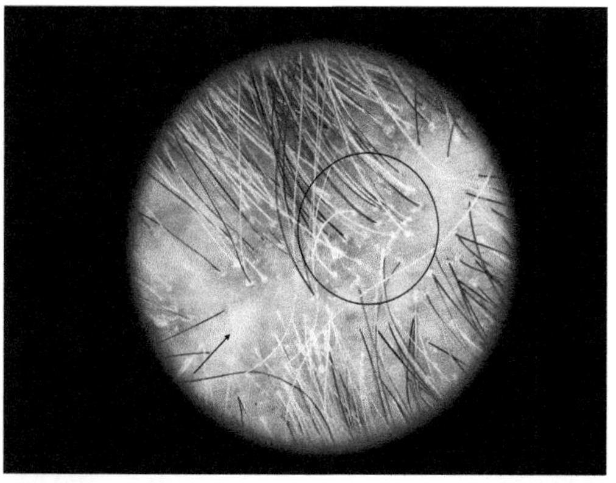

FIGURE 8.42 Trichoscopy of classic lichen planopilaris reveals pink-white and white areas "empty" of follicles (arrow) and areas displaying the characteristic perifollicular, tubular scaling (circle).

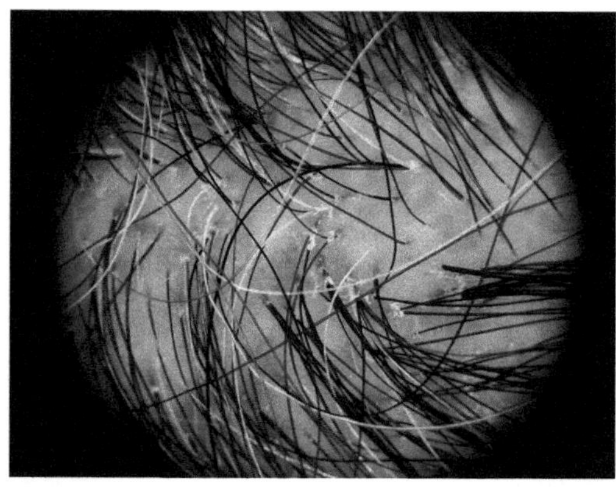

FIGURE 8.43 The typical perifollicular and tubular scaling of lichen planopilaris.

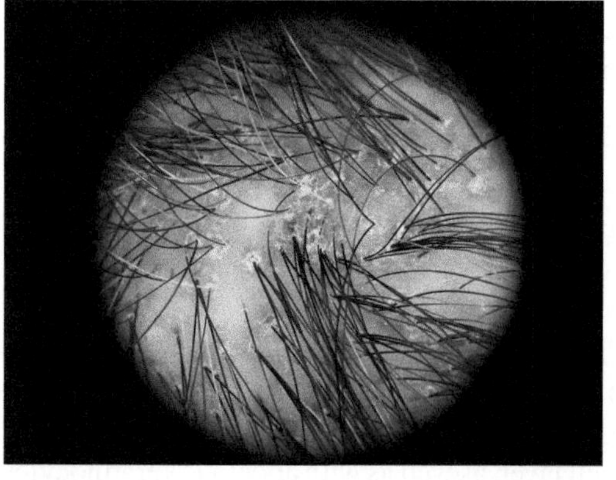

FIGURE 8.44 Subtle perifollicular scale and pink-white areas corresponding to fibrosis of the frontal area in frontal fibrosing alopecia.

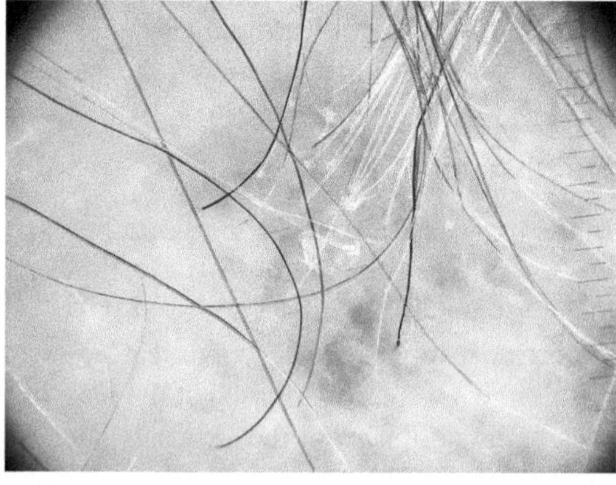

FIGURE 8.45 Subtle erythema and elongated linear vessels around the affected hair follicles in lichen planopilaris.

adherent scaling (Figure 8.47). Depending on the phase of the disease, the lesions can be hyper- (early phase) or hypopigmented (late phase). Progressively, they turn into atrophic, hard in palpation, whitish plaques, lacking follicular openings.

In early stages of the disease, follicular plugs are usually dermatoscopically visible as coarse white-yellow dots in the opening of the infundibulum. Thick arborizing, serpentine, or tortuous branching vessels might also be present (Figures 8.48 and 8.49). Light or dark brown structureless areas, histopathologically corresponding to pigment incontinence, are mainly visible in active lesions (Figure 8.50). A pattern consisting of blue-gray granules ("speckled" pattern) is more common in the dark-skinned population. The presence of red dots that may typically be seen in active plaques is considered a good prognostic factor of hair regrowth. Structureless white areas, thin arborizing vessels, and sparse follicular plugs typify trichoscopy of long-standing DLE plaques.

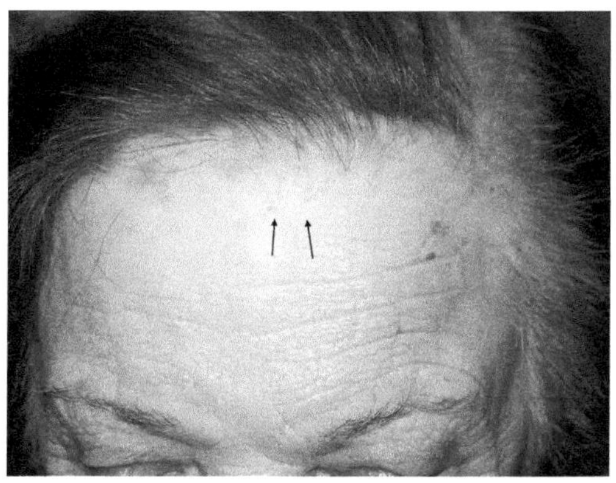

FIGURE 8.46 Solitary, isolated terminal hair in the area of the original hairline.

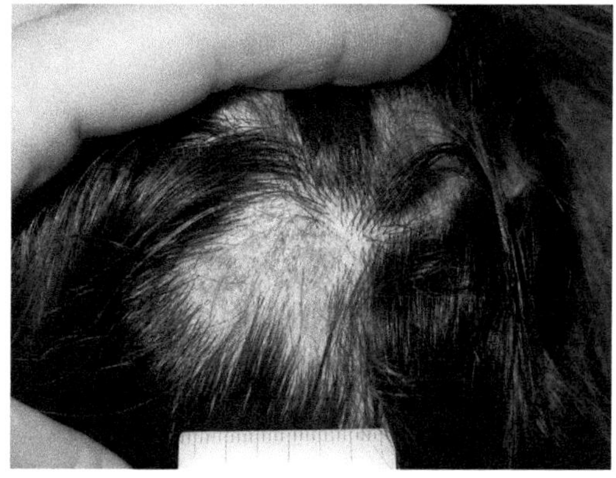

FIGURE 8.47 Clinical presentation of discoid lupus erythematosus of the scalp, with lack of hair follicles and presence of erythema.

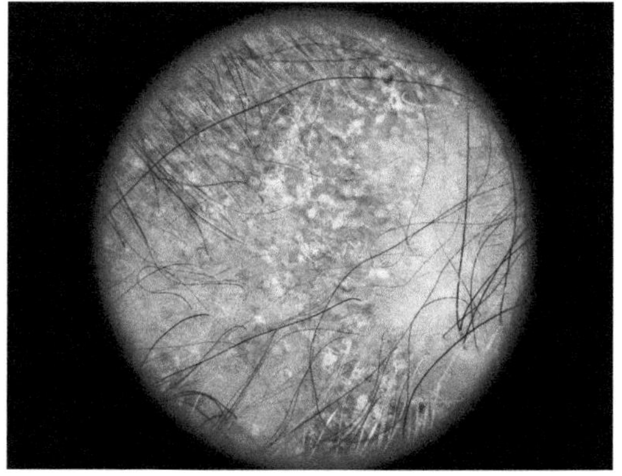

FIGURE 8.48 Dermatoscopy of discoid lupus erythematosus revealing follicular plugs, white scales, tortuous arborizing vessels, and whitish areas.

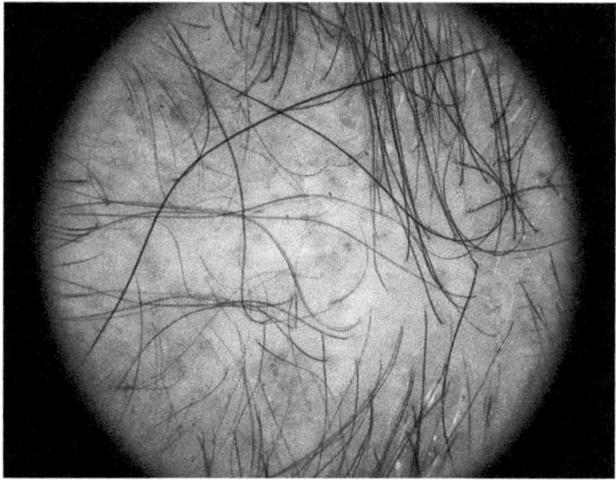

FIGURE 8.49 Follicular plugs, seen as yellow dots, white areas, and some vessels in a case of discoid lupus erythematosus.

8.2.3 Folliculitis Decalvans

Folliculitis decalvans belongs to the group of primary neutrophilic cicatricial alopecias. Recurrent follicular pustules, tufted hairs, and patches of scarring alopecia constitute the characteristic clinical triad of the disease (Figure 8.51).

The most frequent finding in trichoscopy is the presence of alopecia plaques that lack hair shafts and follicular openings ("empty areas") (Figure 8.52). The latter feature is generally considered the hallmark of cicatricial alopecia. Tufting of follicular units is found in a high percentage (~80%) and is recognized as numerous hair shafts (up to 20) emerging from the same follicular orifice (polytrichia or "dolly" hair) (Figures 8.52 and 8.53). Yellow scales and crusts in a perifollicular arrangement are common (Figures 8.53 and 8.54). The use of a dermatoscope facilitates recognition of pustules that are seen as yellow areas around follicular units, with vessels and foci of hemorrhage (Figure 8.54). Perifollicular erythema arranged in a starburst pattern represents an additional trichoscopic feature. In late-phase disease, ivory-white and milky-red structureless areas, without follicular orifices, predominate in dermatoscopy.

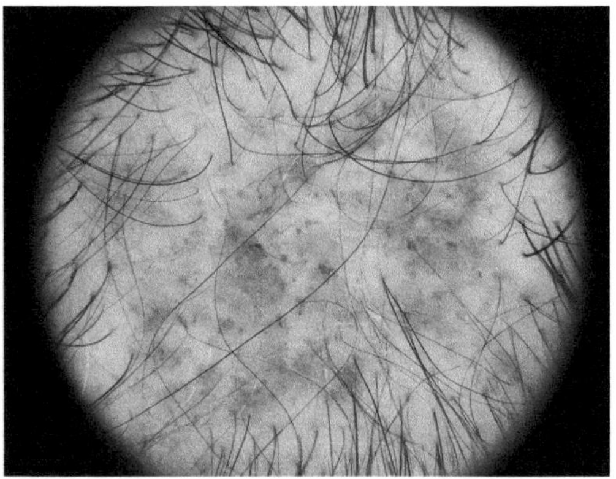

FIGURE 8.50 Dermatoscopy of a lesion of discoid lupus erythematosus revealing a few follicular plugs, linear vessels, and brown-gray areas, the latter corresponding to pigment incontinence.

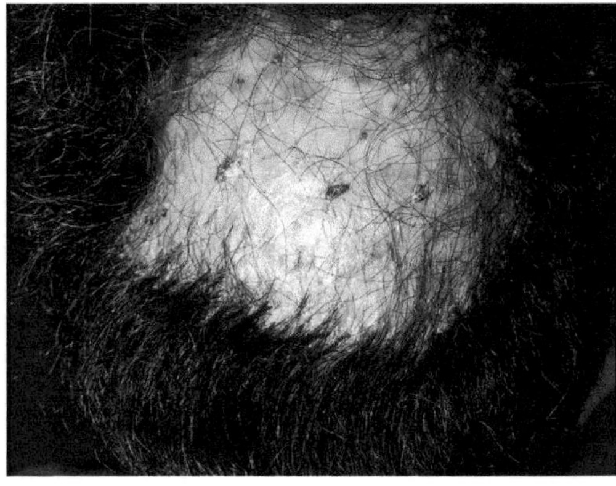

FIGURE 8.51 Clinical presentation of folliculitis decalvans: a plaque of alopecia with perifollicular pustules and tufted hair at the periphery.

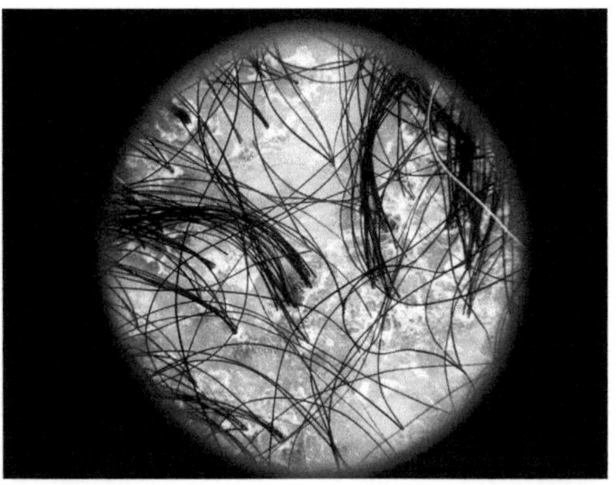

FIGURE 8.52 Dermatoscopy of folliculitis decalvans revealing "empty" areas, perifollicular pustules, tufted hairs, and foci of hemorrhage.

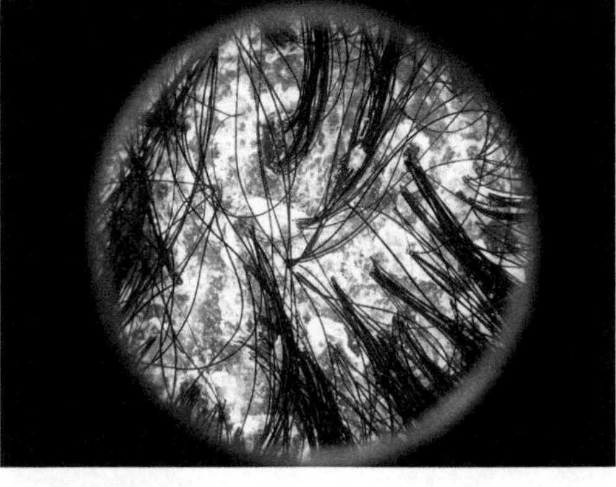

FIGURE 8.53 Prominent tufting of hair follicles, with numerous hair shafts emerging from a single follicle, and intense yellowish perifollicular scale in folliculitis decalvans.

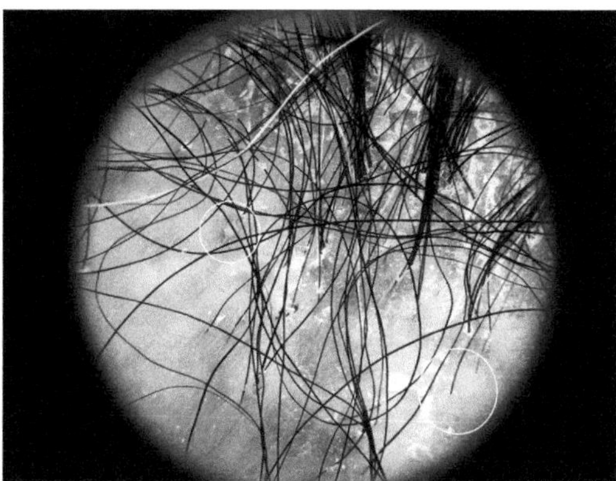

FIGURE 8.54 "Empty" areas, yellow perifollicular scaling and follicular pustules (circles) in folliculitis decalvans.

8.2.4 Dissecting Cellulitis of the Scalp

Dissecting cellulitis is a rare inflammatory disorder that typically affects young male patients of dark skin phototype. On a clinical basis, dissecting cellulitis is characterized by the presence of painful pustules, nodules, and abscesses on the scalp. The inflammatory process gradually expands, leaving behind areas of cicatricial alopecia.

Trichoscopic findings depend on the disease stage. Inflammatory lesions show numerous empty follicular openings, yellow dots, and black dots, while long-standing disease shows a higher number of yellowish/whitish areas and the absence of follicular openings. The latter conforms with the course of the disease, since in the acute phase inflammation disturbs the follicular cycle, resulting in temporary hair loss (empty follicular openings), yellow dots (empty infundibulum, filled with sebum/keratin), and black dots (destroyed hair shafts). A reddish background, mirroring underlying inflammation, is a common feature. Various types of blood vessels can be seen in trichoscopy, including red dots, enlarged branching, and tortuous branching vessels. Correct diagnosis at this stage is essential for the outcome, since alopecia is still reversible. The appearance of short, vellus hair is an early indication of remission. If left untreated, it results in permanent destruction of the follicular units, trichoscopically recognized by the absence of follicular openings on a yellowish/whitish background (Table 8.2).

8.3 Trichoscopy in Children

Congenital anomalies of the hair shaft are rare. Dermatoscopy facilitates the recognition of many of them, including monilethrix, pili torti, trichorrhexis nodosa, trichorrhexis invaginata, and pili annulati. Other hair disorders that are mostly diagnosed during childhood and can be easily diagnosed with the use of dermatoscope are loose anagen hair syndrome, aplasia cutis congenita, and temporal triangular alopecia.

8.3.1 Temporal Triangular Alopecia

Temporal triangular alopecia (TTA) may be present at birth, or it may develop later in life, often within the first 3 years. A unilateral alopecia patch located in the frontotemporal region is the

TABLE 8.2

Basic Trichoscopic Characteristics of Cicatricial Alopecias

Disease	Trichoscopic Characteristics	Description
Lichen planopilaris	Perifollicular and peripilar tubular scale	Silver-white scale surrounding the proximal part of the hair shaft
	White dots	White areas of fibrosis/atrophy, lacking follicular openings
	Subtle erythema and telangiectasia	
Chronic discoid lupus erythematosus	White dots	White areas of fibrosis/atrophy, lacking follicular openings
	Yellow dots	Follicular plugs
	Arborizing vessels	
	Red spots	Red dots
Folliculitis decalvans	Tufted hairs	Numerous hairs (5–20) arising from one follicle
	White dots	White areas around the follicles
	Perifollicular scale	
	Pustules	
Dissecting cellulitis of the scalp	Yellow spots	
	Black dots	
	Reddish background	
	Red dots	
	Arborizing vessels	

clinical hallmark of this entity (Figure 8.55). Interestingly, in histopathology, there is a normal number of hair follicles, with a predominance of vellus hairs.

Dermatoscopy will reveal short, most commonly white, hairs (short upright regrowing, vellus hypopigmented and/or circle hairs), occupying the entire field of alopecia. Empty follicles, or white dots, are not uncommon.

8.3.2 Loose Anagen Hair Syndrome

Loose anagen hair syndrome (LAHS) is a genetically driven disorder, transmitted in an autosomal dominant manner. It typically affects young blonde girls of more than 2 years of age. The main complaint of the parents is that the hair of the child "does not grow." On clinical examination, the hair is thin and sparse, but there are no visible hairless areas. Pull test is usually positive. Microscopic examination of the pulled hairs is extremely useful, since it reveals loose anagen hairs, with no root sheaths and deformed pigmented anagen bulbs. For the diagnosis of LAHS, more than 70% of dysmorphic bulbs should be present in the trichogram.

The trichoscopic features of LAHS include sparse rectangular black granules and the solitary yellow dots. Differential diagnosis includes diffuse alopecia areata.

8.3.3 Aplasia Cutis

Aplasia cutis congenita (ACC) is the result of congenital focal aplasia of the epidermis and dermis. It clinically presents as a smooth, yellowish, solitary area of focal permanent alopecia, and it is usually accompanied by other defects, enabling early diagnosis. The differential

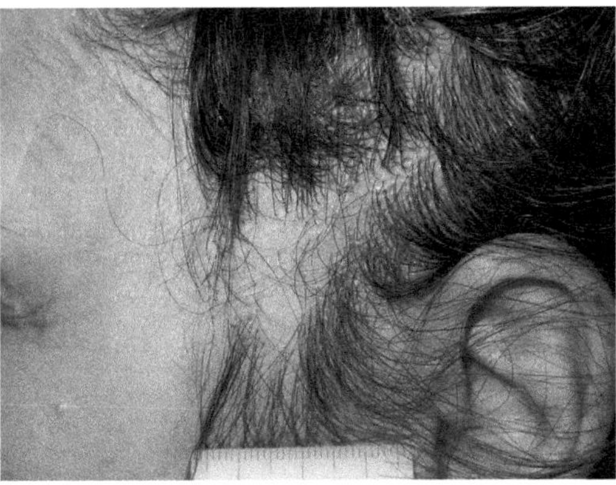

FIGURE 8.55 A unilateral alopecia involving the frontotemporal area of the scalp in a case of triangular temporal alopecia.

diagnosis includes alopecia areata, nevus sebaceous, and cicatricial alopecia secondary to mechanical trauma.

The trichoscopic clue for diagnosis is the elongated anagen hair bulbs, visible through the semitranslucent epidermis. They are located at the hair-bearing margins of the alopecic field arranged in a radial manner (starburst follicular pattern). The center of the lesion is atrophic with prominent vessels and lack of follicular orifices.

8.4 Hair Shaft Deformities

8.4.1 Monilethrix

Monilethrix (also known as "beaded hair") is a rare genodermatosis (autosomal dominant trait) characterized by a hair shaft deformity, resulting in hypotrichosis. Alopecia usually involves the occiput and the nape of the neck (Figure 8.56); however, in severe cases, the entire scalp, the eyebrows/eyelashes, and secondary hair may be affected. The pathognomonic hair shaft dysplasia consists of dystrophic constrictions regularly separated by elliptical nodes of normal thickness, resulting in a beaded appearance of the affected hair shaft (Figure 8.56). The thin part is fragile and easily breaks. Monilethrix is accompanied by follicular hyperkeratosis and perifollicular erythema. Trichoscopy facilitates *in vivo* detection of the characteristic hair shaft dysplasia (Figure 8.57).

8.4.2 Pseudomonilethrix or Pohl-Pinkus Constrictions

Hair in pseudomonilethrix, though clinically similar to monilethrix, does not present with true dystrophic constrictions but with flattened irregular beading. Pseudomonilethrix is a trichoscopic feature of alopecia areata, but it can be present in other types of alopecia, namely, chemotherapy-related alopecia, or as a result of excessive styling, back-combing, and other manipulations that put excessive stress on the hair shaft.

8.4.3 Trichorrhexis Nodosa

Trichorrhexis nodosa is a common congenital, familial, or acquired hair shaft anomaly, characterized by the presence of one or more hypopigmented/white swellings (nodes) on the

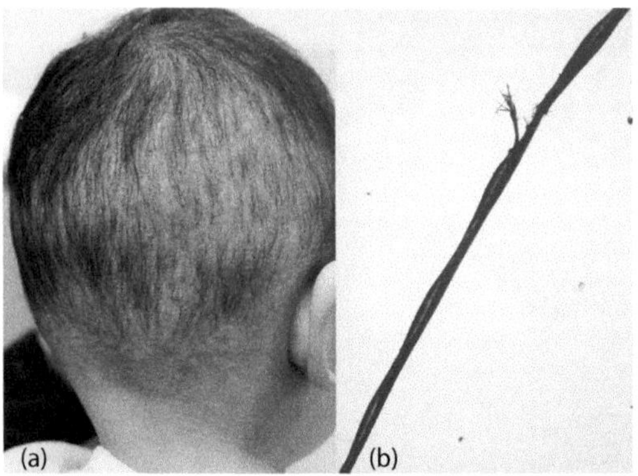

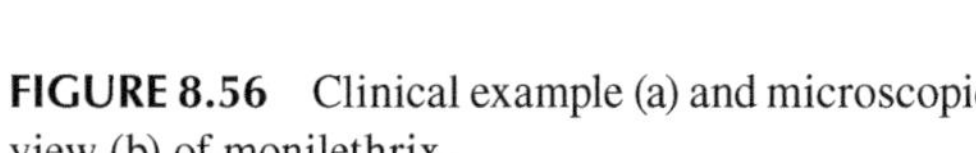
FIGURE 8.56 Clinical example (a) and microscopic view (b) of monilethrix.

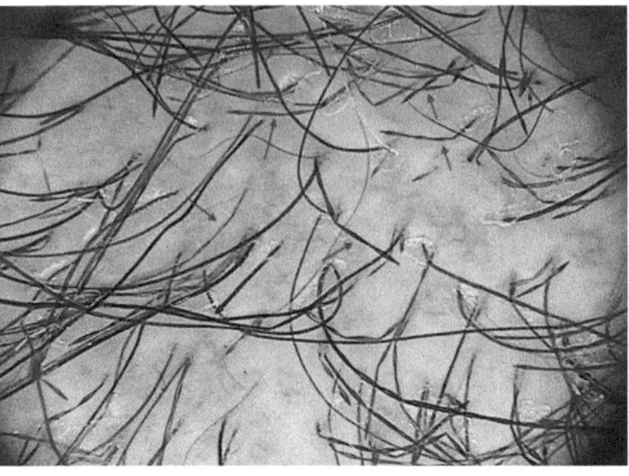

FIGURE 8.57 Trichoscopy of monilethrix. (Courtesy of Dr. Rakowska.)

hair shaft, with loss of cuticle. Trichoscopy highlights the characteristic morphology of the node, in which the cortical fibers splay outward and fracture. Occasionally, the latter gives the node the dermatoscopic appearance of two brooms thrust together end to end (Figure 8.58). Complete rupture of the hair shaft at this site is the rule.

Trichorrhexis nodosa can be seen as part of congenital disorders (e.g., Menkes syndrome and Pollitt syndrome), but acquired development is also common. Mechanical or chemical (due to excessive use of styling products) trauma of the hair shaft as well as intensive rubbing of the scalp are the most usual causes of acquired trichorrhexis nodosa. Adequate management of pruritus results in disease remission, typified by the normal appearance of the shafts.

8.4.4 Trichorrhexis Invaginata

Trichorrhexis invaginata is the pathognomonic hair defect of Netherton syndrome. Netherton syndrome is a rare autosomal recessive genodermatosis.

The deformity leads to cortical softness and subsequent invagination of the fully keratinized distal part of the hair shaft into the softer, abnormally keratinized proximal part (Figure 8.59). The hair of the patients is brittle, dry, and short. With the use of trichoscopy, we observe the characteristic nodular swellings irregularly distributed along the hair shaft (Figure 8.60).

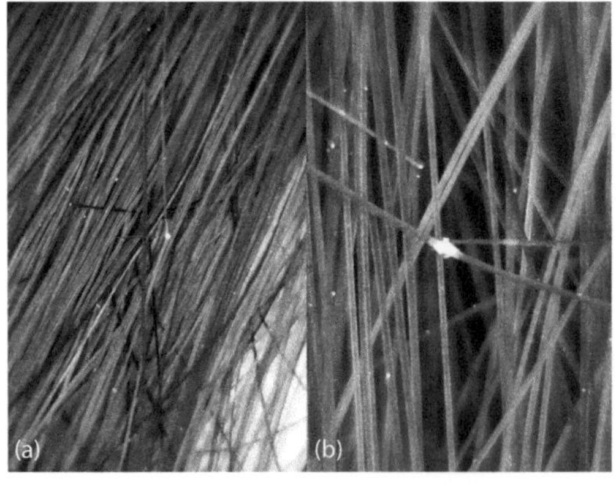

FIGURE 8.58 Trichoscopy of trichorrhexis nodosa in low (a) and higher (b) magnification.

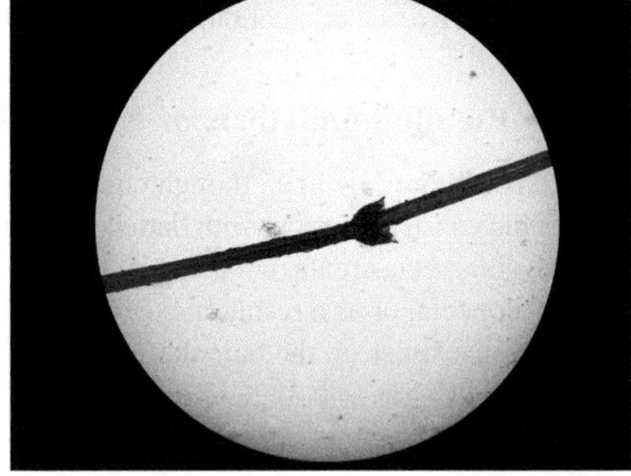

FIGURE 8.59 Microscopic view of trichorrhexis invaginata.

8.4.5 Trichoptilosis

Trichoptilosis is the splitting or fraying of the distal end of the hair shaft into two or more segments (Figures 8.61 and 8.62). It can be seen in various types of alopecia, but it is also common in healthy individuals with long hair. It typically appears as a result of chronic trauma due to excessive hairstyling.

8.4.6 Trichoschisis

Trichoschisis is a rare hair shaft abnormality characterized by sudden hair shaft break across the axis of the shaft. It is usually seen in people who have congenital hair growth disorders, such as trichothiodystrophy. It is associated with low sulfur and cysteine levels in the hair shaft.

8.4.7 Pili Torti

Pili torti (also known as "twisted hairs") is a rare, congenital or acquired hair abnormality, in which the hair shaft is flattened at irregular intervals and twisted 180° along its axis (Figure 8.63).

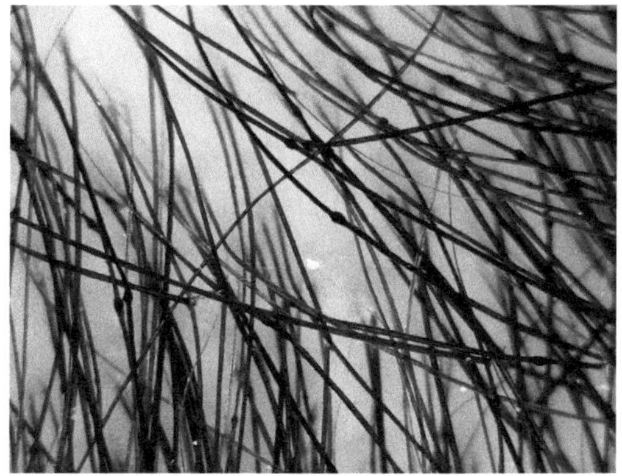

FIGURE 8.60 Trichoscopic view of trichorrhexis invaginata in Netherton syndrome.

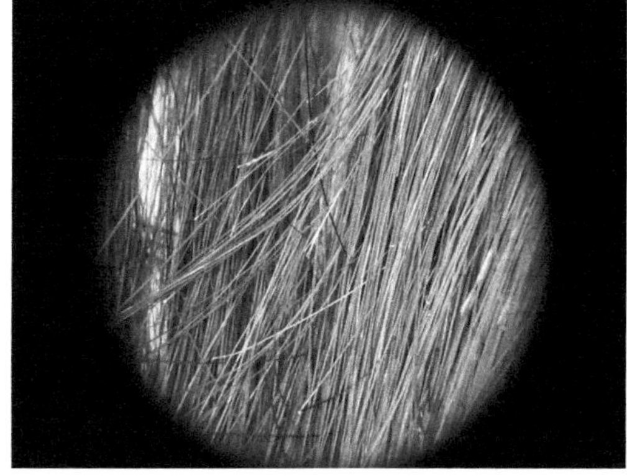

FIGURE 8.61 Dermatoscopy of trichoptilosis reveals the splitting of the distal end of the hair shaft.

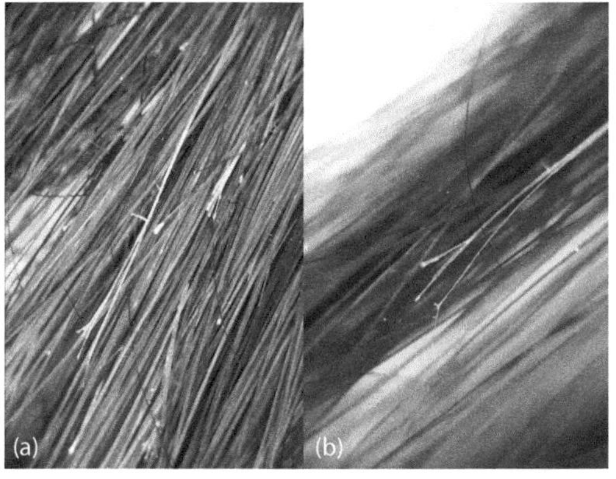

FIGURE 8.62 The previous image of trichoptilosis at higher magnifications (a,b).

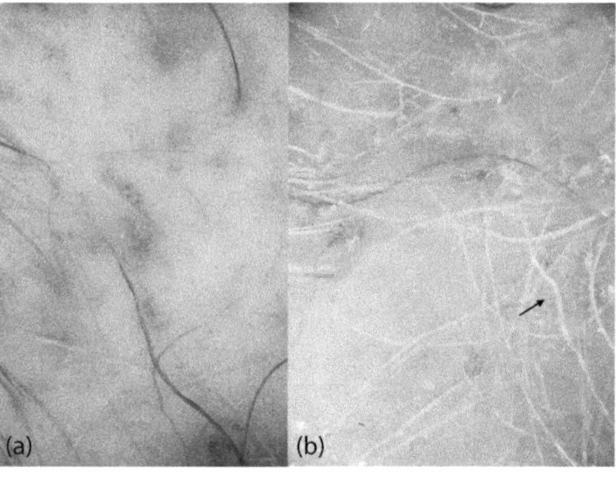

FIGURE 8.63 Trichoscopy of pili torti (a,b). (Courtesy of Dr. Rakowska.)

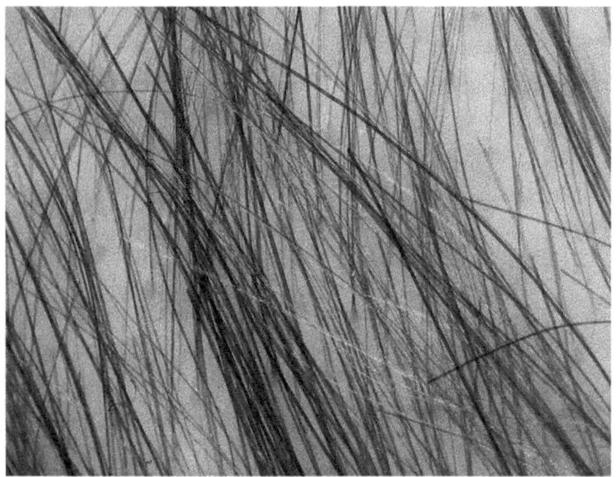

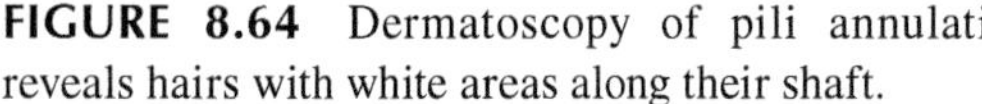

FIGURE 8.64 Dermatoscopy of pili annulati reveals hairs with white areas along their shaft.

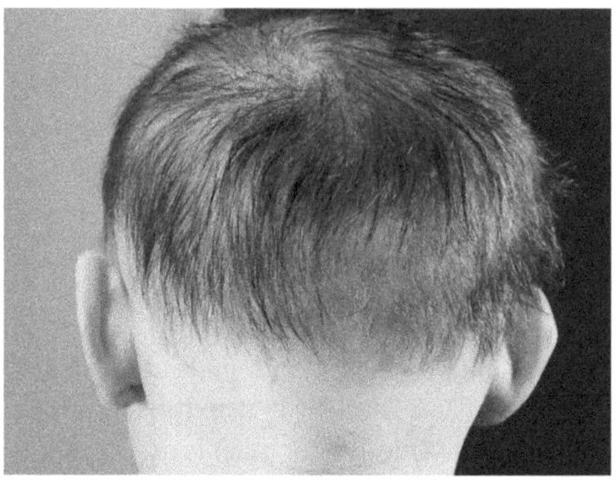

FIGURE 8.65 Clinical aspect of hypotrichosis associated to pili annulati.

The disease is congenital or presents during the first 2 years of life, but it may spontaneously improve after puberty. On the clinical basis, it develops with brittle, fragile, coarse, and lusterless hair as a result of the uneven reflection of light on the twisted hair surface.

8.4.8 Pili Annulati

Pili annulati is a rare autosomal dominant hair disorder. It is typified by the presence of alternating dark and light bands of the hair shafts (Figure 8.64). The light areas are subtle and occupy almost all the hair shaft thickness. The hairs of the affected individuals are normally growing, without any clinical signs of fragility. Hypotrichosis associated with pili annulati is a rare event (Figure 8.65).

BIBLIOGRAPHY

Abedini R, Kamyab Hesari K, Daneshpazhooh M, Ansari MS, Tohidinik HR, Ansari M. Validity of trichoscopy in the diagnosis of primary cicatricial alopecias. *Int J Dermatol.* 2016;55:1106–14.

Abraham LS, Torres FN, Azulay-Abulafia L. Dermoscopic clues to distinguish trichotillomania from patchy alopecia areata. *An Bras Dermatol.* 2010;85:723–6.

Adaimy L, Chouery E, Megarbane H et al. Mutation in WNT10A is associated with an autosomal recessive ectodermal dysplasia: The odonto-onycho-dermal dysplasia. *Am J Hum Genet.* 2007;81:821–8.

Alkhalifah A. Alopecia areata update. *Dermatol Clin.* 2013;31:93–108.

Amer M, Helmy A, Amer A. Trichoscopy as a useful method to differentiate tinea capitis from alopecia areata in children at Zagazig University Hospitals. *Int J Dermatol.* 2017;56:116–20.

Assouly P, Reygagne P. Lichen planopilaris: Update on diagnosis and treatment. *Semin Cutan Med Surg.* 2009;28:3–10.

Bittencourt Mde J, Moure ER, Pies OT, Mendes AD, Depra MM, Mello AL. Trichoscopy as a diagnostic tool in trichorrhexis invaginata and Netherton syndrome. *An Bras Dermatol.* 2015;90:114–6.

Blume-Peytavi U, Blumeyer A, Tosti A et al. S1 guideline for diagnostic evaluation in androgenetic alopecia in men, women and adolescents. *Br J Dermatol.* 2011;164:5–15.

Deloche C, de Lacharriere O, Misciali C et al. Histological features of peripilar signs associated with androgenetic alopecia. *Arch Dermatol Res.* 2004;295:422–8.

Dimino-Emme L, Camisa C. Trichotillomania associated with the "Friar Tuck sign" and nail-biting. *Cutis*. 1991;47:107–10.

Dishop MK, Bree AF, Hicks MJ. Pathologic changes of skin and hair in ankyloblepharon-ectodermal defects-cleft lip/palate (AEC) syndrome. *Am J Med Genet A*. 2009;149A:1935–41.

Duque-Estrada B, Tamler C, Sodre CT, Barcaui CB, Pereira FB. Dermoscopy patterns of cicatricial alopecia resulting from discoid lupus erythematosus and lichen planopilaris. *An Bras Dermatol*. 2010;85:179–83.

Ekiz O, Sen BB, Rifaioglu EN, Balta I. Trichoscopy in paediatric patients with tinea capitis: A useful method to differentiate from alopecia areata. *J Eur Acad Dermatol Venereol*. 2014;28:1255–8.

Elghblawi E. Idiosyncratic findings in trichoscopy of tinea capitis: Comma, zigzag hairs, corkscrew, and Morse code-like hair. *Int J Trichology*. 2016;8:180–3.

Fernandez-Crehuet P, Vano-Galvan S, Martorell-Calatayud A, Arias-Santiago S, Grimalt R, Camacho-Martinez FM. Clinical and trichoscopic characteristics of temporal triangular alopecia: A multicenter study. *J Am Acad Dermatol*. 2016;75:634–7.

Fernandez-Crehuet P, Vano-Galvan S, Molina-Ruiz AM et al. Trichoscopic features of folliculitis decalvans: Results in 58 patients. *Int J Trichology*. 2017;9:140–1.

Guttikonda AS, Aruna C, Ramamurthy DV, Sridevi K, Alagappan SK. Evaluation of clinical significance of dermoscopy in alopecia areata. *Indian J Dermatol*. 2016;61:628–33.

Hernandez-Bel P, Malvehy J, Crocker A, Sanchez-Carazo JL, Febrer I, Alegre V. Comma hairs: A new dermoscopic marker for tinea capitis. *Actas Dermosifiliogr*. 2012;103:836–7.

Hughes R, Chiaverini C, Bahadoran P, Lacour JP. Corkscrew hair: A new dermoscopic sign for diagnosis of tinea capitis in black children. *Arch Dermatol*. 2011;147:355–6.

Inui S, Nakajima T, Itami S. Coudability hairs: A revisited sign of alopecia areata assessed by trichoscopy. *Clin Exp Dermatol*. 2010;35:361–5.

Inui S, Nakajima T, Itami S. Temporal triangular alopecia: Trichoscopic diagnosis. *J Dermatol*. 2012;39:572–4.

Karadag Kose O, Gulec AT. Clinical evaluation of alopecias using a handheld dermatoscope. *J Am Acad Dermatol*. 2012;67:206–14.

Kowalska-Oledzka E, Slowinska M, Rakowska A et al. "Black dots" seen under trichoscopy are not specific for alopecia areata. *Clin Exp Dermatol*. 2012;37:615–9.

Lacarrubba F, Micali G, Tosti A. Absence of vellus hair in the hairline: A videodermatoscopic feature of frontal fibrosing alopecia. *Br J Dermatol*. 2013;169:473–4.

Lacarrubba F, Verzi AE, Micali G. Newly described features resulting from high-magnification dermoscopy of tinea capitis. *JAMA Dermatol*. 2015;151:308–10.

Lanuti E, Miteva M, Romanelli P, Tosti A. Trichoscopy and histopathology of follicular keratotic plugs in scalp discoid lupus erythematosus. *Int J Trichology*. 2012;4:36–8.

Lee DY, Lee JH, Yang JM, Lee ES. The use of dermoscopy for the diagnosis of trichotillomania. *J Eur Acad Dermatol Venereol*. 2009;23:731–2.

Ludwig E. Classification of the types of androgenetic alopecia (common baldness) occurring in the female sex. *Br J Dermatol*. 1977;97:247–54.

Mane M, Nath AK, Thappa DM. Utility of dermoscopy in alopecia areata. *Indian J Dermatol*. 2011;56:407–11.

Mapelli ET, Gualandri L, Cerri A, Menni S. Comma hairs in tinea capitis: A useful dermatoscopic sign for diagnosis of tinea capitis. *Pediatr Dermatol*. 2012;29:223–4.

Mathew J. Trichoscopy as an aid in the diagnosis of trichotillomania. *Int J Trichology*. 2012;4:101–2.

More CB, Bhavsar K, Joshi J, Varma SN, Tailor M. Hereditary ectodermal dysplasia: A retrospective study. *J Nat Sci Biol Med*. 2013;4:445–50.

Naeem M, Jelani M, Lee K et al. Ectodermal dysplasia of hair and nail type: Mapping of a novel locus to chromosome 17p12-q21.2. *Br J Dermatol*. 2006;155:1184–90.

Nikam VV, Mehta HH. A nonrandomized study of trichoscopy patterns using nonpolarized (contact) and polarized (noncontact) dermatoscopy in hair and shaft disorders. *Int J Trichology.* 2014;6:54–62.

Norwood OT. Male pattern baldness: Classification and incidence. *South Med J.* 1975;68:1359–65.

Norwood OT. Incidence of female androgenetic alopecia (female pattern alopecia). *Dermatol Surg.* 2001;27:53–4.

Park J, Kim JI, Kim HU, Yun SK, Kim SJ. Trichoscopic findings of hair loss in Koreans. *Ann Dermatol.* 2015;27:539–50.

Peralta L, Morais P. Photoletter to the editor: The Friar Tuck sign in trichotillomania. *J Dermatol Case Rep.* 2012;6:63–4.

Pinheiro AMC, Mauad EBS, Fernandes LFA, Drumond RB. Aplasia cutis congenita: Trichoscopy findings. *Int J Trichology.* 2016;8:184–5.

Rakowska A, Gorska R, Rudnicka L, Zadurska M. Trichoscopic hair evaluation in patients with ectodermal dysplasia. *J Pediatr.* 2015;167:193–5.

Rakowska A, Maj M, Zadurska M et al. Trichoscopy of focal alopecia in children—New trichoscopic findings: Hair bulbs arranged radially along hair-bearing margins in aplasia cutis congenita. *Skin Appendage Disord.* 2016;2:1–6.

Rakowska A WA, Sikora M, Olszewska M, Rudnicka L. Two different trichoscopic patterns of mid-frontal scalp in patients with frontal fibrosing alopecia and clinical features of androgenetic alopecia. *Przegl Dermatol.* 2017;104:9–15.

Rakowska A, Slowinska M, Czuwara J, Olszewska M, Rudnicka L. Dermoscopy as a tool for rapid diagnosis of monilethrix. *J Drugs Dermatol.* 2007;6:222–4.

Rakowska A, Slowinska M, Kowalska-Oledzka E et al. Trichoscopy of cicatricial alopecia. *J Drugs Dermatol.* 2012;11:753–8.

Rakowska A, Slowinska M, Kowalska-Oledzka E, Olszewska M, Rudnicka L. Dermoscopy in female androgenic alopecia: Method standardization and diagnostic criteria. *Int J Trichology.* 2009;1:123–30.

Rakowska A, Slowinska M, Olszewska M, Rudnicka L. New trichoscopy findings in trichotillomania: Flame hairs, V-sign, hook hairs, hair powder, tulip hairs. *Acta Derm Venereol.* 2014;94:303–6.

Rakowska A, Zadurska M, Czuwara J et al. Trichoscopy findings in loose anagen hair syndrome: Rectangular granular structures and solitary yellow dots. *J Dermatol Case Rep.* 2015;9:1–5.

Rebora A, Guarrera M. Teloptosis and kenogen: Two new concepts in human trichology. *Arch Dermatol.* 2004;140:619–20.

Ross EK, Vincenzi C, Tosti A. Videodermoscopy in the evaluation of hair and scalp disorders. *J Am Acad Dermatol.* 2006;55:799–806.

Rossi A, Fortuna MC, Pranteda G et al. Clinical, histological and trichoscopic correlations in scalp disorders. *Dermatology.* 2015;231:201–8.

Rudnicka L, Olszewska M, Rakowska A. *Atlas of Trichoscopy: Dermoscopy in Hair and Scalp Disease.* London, UK: Springer; 2012.

Rudnicka L, Olszewska M, Rakowska A, Slowinska M. Trichoscopy update 2011. *J Dermatol Case Rep.* 2011;5:82–8.

Rudnicka L, Rakowska A, Kerzeja M et al. Hair shafts in trichoscopy: Clues for diagnosis of hair and scalp diseases. *Dermatol Clin.* 2013;31(4):695–708, x.

Sah DE, Koo J, Price VH. Trichotillomania. *Dermatol Ther.* 2008;21:13–21.

Slowinska M, Rudnicka L, Schwartz RA et al. Comma hairs: A dermatoscopic marker for tinea capitis: A rapid diagnostic method. *J Am Acad Dermatol.* 2008;59:S77–9.

Tosti A, Miteva M, Torres F. Lonely hair: A clue to the diagnosis of frontal fibrosing alopecia. *Arch Dermatol.* 2011;147:1240.

Tosti A, Torres F, Miteva M. Dermoscopy of early dissecting cellulitis of the scalp simulates alopecia areata. *Actas Dermosifiliogr.* 2013;104:92–3.

Tosti A, Torres F, Misciali C et al. Follicular red dots: A novel dermoscopic pattern observed in scalp discoid lupus erythematosus. *Arch Dermatol.* 2009;145:1406–9.

Vazquez-Lopez F, Palacios-Garcia L, Argenziano G. Dermoscopic corkscrew hairs dissolve after successful therapy of *Trichophyton violaceum* tinea capitis: A case report. *Australas J Dermatol.* 2012;53:118–9.

Verzi AE, Lacarrubba F, Micali G. Starburst hair follicles: A dermoscopic clue for aplasia cutis congenita. *J Am Acad Dermatol.* 2016;75:e141–e2.

Verzi AE, Lacarrubba F, Micali G. Heterogeneity of trichoscopy findings in dissecting cellulitis of the scalp: Correlation with disease activity and duration. *Br J Dermatol.* 2017;177(6). doi: 10.1111/bjd.15685

Whiting DA. Possible mechanisms of miniaturization during androgenetic alopecia or pattern hair loss. *J Am Acad Dermatol.* 2001;45:S81–6.

9

Special Clinical Scenarios

9.1 Pigmented Macules on the Face

The differential diagnosis of a pigmented facial macule is one of the most challenging scenarios for clinicians. The latter results from the numerous overlapping clinical and dermatoscopic features of the entities that are included in the differential diagnosis. In other body sites, histopathologic examination after an excisional or partial biopsy would easily resolve any diagnostic dilemma, while on the face, the surgical procedures are limited by practical and cosmetic sequences.

Data from epidemiology and evolution of nevi throughout the lifetime must be encountered during the diagnostic approach of melanocytic lesions. Opposed to the other anatomical sites, early facial melanoma (lentigo maligna) develops later in life, is flat, and grows slowly. In this context, and given that nevi on the face develop earlier in life and transform by age into elevated, dome-shaped, flesh-colored papules (Figure 9.1), they are not included in the differential diagnosis of facial melanoma. Lentigo maligna (Figure 9.2) is associated with chronic, cumulative ultraviolet radiation, is usually found in the elderly, and clinically mimics solar lentigo and pigmented actinic keratosis that are flat and often pigmented. Discrimination of lentigo maligna from the latter entities is challenging on both clinical and dermatoscopic grounds.

The discrepancy in the diagnosis of lentigo maligna is further widened by the various and controversial histopathologic terms that are still used to describe ambiguous melanocytic lesions on the face or other sun-damaged areas, namely, "atypical melanocytic proliferation," "unstable lentigo," etc. From the clinical point of view, this terminology is meaningless for the clinician, since it is not translated into a distinct biologic behavior and management, accordingly. We believe that these vague melanocytic lesions, most probably, represent early melanomas that have not fully developed histopathologic characteristics. Our advice to physicians is either to consider the aforementioned entities as a synonym to lentigo maligna, or to lentiginous melanoma, or to contact the dermatopathologist and seek a reevaluation or a second expert opinion.

The dermatoscopic features of lentigo maligna are analytically described in Chapter 3. The initial dermatoscopic manifestations emerge around the follicular openings and progress with the evolution of the tumor. The diagnostic difficulties of lentigo maligna arise from the following issues:

1. The dermatoscopic features of early stage lentigo maligna (gray dots, asymmetrical pigmentation of follicles) are difficult to recognize and are not constant (Figure 9.3). In the late stage, the typical dermatoscopic features are more evident, but lesions are no longer considered early stage (Figure 9.4).
2. Most of the dermatoscopic features of lentigo maligna are not specific. This means that they are also present in solar lentigo/flat seborrheic keratosis and pigmented actinic keratosis, which represent the main differentials of lentigo maligna (Figures 9.5 and 9.6).

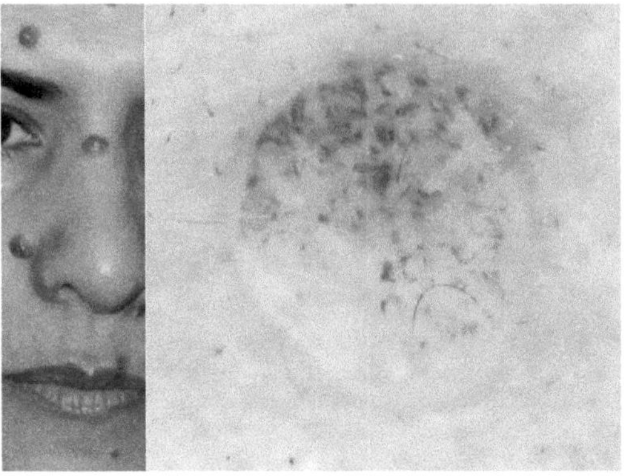

FIGURE 9.1 Typical clinical and dermatoscopic images of nevi in adults. They are dermal nevi and clinically nodular.

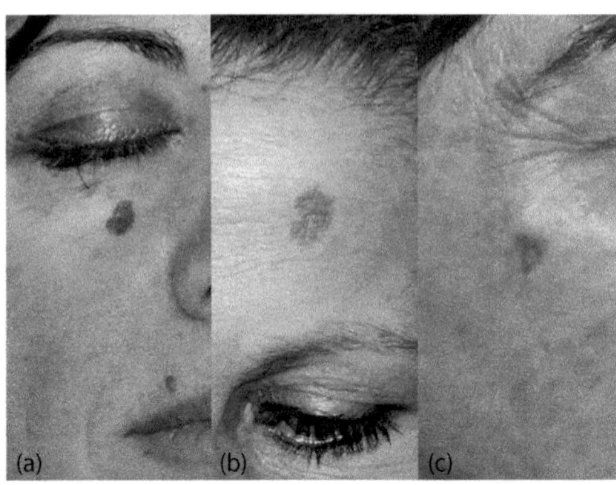

FIGURE 9.2 Differential diagnosis of flat pigmented lesions on the face of adults includes lentigo malignant melanoma (a), pigmented actinic keratosis (b), and flat seborrheic keratosis/solar lentigo (c).

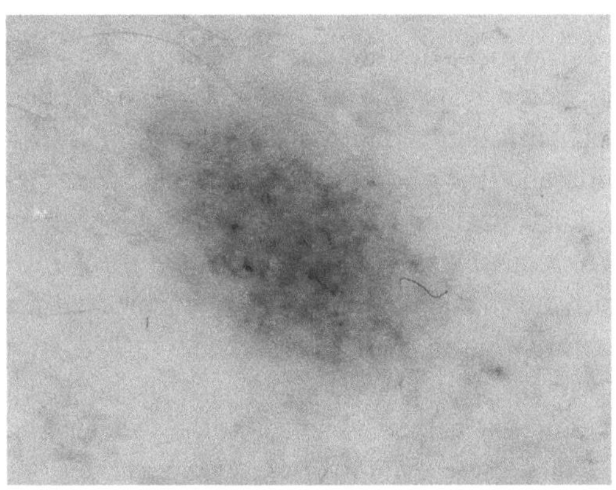

FIGURE 9.3 Early stage of a lentigo maligna melanoma. The dermatoscopic criteria (gray dots/globules) are subtle and difficult to detect.

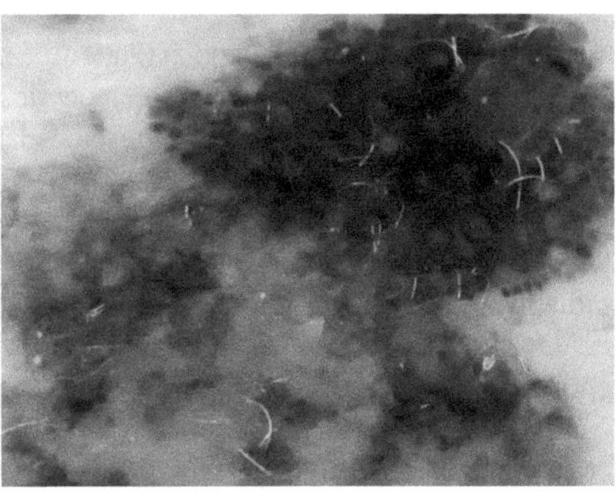

FIGURE 9.4 Advanced stage lentigo maligna melanoma. The dermatoscopic features are now obvious, but at this level the diagnosis is not considered as early.

FIGURE 9.5 Pigmented actinic keratosis dermatoscopically displaying multiple gray dots.

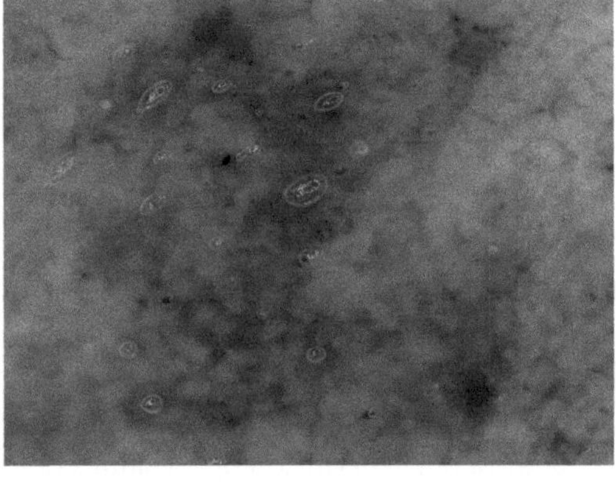

FIGURE 9.6 Gray dots and globules are seen in flat seborrheic keratosis, as well.

Numerous studies intended to detect dermatoscopic criteria for enhancing early detection of lentigo maligna. However, despite the long list of dermatoscopic features attributed to lentigo maligna, our diagnostic accuracy, especially regarding the discrimination from pigmented actinic keratosis, did not significantly improve. A useful clue remains the presence of wide and evident follicular openings that are spared from pigmentation in pigmented actinic keratoses versus the fuzzy (due to presence of atypical melanocytes along the follicular epithelium) follicles seen in lentigo maligna (Figure 9.7).

Recently, a multicenter research group proposed a diagnostic algorithm that reached high sensitivity and specificity for lentigo maligna, as well as improved reproducibility. According to the authors, the diagnostic approach must focus on the recognition of "nonmelanoma" criteria, characterizing solar lentigo/flat seborrheic keratosis and pigmented actinic keratosis. Analytically, the method suggests that if one of the following nonmelanoma dermatoscopic criteria are clearly present all over the lesion, then a biopsy is not necessary, and any treatment can be applied.

Nonmelanoma criteria of solar lentigo:

1. Brown parallel lines, mimicking fingerprints (fingerprinting). They may cross each other perpendicularly, appearing as a network (Figures 9.8 and 9.9). Opposed to the trunk, where the presence of a pigment network indicates a melanocytic lesion, on the face a pigment network indicates a nonmelanocytic lesion, namely, solar lentigo.
2. Sharp demarcation or moth-eaten borders (Figures 9.10 and 9.11).
3. Typical features of seborrheic keratosis, i.e., milia-like cysts or comedo-like openings (Figure 9.12).

Nonmelanoma criteria of pigmented actinic keratosis:

1. Evident/white follicles often filled with keratin plugs. Using nonpolarized light, the rosettes (four dots in a square) can be detected inside the follicles (Figures 9.13 and 9.14).
2. White or brown scales. Brown scales result from pigmented parakeratosis (Figures 9.15 and 9.16).
3. Erythema (Figure 9.15).

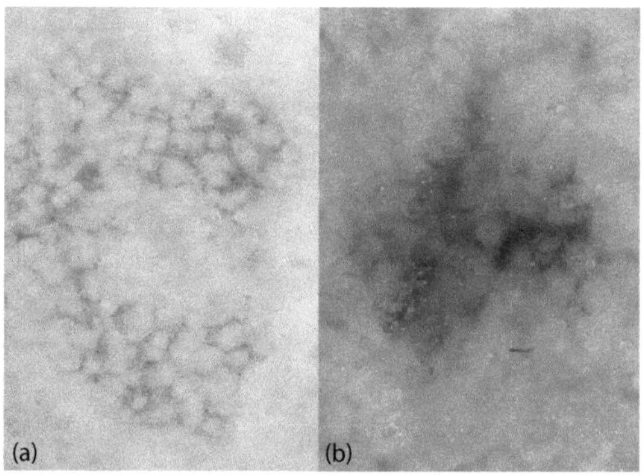

FIGURE 9.7 In pigmented actinic keratosis, (a) the follicular openings are spared from pigmentation, in contrast to what is seen in lentigo maligna (b).

FIGURE 9.8 Brown fine parallel lines resembling fingerprints, indicative of seborrheic keratosis/solar lentigo.

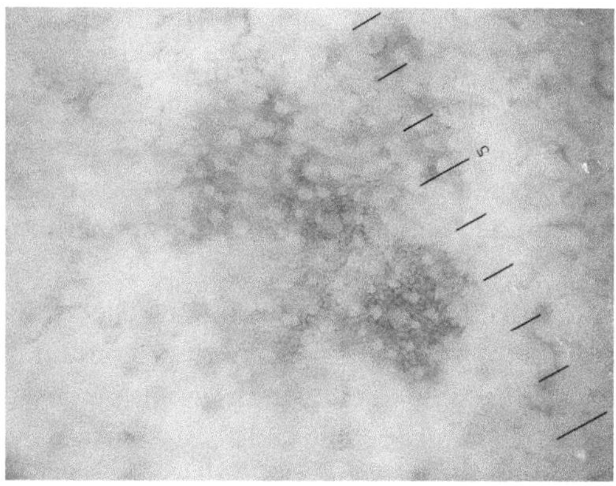

FIGURE 9.9 Typical pigment network in between follicular openings, indicating seborrheic keratosis/solar lentigo.

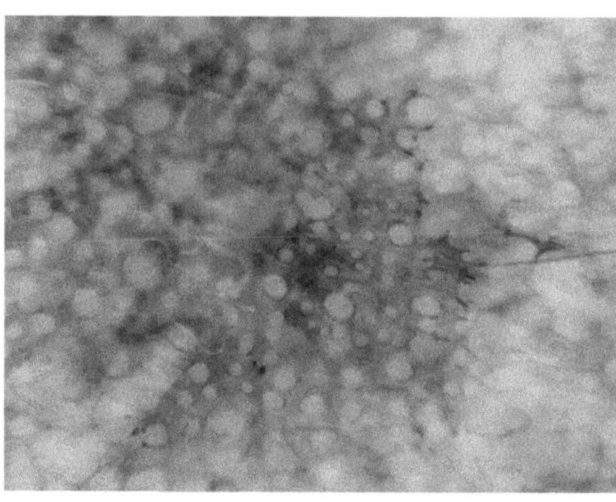

FIGURE 9.10 Sharply demarcated or moth-eaten border, indicating seborrheic keratosis/solar lentigo (1).

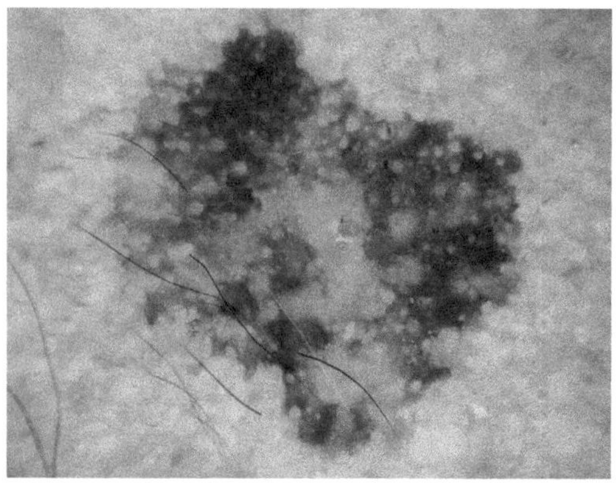

FIGURE 9.11 Sharply demarcated or moth-eaten border, indicating seborrheic keratosis/solar lentigo (2).

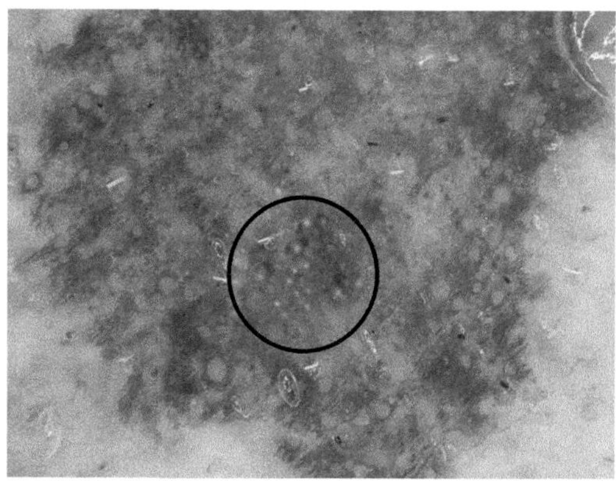

FIGURE 9.12 Milia-like cysts, indicating seborrheic keratosis.

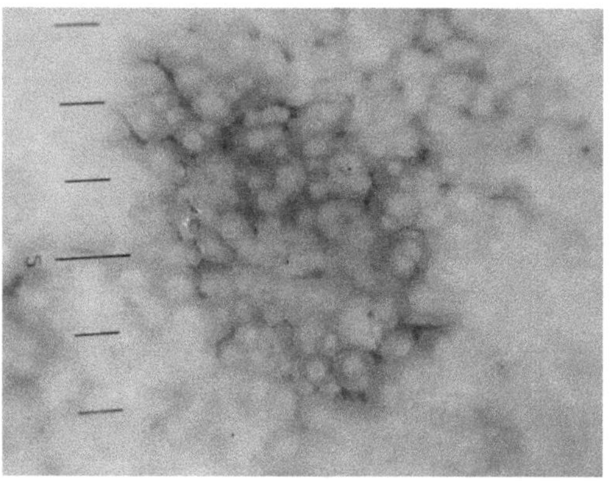

FIGURE 9.13 Wide follicular openings, free of pigment, some plugged with keratin, indicating pigmented actinic keratosis.

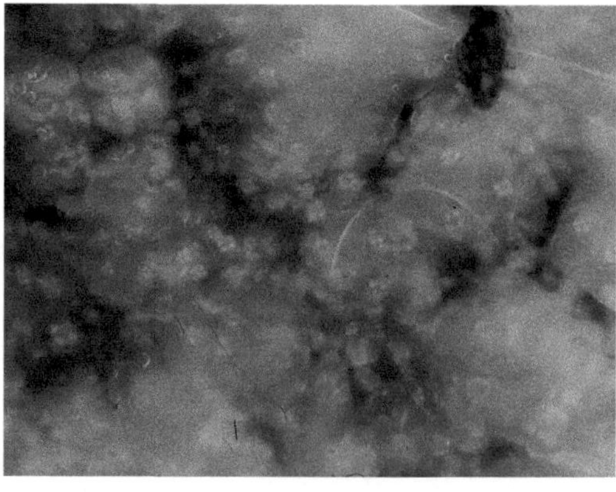

FIGURE 9.14 Rosettes inside wide, nonpigmented follicular openings, indicating pigmented actinic keratosis.

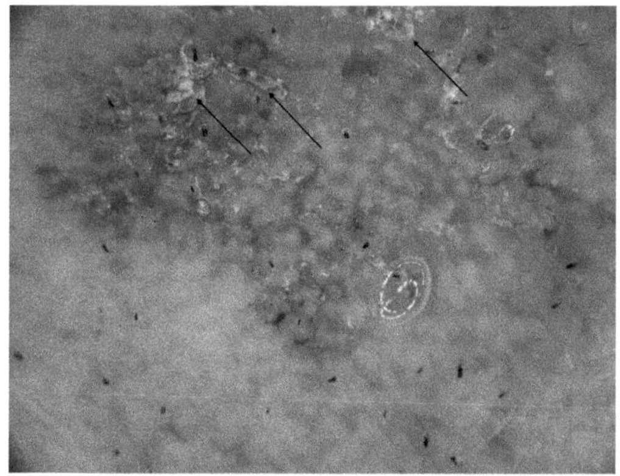

FIGURE 9.15 Fine scaling and erythema, both indicating pigmented actinic keratosis.

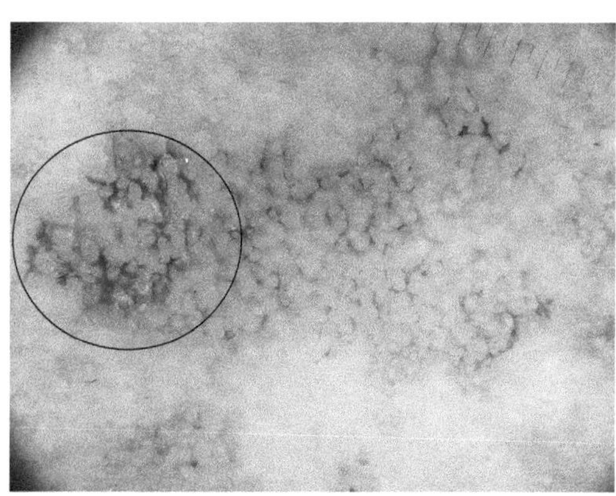

FIGURE 9.16 Brown scales, indicating pigmented actinic keratosis.

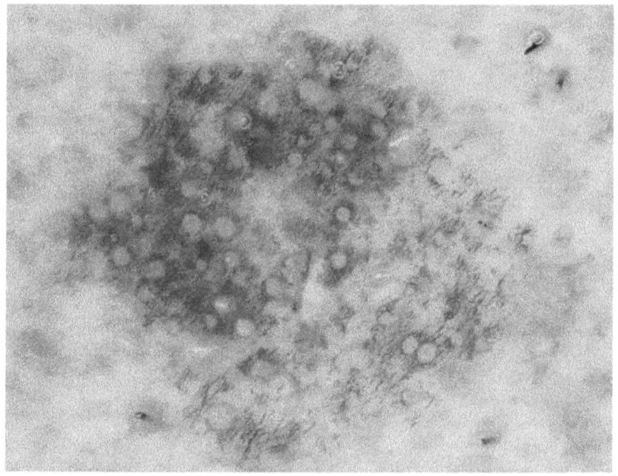

FIGURE 9.17 Brown parallel lines resembling fingerprints distributed throughout the largest part of the lesion are a "key feature" in dermatoscopy, highly indicative of a seborrheic keratosis/solar lentigo.

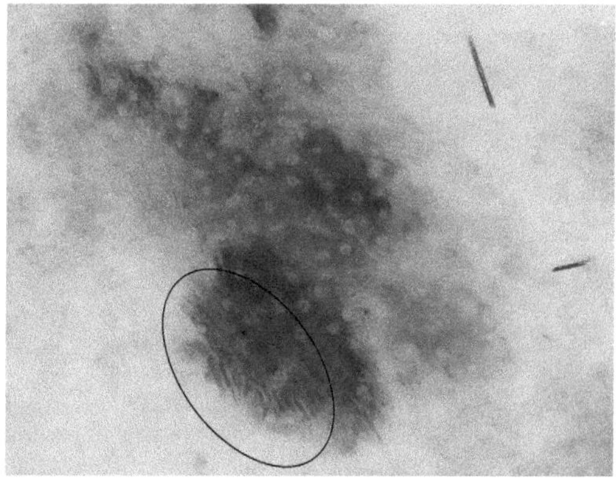

FIGURE 9.18 Brown parallel lines resembling fingerprints seen only in a small part of the lesion (circle). This kind of distribution is not enough for the lesion to be safely classified as seborrheic keratosis/solar lentigo. Indeed, this is a melanoma.

It has to be clarified that for a feature to be evaluated as "present," it must occupy a significant part of the lesion and must attract the visual attention of the examiner, compared to other features (predominant feature) (Figure 9.17). If none of the aforementioned criteria is present, then the lesion should be considered as suspicious for melanoma, even if not displaying any lentigo maligna–associated criterion (Figure 9.18).

Despite the increased specificity and sensitivity of this algorithm, "false-positive" cases are not uncommon. A typical example is lichen planus–like keratosis, which is a seborrheic keratosis or a solar lentigo in regression (Figure 9.19). Misinterpretation of lesions undergoing regression is not unusual even among experts. In this context and considering the overlapping features of regressed melanoma and its benign mimickers, our expert recommendation is to histopathologically examine any doubtful cases showing regression.

Figures 9.20 through 9.30 illustrate clinical examples of the described diagnostic strategy.

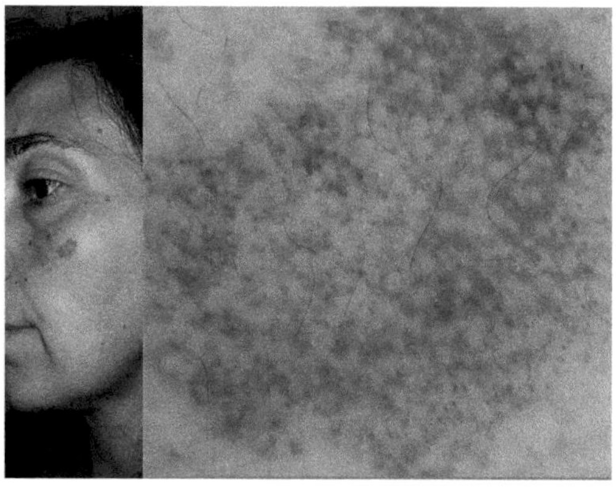

FIGURE 9.19 In this lesion, none of the six nonmelanoma criteria were found; therefore, it is considered suspicious. However, this is a lichen planus–like keratosis.

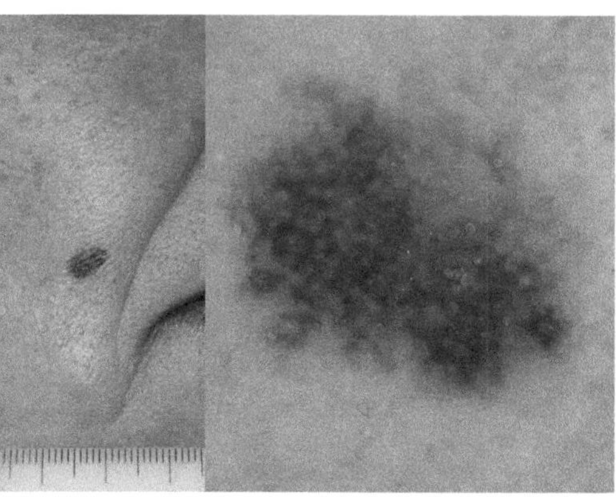

FIGURE 9.20 In this lesion, none of the six nonmelanoma criteria were found; therefore, it is considered suspicious. Although almost none of the dermatoscopic features of lentigo maligna are present, this is a melanoma.

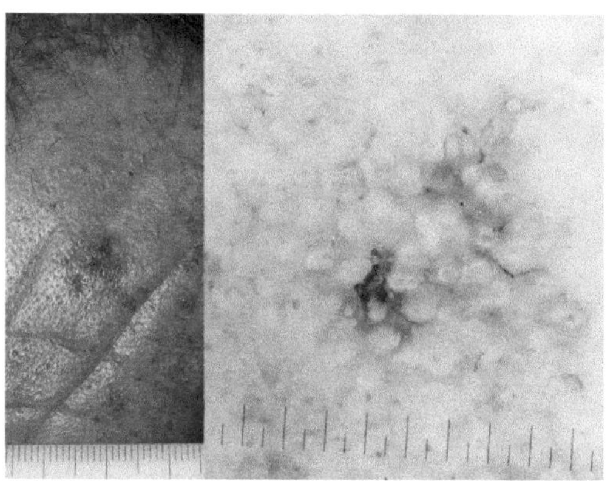

FIGURE 9.21 In this case, one of the six nonmelanoma criteria is prominent, namely, white follicles, highly indicative of a pigmented actinic keratosis.

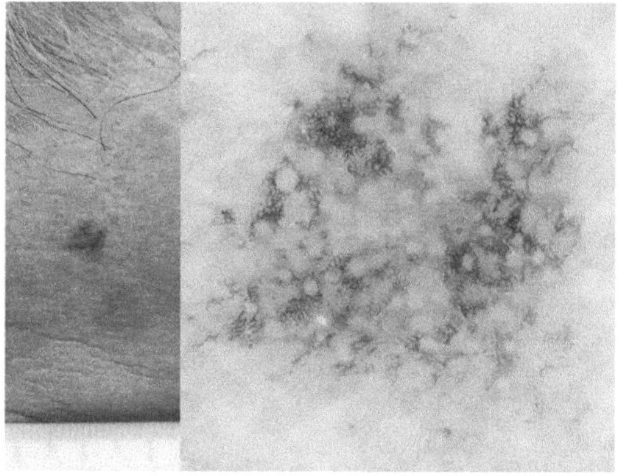

FIGURE 9.22 The clear presence of one of the six nonmelanoma criteria is prominent, namely, typical network between the follicles, which typifies this solar lentigo.

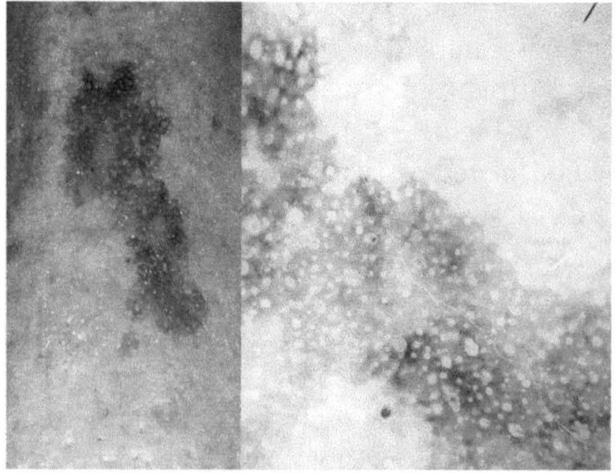

FIGURE 9.23 Although clinically this lesion is quite suspicious, dermatoscopy reveals white circles as the prominent feature. This is a pigmented actinic keratosis.

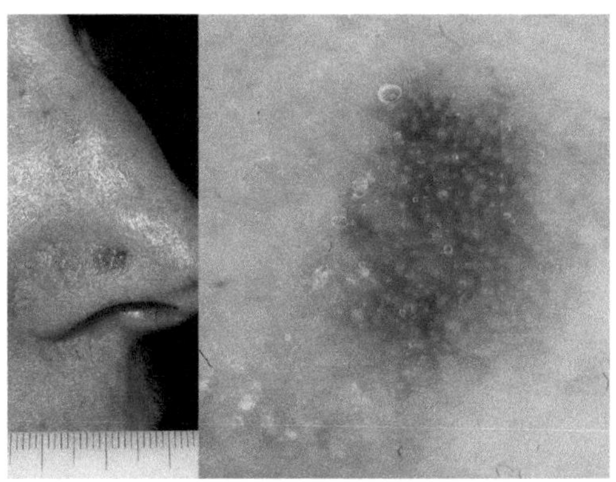

FIGURE 9.24 In this lesion, none of the six nonmelanoma criteria were found; therefore, it is considered suspicious. Although almost none of the dermatoscopic features of lentigo maligna are detected, this is a melanoma.

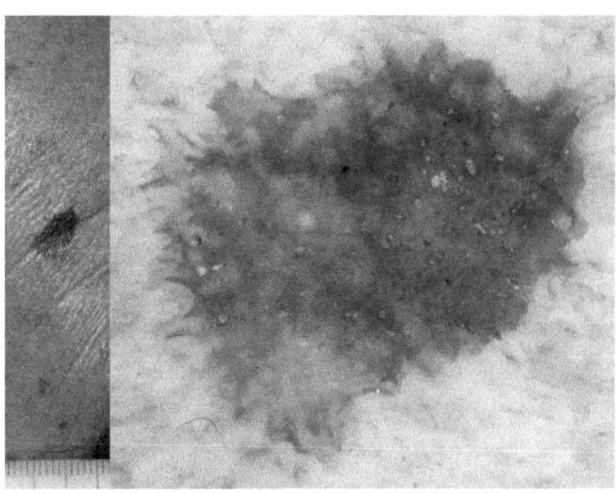

FIGURE 9.25 In this case, one out of six nonmelanoma criteria is prominent: sharp demarcated periphery. This is a seborrheic keratosis.

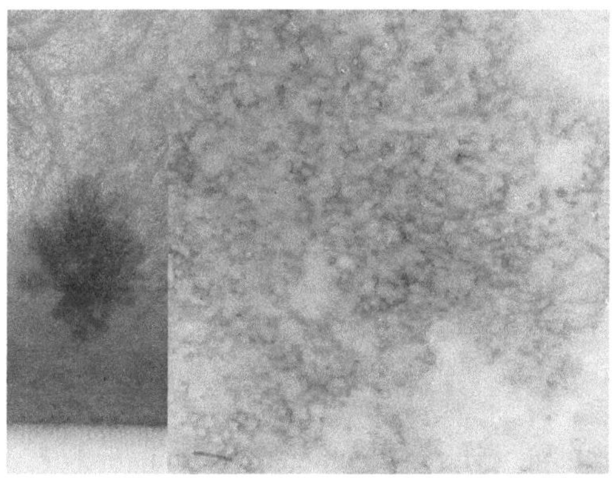

FIGURE 9.26 The presence of nonpigmented follicles and erythema allows for the diagnosis of actinic keratosis.

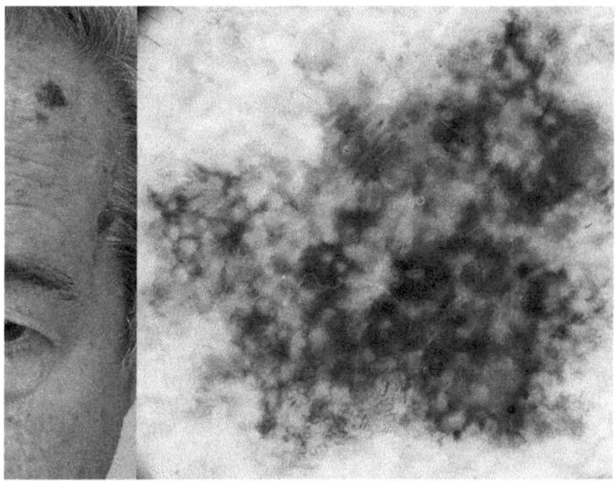

FIGURE 9.27 A typical pigmented network can be seen at the periphery of the lesion. However, it is not a predominant feature in the lesion; therefore, it is insufficient for the safe classification of this lesion as seborrheic keratosis/solar lentigo. Indeed, this is a melanoma.

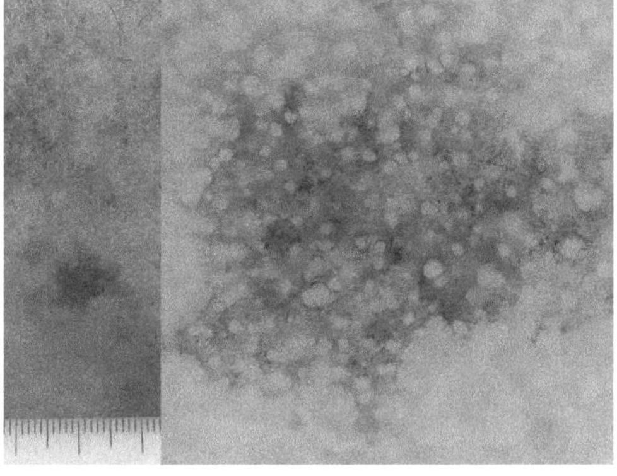

FIGURE 9.28 In this lesion, one out of six nonmelanoma criteria is prominent: typical network between follicles. This is a solar lentigo.

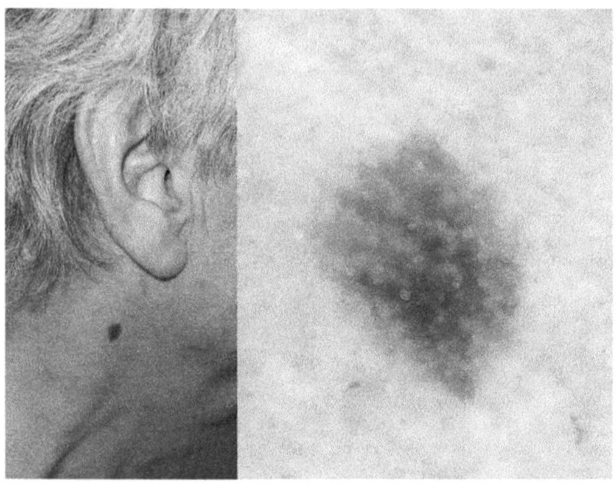

FIGURE 9.29 None of the six nonmelanoma criteria of the algorithm can be identified. Consequently, this lesion must be considered suspicious, although none of the dermatoscopic features of lentigo maligna can be seen. Indeed, this is a melanoma.

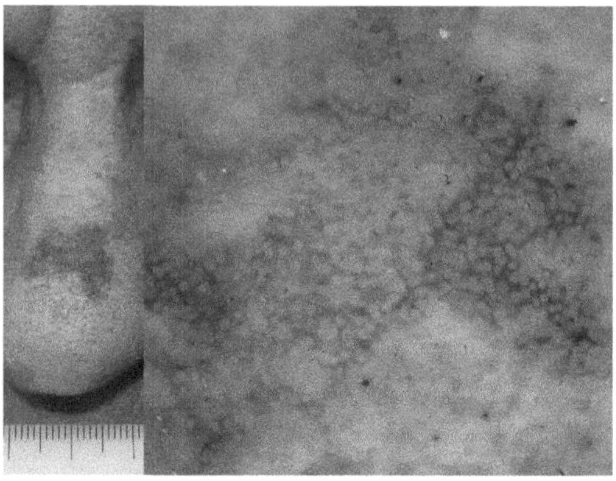

FIGURE 9.30 The presence of nonpigmented follicles and erythema allows for the diagnosis of actinic keratosis.

Management of suspicious lesions includes various options that are scientifically evidence based and clinically meaningful:

1. Excision is definitely the treatment of choice, especially in highly suspicious lesions.
2. Punch or shave biopsy: In general, partial biopsies for diagnosing melanoma are not recommended, since the histopathologic differential diagnosis between a nevus and a melanoma is extremely difficult if only a part of a lesion is examined. However, as already mentioned, in this scenario, a nevus is not included in the differential diagnosis. Therefore, a partial biopsy to determine the melanocytic or nonmelanocytic nature of the lesion is of high value. If the answer is that the lesion is melanocytic, then this is almost equal to a diagnosis of melanoma. An unusual scenario that may result in diagnostic misinterpretation is the coexistence of two different tumors (collision tumor). The possibility of misdiagnosing collision tumors is higher with punch (as compared to shave) biopsies, since the pathologist practically examines only a small part of the existing lesion.
3. Follow-up is a reasonable choice for a lentigo maligna arising in an elderly individual with low life expectancy. Lentigo maligna is the most slowly growing melanoma type, with only a small percentage of them progressing into an invasive phase. Action should be undertaken if a nodular or a popular component appears during follow-up. Radiotherapy or imiquimod also represent reasonable alternatives.

9.2 Diagnosis and Management of Spitzoid-Looking Lesions

For years, the appropriate classification and management of spitzoid-looking lesions has been a subject of debate and diverse approaches among scientists of all specialties dealing with the diagnosis and management of skin tumors. The term *spitzoid*, although widely used, is probably inappropriate. It refers to a heterogenous "group" of lesions, including the classic Spitz nevus and many other tumors sharing common or similar morphological characteristics. In the past, even

Spitz nevus has been a subject of debate regarding its biology and even now its management is problematic.

It is important for physicians to understand the complexity of spitzoid lesions. Let's start from what is already known, as discussed in the following sections.

Facts

1. Spitz nevus is just a type of nevus. Therefore, biologically it is considered to be absolutely benign, despite the unusual dynamic growth in early stages.
2. The same is true for Reed nevus. There is not an absolute agreement if Spitz and Reed nevi are two different types of nevi or a variant of the same type. This disagreement, however, is rather not practically significant, since it is widely accepted that Spitz and Reed nevi are just nevi and therefore benign.
3. It is absolutely clear that melanomas sharing morphological features with Spitz and Reed nevi do exist, and this is the reason why these melanomas are often described as "spitzoid." The morphological similarity between "spitzoid" melanoma and Spitz/Reed nevi can be clinical and/or dermatoscopic and might be partial or absolute: Most spitzoid melanomas, although displaying dermatoscopic features seen in Spitz and Reed nevi (peripheral streaks or pseudopods, inverse network, dotted vessels), can be recognized as melanomas because these features are asymmetrically distributed in the lesion. However, a subgroup of spitzoid melanomas is characterized by perfect morphological symmetry, resulting in a complete morphological overlap with Spitz and Reed nevi.
4. The morphological overlap is not only clinical and dermatoscopic but also histopathologic. There are tumors in which the histopathologic morphology does not allow them to be safely categorized, neither as nevi nor as melanomas. Different terms have been used to describe and group these tumors: Spitz nevus with atypia and metastatic potential, metastatic Spitz tumor, atypical Spitz tumor, atypical Spitz nevus, melanocytic tumor of unknown malignant potential, melanocytoma. It is very unclear if these tumors with "intermediate" histopathologic morphology are also defined by "intermediate" biologic behavior or are either nevi or melanomas difficult to diagnose histopathologically.
5. It is also known that some spitzoid tumors might "metastasize" to the regional lymph nodes, without however having the potential to give late or visceral metastases or cause any other consequence for the general health of the patient. Thus, these lymph node nests should be considered to be deposits rather than "metastases," just like those seen in congenital or blue nevi.

Dermatoscopic Features

Ia. Reed nevus: Reed nevus is dermatoscopically typified by the "starburst" pattern, which consists of a heavily pigmented center (black/black-bluish/dark brown) and symmetrically distributed peripheral streaks or pseudopods that originate from the pigmented center of the lesion and expand radially to the periphery (Figures 9.31 and 9.32). Other dermatoscopic patterns that can be found in Reed nevi are the reticular and homogenous patterns (Figures 9.33 and 9.34). The starburst pattern is indicative of the biological tendency of Reed nevus to rapidly grow peripherally, and it gradually converts to a homogenous or reticular pattern as the nevus stabilizes. At the stage of homogenous or reticular pattern, a Reed nevus cannot be identified as such, since these patterns are very common in other kinds of nevi.

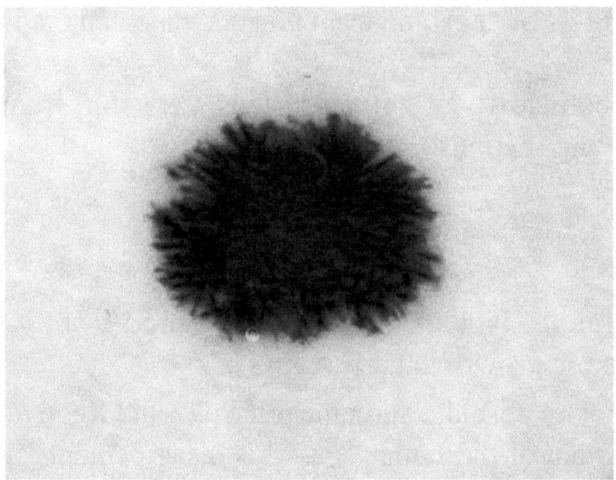

FIGURE 9.31 The dermatoscopic "starburst" pattern, consisting of heavily pigmented center and peripheral streaks that start from the center of the lesion and expand radially to the periphery.

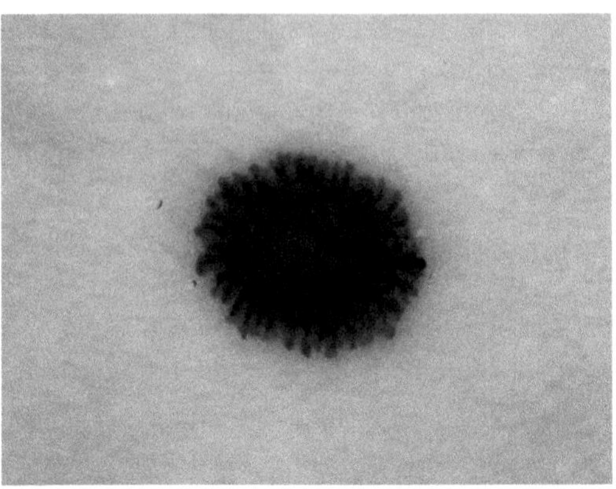

FIGURE 9.32 An image similar to the previous one. The only (and not substantial) difference is the presence of globules at the distal end of the streaks (pseudopods).

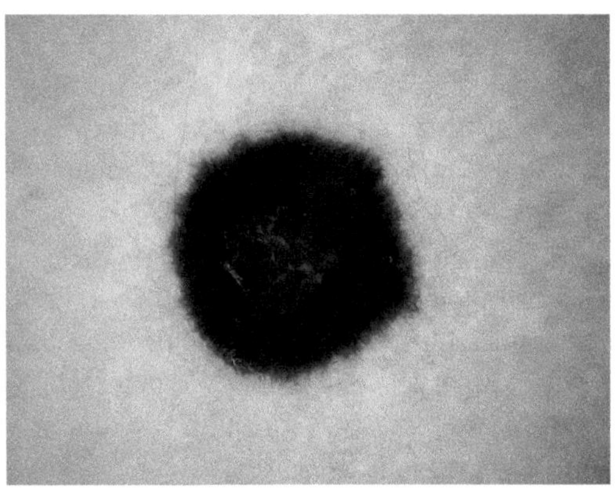

FIGURE 9.33 Homogenous pattern in a Reed nevus. At this stage, this nevus resembles a common "black" nevus seen in dark skin type individuals.

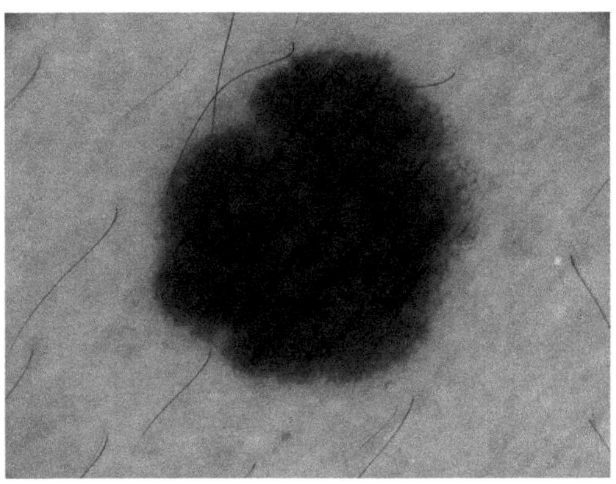

FIGURE 9.34 Reticular pattern in a Reed nevus. Many Reed nevi with a starburst pattern after their stabilization end up looking like this one.

Ib. Pigmented Spitz nevus: The main dermatoscopic pattern of this nevus consists of multiple dark brown or black globules surrounded by white color. Usually, the white color surrounding the globules has the form of a "network" of white lines, and the terms used to describe it are *reticular depigmentation*, *inverse network*, and *white network* (Figures 9.35 and 9.36). If this white network is absent, a pigmented Spitz nevus is very difficult to identify as such, since the globular pattern is much more frequent in other types of nevi. It must be noted that parts of Spitz and Reed nevi are characterized by a multicomponent dermatoscopic pattern; therefore, they morphologically look like melanoma (Figure 9.37).

Ic. Nonpigmented Spitz nevus: Dermatoscopically, the classical Spitz nevus is characterized by multiple dotted or globular vessels that are surrounded by white color ("reticular depigmentation," "inverse network," and "white network"). In nodular Spitz nevi, the vessels can appear as glomerular or as "comma" or "hairpin," and they are again surrounded by white color (Figures 9.38 through 9.40).

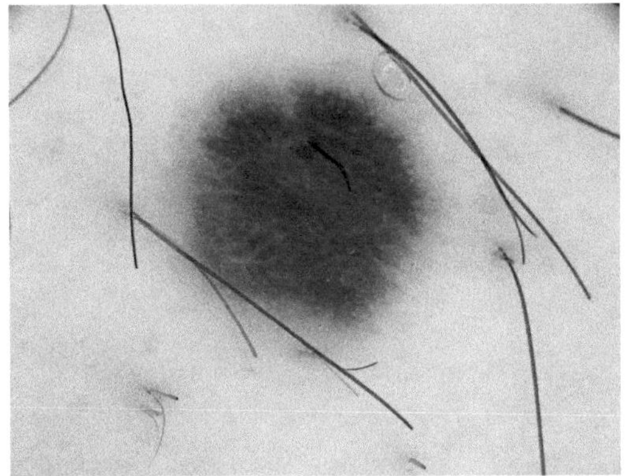

FIGURE 9.35 Multiple brown globules surrounded by a white network. This is the typical pattern of pigmented Spitz nevus.

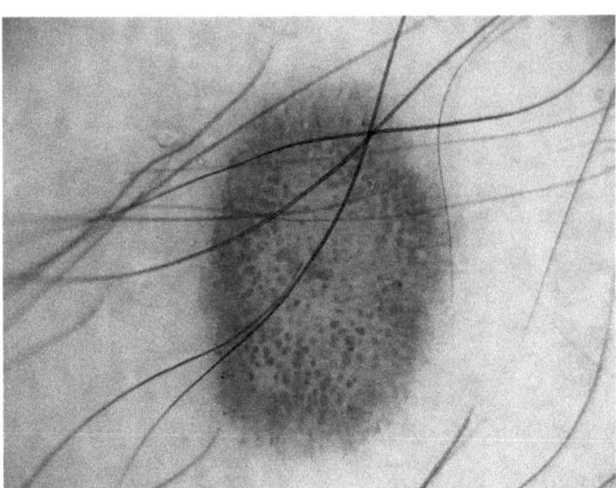

FIGURE 9.36 Multiple brown globules surrounded by a white network in a pigmented Spitz nevus.

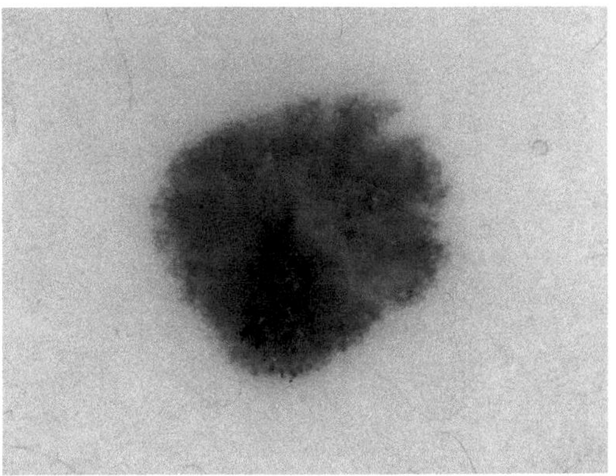

FIGURE 9.37 This is a Reed nevus characterized by a multicomponent pattern and atypical globules. The dermatoscopic aspect is rather suggestive of melanoma than a nevus, and for this reason the excision of the lesion is fully justified.

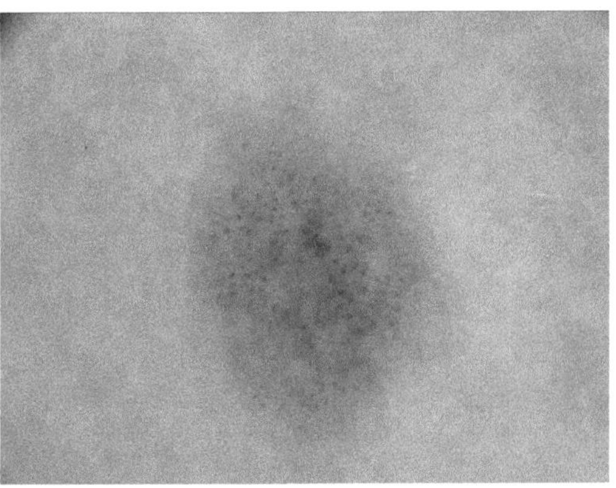

FIGURE 9.38 The dermatoscopic pattern of a classic nonpigmented Spitz nevus consists of multiple dotted vessels that are surrounded by white color.

II. Atypical Spitz nevus: The majority of atypical Spitz nevi (about 80%) is described by dermatoscopic asymmetry and/or a multicomponent pattern (Figures 9.41 and 9.42). This melanoma resemblance does not lead to any clinical problem, since the recommendation and management regarding atypical Spitz nevi are excision. On the contrary, a clinical problem occurs with the remaining 20% of atypical Spitz tumors that appear as red nodules with a dermatoscopic pattern similar to the one of classic nonpigmented Spitz nevus (multiple dotted or circular vessels surrounded by white network) (Figure 9.43). This dermatoscopic overlap is the reason for implying another rule for the management of these kinds of lesions listed at the end of this chapter.

III. Spitzoid melanoma: In general, spitzoid melanoma follows the dermatoscopic rule of asymmetry, resulting from an uneven distribution of colors and structures and/or a multicomponent pattern. Therefore, most spitzoid melanomas are dermatoscopically recognizable (Figure 9.44). However, less frequently, spitzoid melanoma may display a perfect dermatoscopic symmetry,

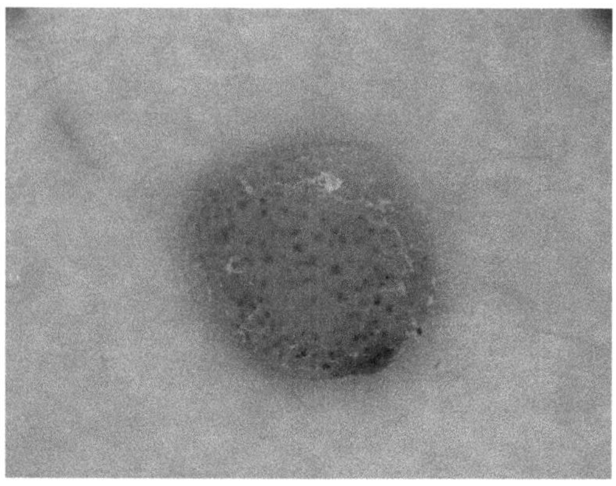

FIGURE 9.39 Spitz nevus: Multiple dotted vessels surrounded by white color.

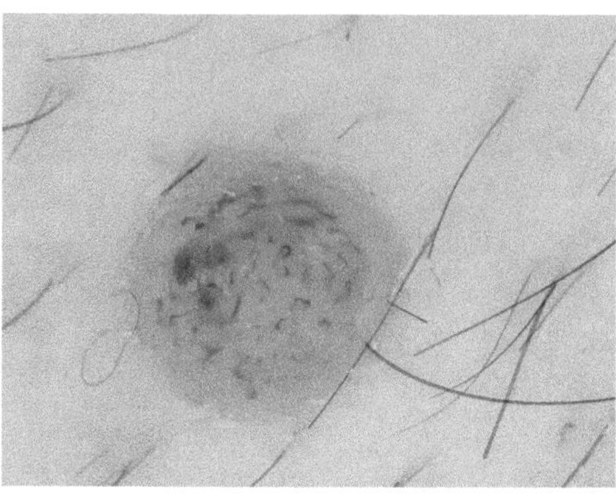

FIGURE 9.40 Dermatoscopy of a nodular Spitz nevus reveals "comma" vessels or "hairpin" vessels or even linear irregular vessels, always surrounded by white color.

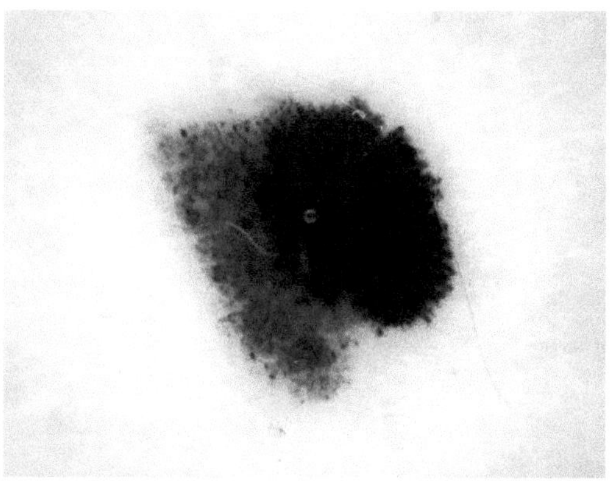

FIGURE 9.41 An atypical Spitz nevus dermatoscopically looking like melanoma.

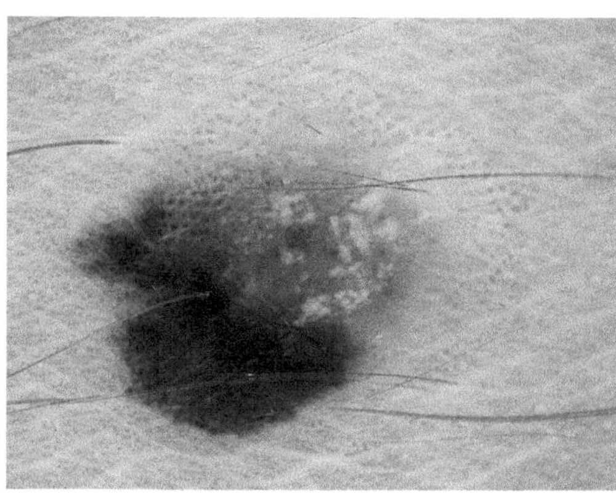

FIGURE 9.42 An atypical Spitz nevus dermatoscopically resembling melanoma.

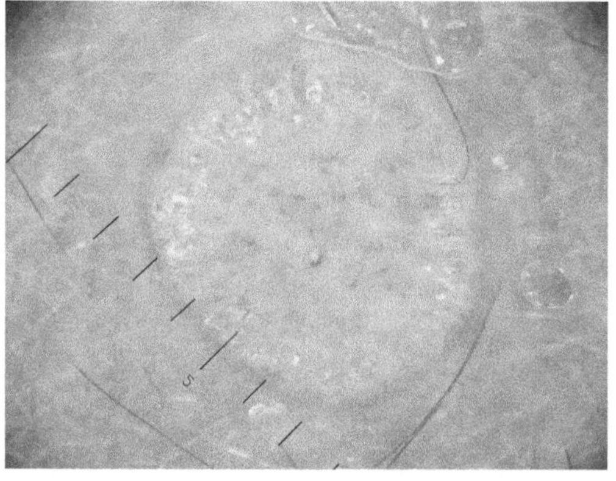

FIGURE 9.43 An atypical Spitz nevus dermatoscopically identical to a nonpigmented Spitz nevus.

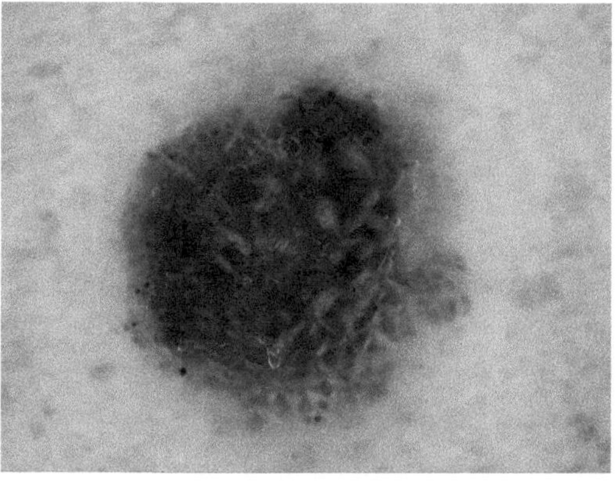

FIGURE 9.44 A spitzoid melanoma is dermatoscopically characterized by a multicomponent pattern, multiple globules, and white shiny lines.

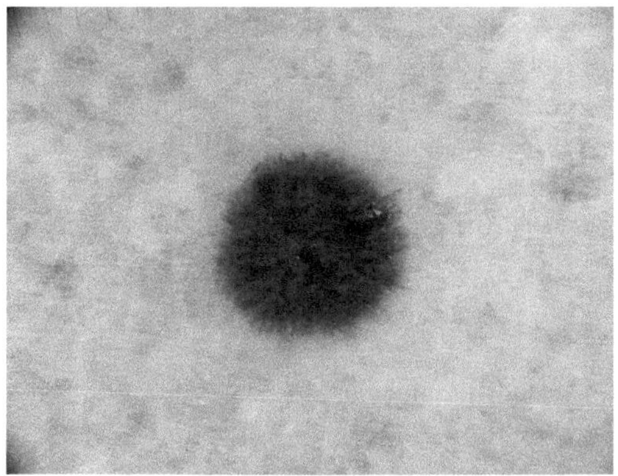

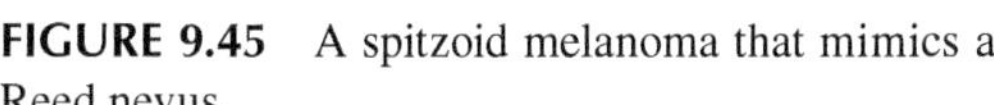

FIGURE 9.45 A spitzoid melanoma that mimics a Reed nevus.

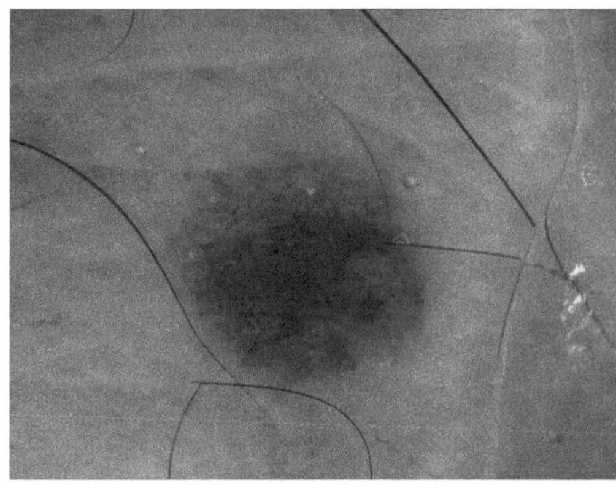

FIGURE 9.46 A spitzoid melanoma with multiple globules surrounded by a white network "masquerading" as a Spitz nevus.

mimicking one of the three previously mentioned patterns of Reed nevi (Figures 9.45 and 9.46). The possibility of a symmetrical "spitzoid" lesion being a melanoma depends strongly on age and remains close to zero until the age of 12–15 years. Afterward, it gradually rises according to age, reaching 50% after the age of 50 years and 100% after the age of 70 years. Obviously, this morphological overlap between Spitz nevi and spitzoid melanoma impacts crucially on the guidelines for the management of spitzoid lesions.

Guidelines for the Management of Spitzoid-Looking Lesions

1. All lesions displaying spitzoid characteristics (i.e., peripheral streaks/pseudopods/reticular depigmentation/dotted vessels) that are distributed asymmetrically should be excised in order to rule out melanoma. All the previously mentioned features, when asymmetrically distributed, should be considered as melanoma-specific criteria.
2. All nodular lesions exhibiting spitzoid features should be excised even in the case of symmetric distribution and irrespective of the age of the patient. This recommendation is based on the fact that 20% of atypical spitzoid tumors appear as symmetric nodules both clinically and dermatoscopically.
3. After the age of 12 years, all dermatoscopically spitzoid-looking lesions, even if they are flat and symmetric, should be excised. This management recommendation is based on the considerable probability of such a lesion to be a melanoma. This possibility increases significantly with age.
4. Flat/raised lesions with symmetrically distributed spitzoid features developing in patients younger than 12 years of age, at the time of the first consultation, can be managed conservatively. This recommendation is based on the extremely low possibility of such a lesion to be a melanoma. Until recently, the general guideline for patients of this age group was the sequential monitoring of the lesion until its morphological stabilization. However, several recent studies suggested that the strategy of monitoring Spitz/Reed nevi is not effective because it will lead to a considerable number of unnecessary excisions. This results from the dynamic biological potential of Spitz/Reed nevi: they often grow very rapidly and occasionally asymmetrically, causing a "false" concern for physicians and parents (Figure 9.21). Therefore, theoretically, flat symmetric spitzoid-looking

lesions in children do not require any particular management. However, in real life, the presence of such a dynamically evolving lesion is likely to create a lot of anxiety for patients and their families, even if evidence suggests that the risk of melanoma is practically zero. Therefore, most probably physicians will continue monitoring spitzoid lesions in children despite the fact that it seems to not be really necessary. It is useful though to inform the patients and their parents that the monitoring procedure is likely to lead to an unnecessary surgical excision.

9.3 Management of Patients with Multiple Common Nevi and/or Clinically Atypical Nevi

A usual clinical scenario is an individual with multiple common nevi (more than 100), as well as patients suffering from atypical nevi syndrome. Both of them represent risk factors for the development of melanoma. The risk in these patients is attributed to their genetic predisposition of developing melanoma that usually arises *de novo* (70%–80%) and less frequently on a preexisting common or "dysplastic" nevus. This means that prophylactic excision of their nevi does not decrease their risk of melanoma, while it increases morbidity and cost. Consequently, the dual goal during the management of these patients is the early detection of possible new melanomas, while minimizing the unnecessary excisions of benign lesions.

Comparative Approach and Digital Imaging and Monitoring

The common practice is to perform a total-body clinical examination using both the naked eye and the dermatoscope during the first visit of the patient. If a single lesion with clinical and/or dermatoscopic features suspicious for melanoma is detected, an immediate surgical excision should be performed. If no suspicious lesion is found, or if more than one suspicious lesion are present (a common scenario in individuals with atypical nevi syndrome), digital imaging/monitoring is indicated, which includes two steps:

1. *Total-body clinical photography*: Clinical imaging is extremely important for the monitoring procedure, since it gives the opportunity to compare clinical images captured in a previous visit with those of the next follow-up visit, contributing this way to the detection of any newly arisen lesion.
2. *Dermatoscopic digital imaging*: In this step, digital dermatoscopic images of all the nevi larger than 2 mm in diameter should be captured and stored topographically (body mapping), using compatible software. The software is designed to facilitate the comparative evaluation of the lesions and to highlight lesions with a totally different, as compared to others, dermatoscopic pattern ("ugly duckling sign"). The value of the comparative approach is based on the observation that in each individual the majority of its nevi display a similar dermatoscopic pattern, while melanoma displays different characteristics that are helpful to distinguish it among the multiple, similar-looking, benign lesions (Figure 9.47). The comparison helps us detect the morphologically different, rather than the most "atypical," lesion (Figure 9.48). If a lesion that significantly differs from the others is found, immediate excision, or short-term (3–4 months) follow-up should be performed. It must be underlined though, that only flat lesions are good candidates for follow-up, whereas a doubtful nodule should never be monitored but instead excised. This is also the case in lesions undergoing regression.

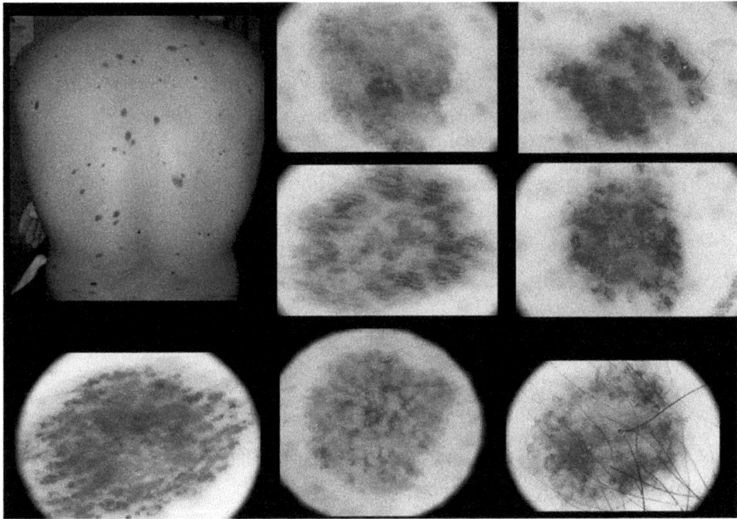

FIGURE 9.47 A patient with multiple nevi that all display dermatoscopic atypia, but their patterns are similar. No lesion looks different from the others.

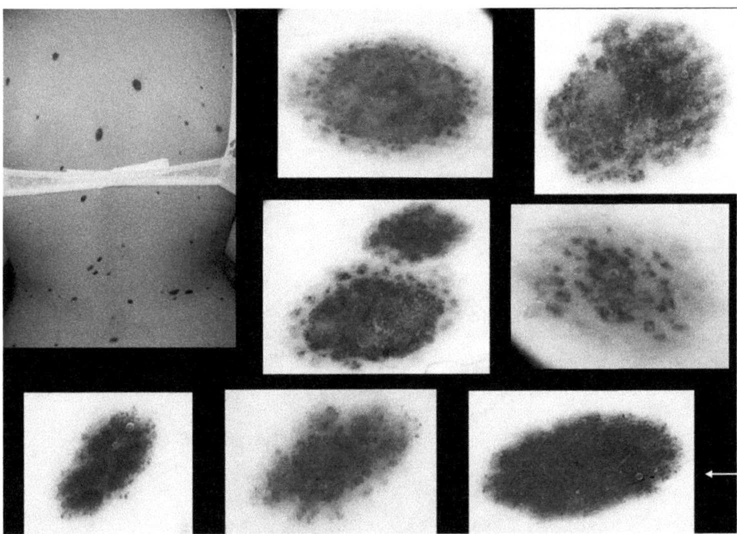

FIGURE 9.48 This is a patient with multiple atypical nevi. All but one lesion (arrow) share a similar dermatoscopic pattern. This lesion was excised, and the diagnosis was melanoma.

Apart from individuals with multiple (greater than 100) nevi, or "atypical nevi syndrome," other indications for digital monitoring are those with a personal or family history of melanoma, as well as immunocompromised patients.

Prospective Monitoring

After completion of the aforementioned procedure, and in case there are no suspicious lesions posing diagnostic dilemmas, the next visit should be scheduled. The time interval between two sequential "mole mapping" visits is not prefixed, and it is usually individualized based on the risk factors of each patient. A reasonable time interval for digital monitoring is once per year.

During the follow-up visit, total-body clinical and dermatoscopic imaging should be performed, as well as comparative evaluation of the new photos with the previous ones. It has been shown that 10% of all melanomas diagnosed via digital monitoring do not display any melanoma-specific morphological criteria at the time of diagnosis, and their detection is based exclusively on the changes found during the prospective follow-up. Morphological changes that raise the suspicion of melanoma and justify the excision of a lesion are as follows:

1. The presence of a new pigmented lesion in an individual over 50 years of age that does not display dermatoscopic characteristics suggestive of seborrheic keratosis or solar lentigo but exhibits features of a melanocytic tumor (i.e., pigment network or globules). This recommendation is based on the epidemiology of melanocytic tumors and more specifically on the extremely low possibility of the appearance of new nevi after the age of 50 years (Figures 9.49 and 9.50).
2. Any dermatoscopic change of a melanocytic lesion during a short-term follow-up (3 months). It is well known that contrary to melanoma, nevi do not change rapidly. This means that evolution of a melanocytic lesion within 3 months is by definition suspicious (Figure 9.51).

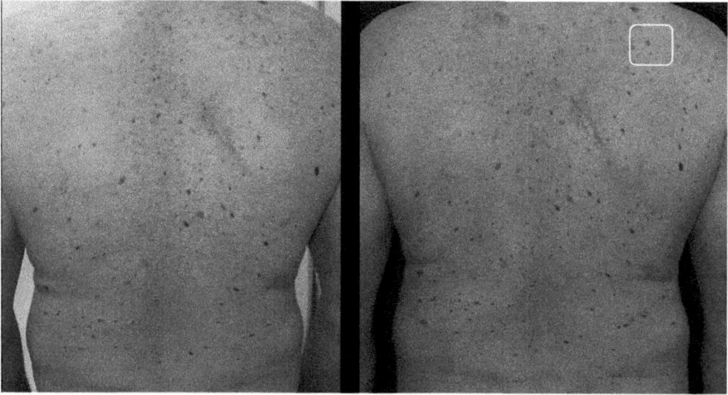

FIGURE 9.49 The total-body photography of a 60-year-old patient in the follow-up visit revealed a new lesion that did not preexist.

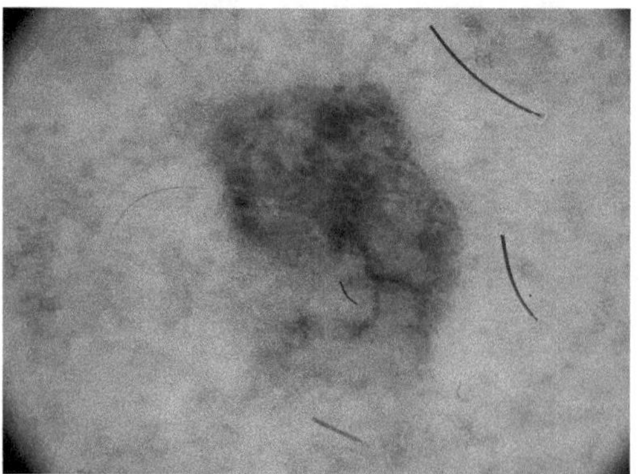

FIGURE 9.50 The lesion of Figure 9.49 displays dermatoscopic features suggestive of a melanocytic tumor (globules). Histopathology confirmed the diagnosis of melanoma.

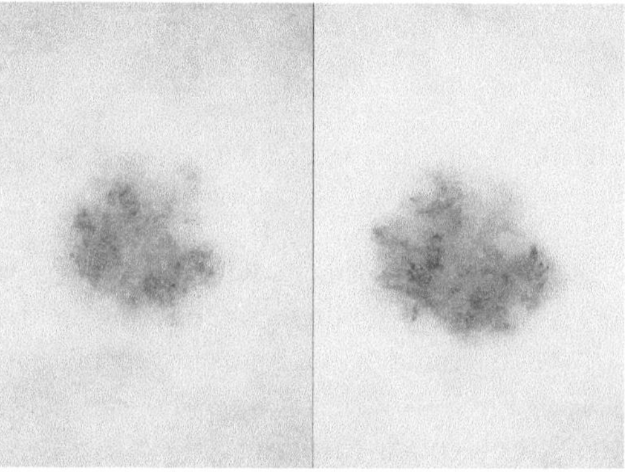

FIGURE 9.51 The prominent increase in size of this lesion in a period of 3 months necessitates its excision.

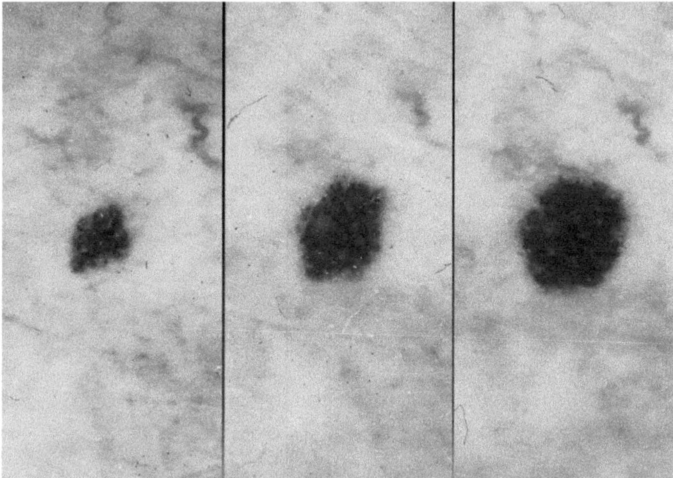

FIGURE 9.52 In a 65-year-old patient, a gradual increase in the size of a lesion in a period of 6 and 12 months is observed. The excision of the lesion is mandatory.

3. Any change in the dermatoscopic image of a melanocytic lesion in a patient over the age of 40 years, with the exception of a symmetric (from the center to the periphery), gradual regression of the lesion (Figure 9.52). This recommendation is based on the knowledge of the biologic evolution of nevi throughout the lifetime. Analytically, after the age of 40 years, nevi stop growing and they remain stable. After the fifth decade, the majority of the acquired nevi gradually involute and disappear.
4. The asymmetric growth of a lesion in any age. This recommendation is based on the observation that benign melanocytic nevi, even during their phase of evolution (early in life), grow in a symmetric manner toward all directions. Opposed to that, melanomas are characterized by asymmetric growth (Figure 9.53).

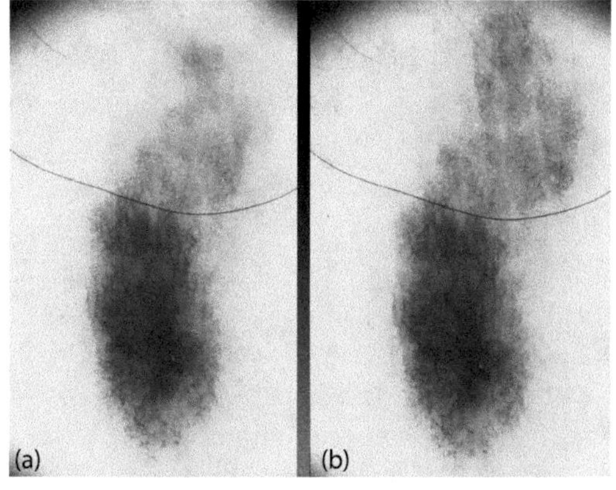

FIGURE 9.53 The asymmetric growth of a lesion, irrespective of age, is suspicious of melanoma, (a) earlier (b) later.

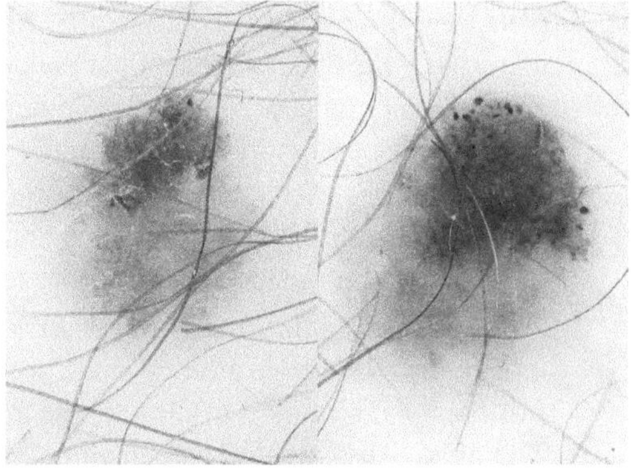

FIGURE 9.54 A lesion that exhibits dermatoscopic criteria (globules) that did not preexist is suspicious for melanoma.

5. The development of dermatoscopic criteria that did not preexist, such as radial lines or globules (Figure 9.54). The only exception is the development of a central hyperpigmented area without any structures, which results after ultraviolet exposure, and it is an expected physical phenomenon.

9.4 Seven Rules to Not Miss Melanoma

Our dual goal in everyday clinical practice should be the detection of all possible melanomas, while minimizing the unnecessary surgical excisions of benign lesions. The number of benign lesions excised in the effort to detect melanoma varies according to the training of the physician. The proportion of benign/malignant lesions has been reported to be 20–40/1 and 5–15/1 for a nontrained and a trained physician, respectively. As a result, the expertise of a dermatologist is not judged only by the number of melanomas they manage to diagnose but also by the number of benign lesions they recognize.

Most melanomas can be easily diagnosed by the ABCD clinical rule and the help of dermatoscopy. However, melanomas lacking clinical and dermatoscopic criteria exist. These "featureless" melanomas resemble benign lesions and may escape detection. In order to minimize this risk, a more holistic approach should be applied, taking into consideration not only the morphology of the tumor but also the epidemiological characteristics of the patient. Seven simple and practical rules are analyzed, aiming to help clinicians minimize the risk of missing melanoma.

1. *Examination of All Lesions.* The most important advantage of dermatoscopy is the fact that it can reveal clinically "occult" melanomas. In order to benefit from it, we should dermatoscopically examine all lesions, even those that are not clinically suspicious. If dermatoscopy is applied only on tumors that are suspicious from a clinical aspect, then, by definition, the "innocent" looking melanomas will never be examined and recognized. In contrast, the dermatoscopic examination is particularly useful for the detection of clinically inconspicuous melanomas, because the dermatoscopic criteria of melanoma almost always precede the clinical ones (Figure 9.55). This rule is particularly relevant for the management of patients with multiple melanocytic lesions among which a melanoma might be "hiding." The dermatoscopic examination of all lesions usually allows for the recognition of the suspicious one (Figure 9.56). An argument against this rule is that it is extremely time-consuming. However, it has been proven that with the appropriate training and experience and by using polarized noncontact dermatoscopy, the additional time needed is no more than 2 minutes.
2. *Total-Body Examination of High-Risk Patients.* It is well-known that a number of melanomas are located on covered body areas (Figure 9.57). As a consequence, the full-body examination of all patients and especially the high-risk ones is mandatory. The high-risk patient groups include older individuals (>60 years), individuals with fair skin type, and those with a history of skin cancer. At a younger age, the presence of multiple melanocytic nevi (>50) is considered as the strongest risk factor for melanoma development. It has been found that individuals with 20 or more nevi on the arms are very likely to have a high total nevus count; thus, a total-body examination is mandatory (Figure 9.58). Therefore, a simple inspection of the arms can help clinicians recognize this high-risk group.

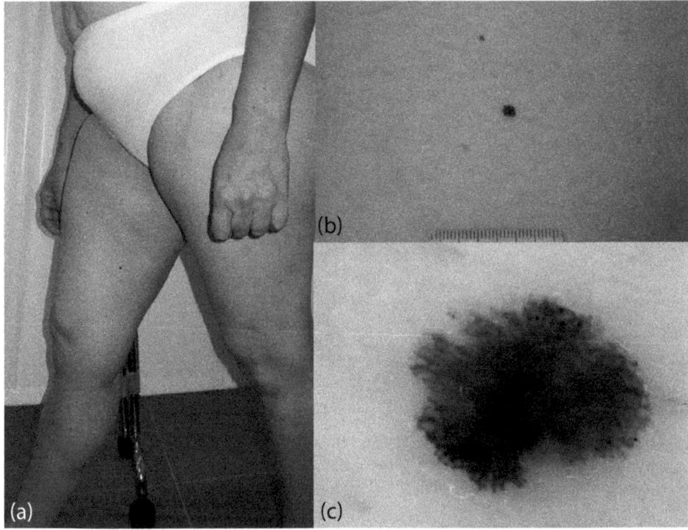

FIGURE 9.55 This is a small lesion (diameter 2 mm) in the inner surface of the thigh of a 65-year-old patient (a), which clinically is not suspicious (b). However, the dermatoscopic examination (c) uncovered its morphological asymmetry by revealing atypical network and globules.

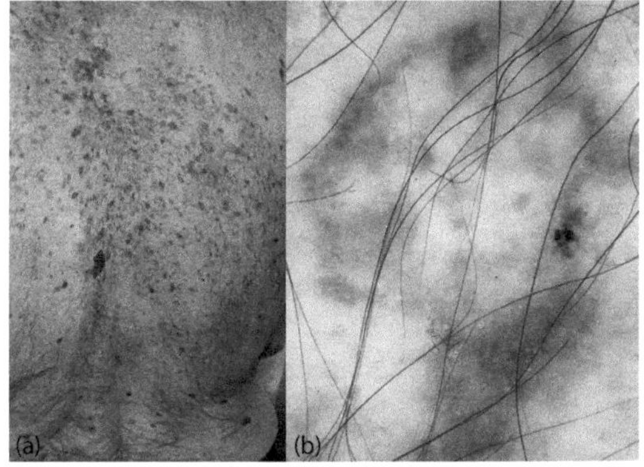

FIGURE 9.56 This is a melanoma "hidden" among multiple nevi and seborrheic keratoses (a). However, if dermatoscopically examined, the diagnosis becomes feasible (b).

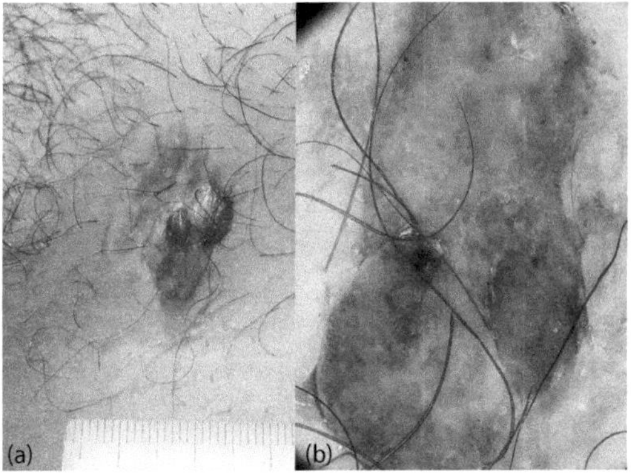

FIGURE 9.57 This is a melanoma located in the inguinal fold. Both in terms of clinical (a) and dermatoscopic (b) examination, its diagnosis is not difficult; however, it could have escaped detection without total-body examination.

In summary, total-body examination is recommended for everybody, but its application is mandatory for individuals belonging to the following categories: (a) those with a personal history of any kind of skin cancer or family history of melanoma (first-degree relatives), (b) individuals older than 50 years with more than 20 nevi in the arms, and (c) individuals older than 50 years with clinical signs of photoaging.

3. *Use of the 10-Second Rule in Single Lesions.* The majority of benign and malignant tumors are characterized by morphological patterns that are easily recognizable if one has seen them several times in the past. The dermatoscopic recognition of these common patterns, after adequate training and cxperience, requires only a few seconds.

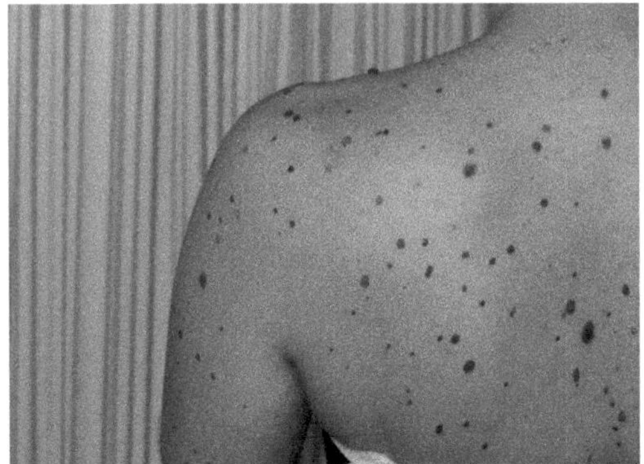

FIGURE 9.58 The presence of more than 20 nevi on the arms is indicative of the presence of multiple nevi also on the trunk.

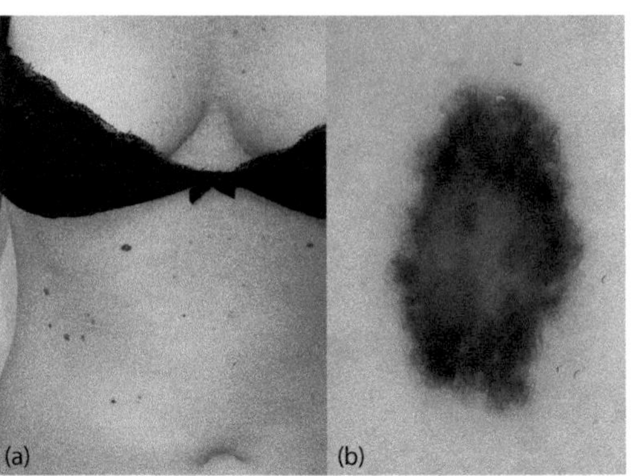

FIGURE 9.59 A clinically atypical pigmented lesion (a). This lesion exhibits central hypopigmentation and focal hyperpigmentation at the periphery (b). These criteria are not enough to definitely diagnose either a nevus or a melanoma. However, given the fact that it is the only atypical lesion of this patient, its immediate excision is the safest choice.

This notion has led to the "10-second rule," which suggests that lesions requiring more time to be diagnosed should be considered as morphologically equivocal. The management of these lesions includes two options, immediate excision or short-term follow-up in 3–4 months in order to evaluate the morphological evolution (Figure 9.59).

4. *Comparative Examination and Monitoring of Multiple Lesions.* The diagnostic approach and management of patients with multiple nevi are discussed in detail in Section 9.3.
5. *Excision of Doubtful Nodular Lesions.* Clinically, nodular melanomas usually deviate from the classic ABCD clinical rule and often mimic benign tumors (dermal nevi, vascular tumors, seborrheic keratosis, or dermatofibroma). In addition, the classic dermatoscopic criteria of superficial spreading melanoma are usually absent (see Chapter 3). For these reasons, the only safe strategy to manage nodular lesions is summarized as follows:

   When evaluating a nodular lesion, one should look for dermatoscopic criteria suggestive of benign tumors, and when a definite specific diagnosis of a benign tumor is not feasible, then the lesion must be excised. Follow-up of nodular lesions is strongly discouraged.

6. *Combination of Dermatoscopy with Clinical and Epidemiological Parameters.* The clinical diagnostic approach of melanocytic lesions is based on the coevaluation of clinical and dermatoscopic morphology, the characteristics of the patient, and the epidemiology of the tumors. Usually, these parameters are in accordance one to each other. For example, the lesion in Figure 9.60 looks both clinically and dermatoscopically like a nevus, and the age of the individual is 25 years. Therefore, clinical morphology, dermatoscopic morphology, and epidemiological characteristics are all in accordance to the diagnosis of a nevus. In contrast, when the aforementioned parameters lead to contradicting conclusions, the lesions must be treated with caution. For example, the lesion in Figure 9.61 clinically and dermoscopically resembles a nevus. However, the age of the patient (85 years old) and the history of the recent appearance of the lesion are not compatible with the diagnosis of a nevus. This "disharmony" between clinical and

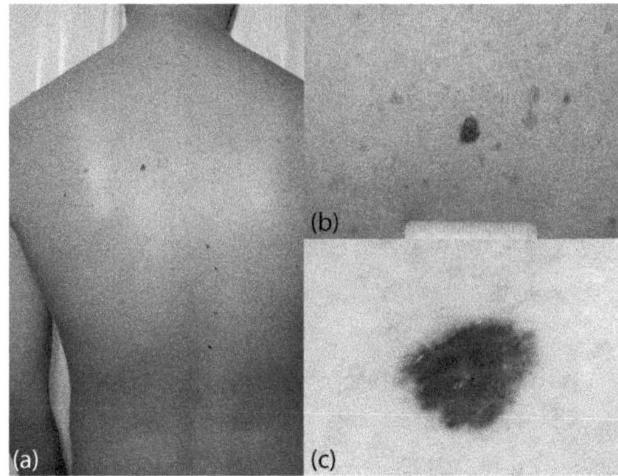

FIGURE 9.60 This is a rather small and symmetrical melanocytic tumor in clinical terms (a,b), which on dermatoscopy is characterized by central hyperpigmentation and peripheral network (c). Overall and given the age of the patient (25 years), the diagnosis of a nevus is quite confident.

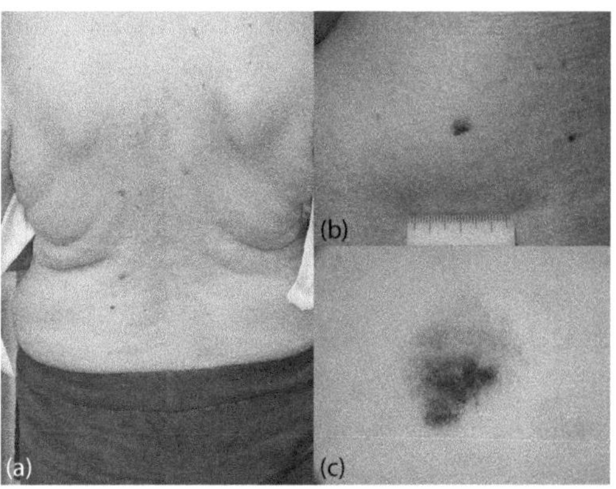

FIGURE 9.61 Clinically, this is a rather small melanocytic tumor (a,b) that dermatoscopically is characterized by a pigmented network with mild atypia (c). The morphology could be compatible with the diagnosis of a nevus, but the fact that the patient is 85 years old and this lesion did not exist in the previous examination renders the lesion suspicious for melanoma.

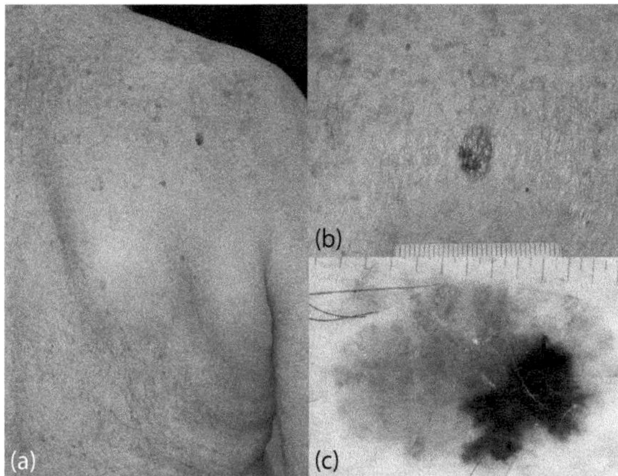

FIGURE 9.62 The clinical (a,b) and the dermatoscopic image of the lesion (c) is highly suggestive of a melanoma developing on a preexisting nevus. However, the first histopathologic report concluded the diagnosis of a nevus. A clinicopathologic consultation revealed that due to some technical sectioning issues, the histopathologic diagnosis of melanoma could not be made in the first place.

epidemiological data should raise concern, although clear-cut dermatoscopic criteria of melanoma are not present.

7. *Combination of Clinical and Histopathologic Criteria.* Histopathologic examination is considered as the gold standard for the diagnosis of melanocytic lesions. Histopathology, however, is not free of limitations, such as technical failures and misinterpretations. Apart from technical issues, which are not rare, there are some lesions that are per se histopathologically equivocal. Characteristic examples are the spitzoid tumors, who se evaluation is practically impossible without considering

the age of the patient. Clinicians should consider that, as a rule, a clinically and dermatoscopically difficult lesion will also be difficult in terms of histopathology, especially if the pathologist does not have adequate clinical information. In conclusion, the histopathologic reports should be interpreted within the context of clinical information. Lesions lacking a satisfactory clinicopathologic correlation must be managed with caution (Figure 9.62).

BIBLIOGRAPHY

Akay BN, Kocyigit P, Heper AO, Erdem C. Dermatoscopy of flat pigmented facial lesions: Diagnostic challenge between pigmented actinic keratosis and lentigo maligna. *Br J Dermatol.* 2010;163:1212–7.

Carrera C, Scope A, Dusza SW et al. Clinical and dermoscopic characterization of pediatric and adolescent melanomas: Multicenter study of 52 cases. *J Am Acad Dermatol.* 2018;78:278–88.

Coit DG, Andtbacka R, Anker CJ et al. Melanoma, version 2.2013: Featured updates to the NCCN guidelines. *J Natl Compr Canc Netw.* 2013;11:395–407.

Forman SB, Ferringer TC, Peckham SJ et al. Is superficial spreading melanoma still the most common form of malignant melanoma? *J Am Acad Dermatol.* 2008;58:1013–20.

Lallas A, Apalla Z, Chaidemenos G. New trends in dermoscopy to minimize the risk of missing melanoma. *J Skin Cancer.* 2012;7:1–5.

Lallas A, Apalla Z, Ioannides D et al. Update on dermoscopy of Spitz/Reed naevi and management guidelines by the International Dermoscopy Society. *Br J Dermatol.* 2017;177:645–55.

Lallas A, Argenziano G, Moscarella E et al. Diagnosis and management of facial pigmented macules. *Clin Dermatol.* 2014;32:94–100.

Lallas A, Moscarella E, Longo C et al. Likelihood of finding melanoma when removing a Spitzoid-looking lesion in patients aged 12 years or older. *J Am Acad Dermatol.* 2015;72:47–53.

Lallas A, Tschandl P, Kyrgidis A et al. Dermoscopic clues to differentiate facial lentigo maligna from pigmented actinic keratosis. *Br J Dermatol.* 2016;174:1079–85.

Lallas A, Zalaudek I, Apalla Z et al. Management rules to detect melanoma. *Dermatology.* 2013;226:52–60.

McGovern VJ, Cochran AJ, Van der Esch EP et al. The classification of malignant melanoma, its histological reporting and registration: A revision of the 1972 Sydney classification. *Pathology.* 1986;18:12–21.

Moscarella E, Lallas A, Kyrgidis A et al. Clinical and dermoscopic features of atypical Spitz tumors: A multicenter, retrospective, case-control study. *J Am Acad Dermatol.* 2015;73:777–84.

Pock L, Drlík L, Hercogová J. Dermatoscopy of pigmented actinic keratosis – A striking similarity to lentigo maligna. *Int J Dermatol.*2007;46:414–6.

Pralong P, Bathelier E, Dalle S et al. Dermoscopy of lentigo maligna melanoma: Report of 125 cases. *Br J Dermatol.* 2012;167:280–7.

Schiffner R, Schiffner-Rohe J, Vogt T et al. Improvement of early recognition of lentigo maligna using dermatoscopy. *J Am Dermatol.* 2000;42:25–32.

Tschandl P, Gambardella A, Boespflug A et al. Seven non-melanoma features of facial lesions: A dermatoscopy algorithm to rule out melanoma. *Acta Derm Venereol.* 2017;97:1219–24.

Tschandl P, Rosendahl C, Kittler H. Dermatoscopy of flat pigmented facial lesions. *J Eur Acad Dermatol Venereol.* 2015;29:120–7.

Welch HG, Black WC. Overdiagnosis in cancer. *J Natl Cancer Inst.* 2010;102:605–13.

Zalaudek I, Grinschgl S, Argenziano G et al. Age-related prevalence of dermoscopy patterns in acquired melanocytic naevi. *Br J Dermatol.* 2006;154:299–304.

Zalaudek I, Lallas A, Longo C et al. Problematic lesions in the elderly. *Dermatol Clin.* 2013;31:549–64; vii–viii.

Index

A

AA, *see* Alopecia areata
ABCD clinical rule, 41; *see also* Melanoma
Acanthoma, clear cell, 85, 86; *see also* Benign nonmelanocytic skin tumors
ACC, *see* Aplasia cutis
Acquired perforating dermatoses, 124; *see also* Inflammatory skin diseases
Acral melanoma (AM), 52; *see also* Melanoma
  and acral nevus, 54
  advanced palmar, 53
  advanced plantar, 54
  dermatoscopic features, 53
  diagnostic algorithm, 56
  early plantar melanoma, 53
  palmar nevus, 54
  parallel ridge pattern, 56
  subungual hemorrhage, 54
Acral nevus, 24, 26; *see also* Nevus
  and acral melanoma, 54
  congenital, 27
  double-line pattern, 55
  fibrillar pattern, 55
  lattice-like pattern, 55
  parallel furrow pattern of, 55
  peas-in-a-pod pattern, 55
Actinic keratoses (AKs), 68, 96, 116, 175; *see also* Keratinocyte skin cancer
  field cancerization, 96
  grade I, 97
  grade II, 97, 98
  grade III, 97, 98
  multiple, 97
  nonmelanoma criteria of pigmented, 171
  pigmented, 53, 98, 99
  progression into invasive SCC, 104
  rosettes in, 98
  strawberry pattern, 96
Actinic lentigo, *see* Solar lentigo
Adnexal tumors, 84; *see also* Benign nonmelanocytic skin tumors
  eccrine poroma, 84, 85
  sebaceous hyperplasia, 84, 85
AFX, *see* Atypical fibroxanthoma
AGA, *see* Androgenetic alopecia
AKs, *see* Actinic keratoses
Alopecia, 144; *see also* Trichoscopy
  christmas tree pattern, 145
  noncicatricial, 144–154
  primary cicatricial, 154–159
  temporal triangular, 159–160
  trichoscopy, 144
Alopecia areata (AA), 147; *see also* Noncicatricial alopecias
  broken hairs and black dots, 150, 151
  circle hairs in, 150
  clinical presentation, 147
  diffuse, 149
  exclamation mark hairs in, 149, 150
  patch-type, 149
  pigtail hairs and yellow dots, 150
  trichoscopic diagnosis of, 148
AM, *see* Acral melanoma
Amelanotic melanoma, 66; *see also* Melanoma
  actinic keratosis, 68
  dermal sarcoma, 70
  dermatoscopic detection, 68
  dermatoscopic features, 67
  flat, 67, 69
  intraepidermal carcinoma, 68
  lichen planus–like keratosis, 69
  nodular, 64, 67, 69
  poorly differentiated squamous cell carcinoma, 69
  superficial basal cell carcinoma, 68
Androgenetic alopecia (AGA), 144; *see also* Trichoscopy
Androgenetic alopecia, 144; *see also* Noncicatricial alopecias
  christmas tree alopecia pattern, 145
  clinical examples of, 145
  frontal and occipital areas in, 147
  with perifollicular hyperpigmentation and vellus hair, 146
  trichoscopy, 146, 148, 149
Angiokeratoma, 62, 81; *see also* Vascular tumors
Angioma, cherry, 80
Angiosarcoma, 108; *see also* Malignant vascular tumors
Anogenital warts, 136; *see also* Human papillomavirus
  clinical aspect, 136
  diagnosis, 137
  multiple white-colored warts, 136
  white halos around vessels, 137
Aplasia cutis (ACC), 160–161; *see also* Trichoscopy in children
Asymmetric lesion growth, 185
Atypical
  mole syndrome, 20
  nevus on glans, 29
  pigmented lesion, 188
Atypical fibroxanthoma (AFX), 107; *see also* Malignant nonmelanocytic tumors

B

Balloon cell nevus, 35
Basal cell carcinoma (BCC), 89; *see also* Malignant nonmelanocytic tumors
  before and after treatment with imiquimod, 95, 96
  dermatoscopic criteria of, 94
  dermatoscopic pattern of, 89

Basal cell carcinoma (BCC) (*Continued*)
with evident vessels, 15
fibroepithelioma of Pinkus, 92
histopathologic subtype, 90–94
mixed, 93
nodular, 90, 95
nonpigmented, 89, 90–93
palmar pits, 95
pigmented, 42, 89–90, 92, 93
response to treatment, 94–96
sclerodermiform, 91
superficial, 68, 91, 93
Basosquamous carcinoma (BSC), 105; *see also* Malignant nonmelanocytic tumors
BCC, *see* Basal cell carcinoma
BD, *see* Bowen's disease
Beaded hair, *see* Monilethrix
Benign melanosis, 62, 63
Benign nonmelanocytic skin tumors, 75
clear cell acanthoma, 86
common adnexal tumors, 84–85
epithelial skin tumors, 75–80
tumors of fibrous tissue, 82–84
vascular tumors, 80–82
Benign tumors, 188
Blue gray nests, 8
Blue nevus, 19, 32
Bowen's disease (BD), 99–100; *see also* Keratinocyte skin cancer
BRAAFF algorithm, 56, 57; *see also* Melanoma
Branched vessels, 10, 11
BSC, *see* Basosquamous carcinoma

C

Cancer, keratinocyte skin, 96–104
Carcinoma
basal cell, 89–96
basal cell pigmented nodular, 92
basosquamous, 105
intraepidermal, 68
Merkel cell carcinoma, 106–107
nodular basal cell, 90, 95
nonpigmented basal cell, 90–93
pigmented basal cell, 42, 93
poorly differentiated squamous cell, 69
squamous cell, 100–103
superficial basal cell, 68, 91, 93
CCA, *see* Clear cell acanthoma
Central nervous system (CNS), 39
Cherry angioma, 80; *see also* Vascular tumors
Christmas tree alopecia pattern, 145
Cicatricial alopecias, primary, 154; *see also* Trichoscopy
discoid lupus erythematosus, 156–157, 158
dissecting cellulitis of scalp, 159
folliculitis decalvans, 158, 159
lichen planopilaris, 154–156
trichoscopic characteristics of, 160
Clear cell acanthoma (CCA), 85, 86; *see also* Benign nonmelanocytic skin tumors
Clinically atypical nevus, 182; *see also* Nevus
asymmetric lesion growth, 185
comparative approach and monitoring, 182–183
multiple atypical nevi, 183
multiple nevi with dermatoscopic atypia, 183
new pigmented lesion, 184
prospective monitoring, 183–186
regression of lesion, 185
Clinically atypical pigmented lesion, 188
Clinical scenarios, 169
melanoma detection rules, 186–190
multiple common nevi and/or atypical nevi management, 182–186
pigmented macules on face, 169–176
spitzoid-looking lesion management, 176–182
CM, *see* Conventional melanoma
CNS, *see* Central nervous system
Coagulated blood, 2
Coma hairs, 153
Combined nevus, 32–33; *see also* Nevus
Comma vessels, 11, 21; *see also* Nevus
Common adnexal tumors, 84–85
Common nevus, 19
Condyloma acuminatum, 136
Congenital acral nevus, 27
Congenital nevus, 23–24; *see also* Subungual melanoma
acral, 27
subungual, 59
Conventional melanoma (CM), 39; *see also* Melanoma
acral melanoma, 52–56
dermatoscopy, 40
differential diagnosis of, 40
facial melanoma, 48–52
mucosal melanoma, 60–63
subungual melanoma, 56–60
of trunk and extremities, 40–48
Corkscrew hairs, 153
Cutaneous granulomas, 3, 6
Cysts, multiple shiny milia-like, 12

D

Darier disease, 124; *see also* Inflammatory skin diseases
Demodex folliculorum, 140
Demodicosis, 139–140; *see also* Infectious skin diseases
Dermal
nevus, 25
sarcoma, 70
Dermatitis, 113; *see also* Inflammatory skin diseases
dermatoscopic image of, 114
diffuse, yellow, superficial scales in, 114
yellow clod sign, 113
Dermatofibroma (DF), 82–84
Dermatoscope, 1
Dermatoscopic ABCD rule, 47; *see also* Melanoma
Dermatoscopy, 1
basal cell carcinoma with evident vessels, 15
branched vessels, 11
cerebriform pattern consisting of gyri and sulci, 9
coagulated blood, 2
colors, 1–5, 6
comma vessels, 11

concentric structures, 9
cutaneous granulomas, 3, 6
dermatoscope, 1
dermatoscopic criteria, 14
device, 1
extracted hemoglobin in purple, 5
extravasated hemoglobin in hemorrhage, 5
extravasated plasma serum, 6
fibrosis, 2
fingerprinting, 9
hairpin vessels, 11
hemoglobin in blood vessels, 5
hypergranulosis, 6
keratoacanthoma, 6
large ulceration, 12
leaf-like areas, 8
light modes, 13–15
linear irregular vessels, 11
linear vessels, 10
location and color of hemoglobin, 4
melanin, 2, 3, 4
melanoma, 14
multiple aggregated globules, 8
multiple glomerular vessels, 10
multiple gray dots, 8
multiple peripheral streaks and pseudopods, 8
multiple round and ovoid bluegray nests, 8
multiple round or ovoid comedy-like openings, 9
multiple sharply demarcated vascular lacunes, 12
multiple shiny milia-like cysts, 12
multiple superficial small erosions, 12
multiple vessels as dots, 10
nonpigmented structures, 9–13
parameters, 1
pigmented structures, 3, 7–9
rosettes, 13
seborrheic keratosis, 14
sebum, 3, 5
spoke wheel areas, 8
structures, 5, 7–13
vessels, 2
white area without identifiable morphological structures, 10
white circles surrounding follicular openings, 12
white halos surrounding vascular structures, 12
white shiny blotches/strands, 13
white shiny streaks, 13
Dermatoses, acquired perforating, 124; *see also* Inflammatory skin diseases
DF, *see* Dermatofibroma
Diagnostic algorithm for acral melanoma, 56
Digital dermatoscopic devices, 1
Discoid lupus erythematosus (DLE), 116–117, 120, 156; *see also* Cicatricial alopecias, primary; Inflammatory skin diseases
clinical presentation of, 157
dermatoscopy of, 157
follicular plugs, 157, 158
isolated terminal hair, 157
Dissecting cellulitis of scalp, 159; *see also* Cicatricial alopecias, primary
DLE, *see* Discoid lupus erythematosus

E

Eccrine poroma, 84, 85; *see also* Adnexal tumors
Eclipse nevus, 24, 25; *see also* Nevus
Eczematous nevus, 33, 34; *see also* Nevus
Epithelial skin tumors, 75; *see also* Benign nonmelanocytic skin tumors
ink-spot lentigo, 75, 77
lichen planus–like keratosis, 80
seborrheic keratosis, 77–79
solar lentigo, 75, 76
tumors of fibrous tissue, 82–84
vascular tumors, 80–82
Erosions, superficial small, 12
Erythema and elongated linear vessels, 156
Extravasated plasma serum, 6

F

Facial melanoma, 48–52; *see also* Lentigo maligna; Melanoma
challenges in differential diagnoses, 52
dermatoscopic features, 50
differential diagnosis of facial macule, 50
nevus on elderly, 50
pigmented actinic keratosis, 53
pseudonetwork, 50
seborrheic keratosis, 53
Facial nevus, 24
Featureless melanomas, 186
Female pattern hair loss (FPHL), 144; *see also* Androgenetic alopecia; Trichoscopy
FFA, *see* Frontal fibrosing alopecia
Fibroepithelioma of Pinkus, 92
Fibrosis, 2
Fibrous histiocytoma, malignant, 107
Fibroxanthoma, atypical, 107; *see also* Malignant nonmelanocytic tumors
Field cancerization, 96
Flat seborrheic keratosis, 170
Focal hemorrhage, 153; *see also* Trichotillomania
Follicular; *see also* Discoid lupus erythematosus
plugs, 157, 158
pustules, 159
Folliculitis decalvans, 158; *see also* Cicatricial alopecias, primary
clinical presentation of, 158
dermatoscopy of, 158
perifollicular scaling and follicular pustules, 159
tufting of hair follicles, 158
FPHL, *see* Female pattern hair loss
Frontal fibrosing alopecia (FFA), 154; *see also* Cicatricial alopecias, primary
clinical presentation of, 155
subtle erythema and elongated linear vessels, 156
subtle perifollicular scale and pink-white areas, 156

G

Genital wart, 136; *see also* Anogenital warts
Genodermatosis, 161
Globular nevus, 20

Globules
multiple aggregated, 8
multiple small, 21
Graham-Little-Piccardi-Lassueur syndrome, 155; *see also* Lichen planopilaris
Granuloma annulare, 118, 119; *see also* Granulomatous skin diseases
Granulomatous skin diseases, 117; *see also* Inflammatory skin diseases
lupus vulgaris, 118
necrobiosis lipoidica, 118–119
sarcoidosis, 118
Gray dots, multiple, 8
Grover's disease, 124, 125; *see also* Inflammatory skin diseases

H

Haemorrhage, focal, 153; *see also* Trichotillomania
Hair
coiled and hook hairs, 152
flame, 152
hair dust, 152
pulling disorder, *see* Trichotillomania
regrowing, 144
shaft, 143
tufting of follicles, 158
vellus, 143, 144
Hairpin vessels, 11, 102
Hair shaft deformities, 161; *see also* Trichoscopy
monilethrix, 161, 162
pili annulati, 164
pili torti, 163–164
pseudomonilethrix, 161
trichoptilosis, 163
trichorrhexis invaginata, 162, 163
trichorrhexis nodosa, 161–162
trichoschisis, 163
Hair shaft deformities, 161–164
normal hair shaft, 143
Hairs, regrowing, 144; *see also* Trichoscopy
Halo nevus, 33, 34, 35; *see also* Nevus
Hemoglobin
in blood vessels, 5
extracted, 5
in hemorrhage, 5
location and color of, 4
Hemorrhage, subungual, 54
Histiocytoma, malignant fibrous, 107
HPV, *see* Human papillomavirus
Human papillomavirus (HPV), 136; *see also* Viral infections
anogenital warts, 136–137
common, plane, and palmoplantar warts, 137–139
Hutchinson sign, 57; *see also* Subungual melanoma
Hypergranulosis, 6
Hyperpigmented facial nevus, 25
Hyperpigmented nevus, 26; *see also* Nevus
facial, 25
Hyperplasia, sebaceous, 84, 85
Hypopigmented nevus, 22; *see also* Nevus

I

i-Hairs, 155
Infectious skin diseases, 131
demodicosis, 139–140
leishmaniasis, 140–141
parasitoses, 131–134
tick bites, 139
tinea corporis, 141
viral infections, 134–139
Inflammatory skin diseases, 111
acquired perforating dermatoses, 124
Darier disease, 124
dermatitis, 113–114
discoid lupus erythematosus, 116–117, 120
granulomatous skin diseases, 117–119
Grover's disease, 124, 125
lichen planus, 113–115
lichen sclerosus, 117
lymphomatoid papulosis, 126
mastocytosis, 122
morphea, 117
mycosis fungoides, 125
parameters to examine, 111
pigmented purpuric dermatoses, 122, 123
pityriasis lichenoides et varioliformis acuta, 123
pityriasis rosea, 115
pityriasis rubra pilaris, 122, 123
porokeratosis, 120, 121
principles, 111
prurigo nodularis, 123–124
psoriasis, 111–113
rosacea, 119, 120
trizonal concentric pattern, 124
urticarial vasculitis, 121
Ink-spot lentigo, 75, 77; *see also* Epithelial skin tumors
Intradermal nevus, 21; *see also* Nevus
Intraepidermal carcinoma, 68; *see also* Bowen's disease
Ixodes ricinus (Tick), 139

K

Kaposi sarcoma (KS), 107, 108; *see also* Malignant vascular tumors
Keratin mass
amorphous white-yellow, 101
blood spots in, 103
Keratinocyte skin cancer, 96; *see also* Malignant nonmelanocytic tumors
actinic keratosis, 96–99
AK into invasive SCC, 104
Bowen's disease, 99–100
squamous cell carcinoma, 100–103
Keratoacanthoma, 6
Keratosis; *see also* Pigmented macules on face
flat seborrheic, 170
lichen planus–like, 69, 173, 174
seborrheic, 14, 42, 171, 172, 173, 175
KS, *see* Kaposi sarcoma

L

LAHS, *see* Loose anagen hair syndrome
Leishmaniasis, 140–141; *see also* Infectious skin diseases
Lentigo, ink-spot, 75, 77
Lentigo maligna (LM), 48, 49, 50, 51, 52, 75, 169, 175; *see also* Facial melanoma; Pigmented macules on face
  advanced, 49, 51
  advanced stage, 170
  dermatoscopic features of, 169
  dermatoscopic progression model of, 52
  discrepancy in diagnosis, 169
  early, 49, 170
  flat pigmented lesions on face, 170
  gray follicular circles, 51
  sequential criteria of, 50
Lentigo maligna melanoma (LMM), 39, 48; *see also* Melanoma
  dermoscopic criteria for, 51
Lesions; *see also* Spitzoid-looking lesion
  comparative examination, 188
  excision of nodular, 188
  on face, 170
  management, 176–182
  in patient under treatment with biologic agent, 113
  psoriatic scalp, 112
Lichen planopilaris (LPP), 154; *see also* Cicatricial alopecias, primary
  clinical presentation of, 155
  Graham-Little-Piccardi-Lassueur syndrome, 155
  perifollicular and tubular scaling of, 156
  trichoscopic feature in, 155–156
  trichoscopy of classic, 156
Lichen planus (LP), 80, 113; *see also* Inflammatory skin diseases
  blue-gray granules in chronic, 115
  located on palms and soles, 114
  Wickham striae, 115
Lichen planus-like keratosis (LPLK), 69, 75, 80, 173, 174; *see also* Epithelial skin tumors; Pigmented macules on face
Lichen sclerosus (LS), 117; *see also* Inflammatory skin diseases
Linear-irregular vessels, 11, 102
Linear vessels, 10
  irregular, 11, 102
LM, *see* Lentigo maligna
LMM, *see* Lentigo maligna melanoma
Loose anagen hair syndrome (LAHS), 160; *see also* Trichoscopy in children
LP, *see* Lichen planus
LPLK, *see* Lichen planus-like keratosis
LPP, *see* Lichen planopilaris
LS, *see* Lichen sclerosus
Lupus erythematosus, discoid, 156–157, 158
Lupus vulgaris, 118; *see also* Granulomatous skin diseases
Lymphomatoid papulosis, 126; *see also* Inflammatory skin diseases

M

Macules on face, pigmented, 169–176
Male pattern hair loss (MPHL), 144; *see also* Androgenetic alopecia; Trichoscopy
Malignant fibrous histiocytoma (MFH), 107; *see also* Malignant nonmelanocytic tumors
Malignant nonmelanocytic tumors, 89
  atypical fibroxanthoma, 107
  basal cell carcinoma, 89–96
  basosquamous carcinoma, 105
  keratinocyte skin cancer, 96–104
  malignant fibrous histiocytoma, 107
  malignant vascular tumors, 107–108
  Merkel cell carcinoma, 106–107
Malignant vascular tumors, 107; *see also* Malignant nonmelanocytic tumors
  angiosarcoma, 108
  kaposi sarcoma, 107, 108
Mastocytosis, 122; *see also* Inflammatory skin diseases
MC, *see* Molluscum contagiosum
MCC, *see* Merkel cell carcinoma
Melanin, 2, 3, 4
Melanocytic
  nevus, 17
  tumor, 189
  tumors of nail apparatus, 28
Melanoma, 14, 39
  acral, 52–56
  in advanced stage, 41
  algorithm, 46
  amelanotic, 66–70
  atypical pigment network, 43
  blue-white veil, 45
  characteristics, 41
  checklist, 47
  classifications, 39
  clinical types of, 39–40
  conventional, 40
  dermatoscopic criteria for, 43
  dermatoscopic features, 42
  dermatoscopic rule, 47
  detected using BRAAFF algorithm, 57
  detection rule, 41
  early stage, 40
  eccentrically located blotch, 44
  facial melanoma, 48–52
  in situ, 48, 49
  in later stage, 41
  Menzies' method, 47
  mucosal melanoma, 60–63
  nodular melanoma, 63–66
  pattern analysis algorithm, 42, 46
  peripheral streaks and pseudopods, 44
  pigmented basal cell carcinoma, 42
  plantar, 57, 58
  polymorphous vascular pattern, 45
  regression in, 44
  seborrheic keratosis, 42
  streaks visible with polarized light, 45
  subungual melanoma, 56–60
  of trunk and extremities, 40–48

Melanoma detection rules, 186
  atypical pigmented lesion, 188
  clinical and histopathologic criteria, 189–190
  comparative examination and multiple lesion monitoring, 188
  dermatoscopic examination, 186, 187
  dermatoscopy and epidemiological parameters, 188–189
  featureless melanomas, 186
  lesion examination, 186
  multiple nevi, 188
  nodular lesion excision, 188
  small melanocytic tumor, 189
  10-second rule in single lesions, 187–188
  total-body examination, 186–187
Melanoma, nodular amelanotic, 64, 67, 69
Melanosis, 61; *see also* Melanoma
  benign, 62, 63
  of mucosa, 62
Menzies' method, 47; *see also* Melanoma
Merkel cell carcinoma (MCC), 106–107; *see also* Malignant nonmelanocytic tumors
Meyerson phenomenon, 33; *see also* Nevus
MF, *see* Mycosis fungoides
MFH, *see* Malignant fibrous histiocytoma
Milia-like cysts, shiny, 12
Mole syndrome, atypical, 20; *see also* Nevus
Molluscum contagiosum (MC), 134; *see also* Viral infections
  clinical aspect of, 135
  dermatoscopic aspect of, 135
  differential diagnosis of, 135
Monilethrix, 161, 162; *see also* Hair shaft deformities
Morphea, 117; *see also* Inflammatory skin diseases
Morse-code hairs, 154
MPHL, *see* Male pattern hair loss
Mucosal melanoma, 60; *see also* Melanoma
  angiokeratoma, 62
  benign melanosis, 62, 63
  differential diagnoses of, 61
  in lower lip, 62
  melanosis of mucosa, 62
  nevus, 62
  parallel lines pattern, 62
  structureless pattern, 62
Mucosal nevus, 28
Multiple
  aggregated globules, 8
  atypical nevi, 183
  common nevi, 182–186
  gray dots, 8
  nevi with dermatoscopic atypia, 183
  peripheral streaks and pseudopods, 8
  round and ovoid bluegray nests, 8
  round or ovoid comedy-like openings, 9
  sharply demarcated vascular lacunes, 12
  shiny milia-like cysts, 12
  superficial small erosions, 12
  vessels as dots, 10
Mycosis fungoides (MF), 125; *see also* Inflammatory skin diseases

N

Necrobiosis lipoidica, 118–119; *see also* Granulomatous skin diseases
Netherton syndrome, 162
Nevus, 17; *see also* Pigmented macules on face
  acral, 24, 26
  acral congenital, 27
  atypical, 20, 29
  balloon cell, 35
  blue, 19, 32
  classifications of, 17
  cobblestone pattern, 21, 23
  combined, 32–33
  comma vessels, 21
  common, 19
  congenital, 23–24
  congenital acral, 27
  dermal, 25
  dermatoscopic pattern of, 18
  double-line parallel furrow pattern, 26
  eclipse, 24, 25
  eczematous, 33, 34
  on elderly face, 50
  evolution of spitz, 31–32
  facial, 24
  fibrillar pattern, 27
  on glans, 29
  globular, 18, 20, 22
  with globules, 21
  halo, 33, 34, 35
  hyperpigmented, 25, 26
  hypopigmented, 22
  intradermal, 21
  lattice-like pattern, 27
  linear branched vessels, 22
  melanocytic, 17
  mucosal, 28
  multiple, 188
  multiple common, 182–186
  multiple small globules, 21
  nonpigmented spitz, 29–30
  palmar, 54
  papillomatous dermal, 25
  parallel furrow pattern, 26
  perifollicular hypopigmentation, 23
  pigmented spitz, 30, 31
  pigment network in, 19
  recurrent, 36
  reed, 30–31, 32
  reticular pattern, 18, 19, 20, 22
  scalp, 24, 25
  sclerosing, 36
  special types, 33
  spitz, 29, 31–32
  starburst pattern, 18
  subungual, 28
  target globules of congenital, 24
  target network of congenital, 23
  traumatized, 33, 34
  of trunk and extremities, 19
  vulvar, 29

Nits, 133, 134; *see also* Parasitoses
NM, *see* Nodular melanoma
Nodular
amelanotic melanoma, 64, 67, 69
basal cell carcinoma, 90, 95
lesion excision, 188
pigmented basal cell carcinoma, 92
Nodular melanoma (NM), 39, 63; *see also* Melanoma
advanced, 63, 64
atypical and irregular linear vessels, 66
blue and black color, 65, 66
characteristics of, 63
dermatoscopic criteria, 65
dermatoscopic features, 64
differential diagnosis of, 64
nodular amelanotic melanoma, 64
polymorphous vascular pattern, 66
with verrucous hyperkeratotic surface, 65
Noncicatricial alopecias, 144; *see also* Trichoscopy
alopecia areata, 147–151
androgenetic alopecia, 144–147
tinea capitis, 153–155
trichotillomania, 151–153
Nonpigmented; *see also* Pigmented
basal cell carcinoma, 90–93
spitz nevus, 29–30
structures, 89

O

Ovoid comedo-like openings, 9

P

PAK, *see* Pigmented actinic keratosis
Palmar
melanoma, 53
nevus, 54
Palmarpits, 95
Palmoplantar warts, 137; *see also* Human papillomavirus
clinical aspect of, 138
dermatoscopic examination, 139
dermatoscopic pattern of, 138
hemorrhages and red spots, 138
multiple tiny red dots, 138
Papillomatous dermal nevus, 25; *see also* Nevus
Papulosis, lymphomatoid, 126; *see also* Inflammatory skin diseases
Parallel furrow pattern (PFP), 54
Parallel ridge pattern (PRP), 54
Parasitoses, 131; *see also* Infectious skin diseases; Phthiriasis
jet with contrail pattern, 132
nits, 133, 134
pediculosis, 131, 133
pseudonits, 132
scabies, 131, 132
Pediculosis, 131, 133; *see also* Parasitoses
Pediculus humanus capitis, 133; *see also* Parasitoses
Perforating dermatoses, acquired, 124; *see also* Inflammatory skin diseases
Perifollicular scaling, 159
and pink-white areas, 156
Peripheral streaks and pseudopods, multiple, 8
PFP, *see* Parallel furrow pattern
Phthiriasis; *see also* Parasitoses
of body, 133–134
pubis, 134
of scalp, 132–133
Pigmented; *see also* Nonpigmented
basal cell carcinoma, 93
network, 172, 175
nodular basal cell carcinoma, 92
purpuric dermatoses, 122, 123
spitz nevus, 30, 31
structures, 3
Pigmented actinic keratosis (PAK), 49, 170, 172, 173, 174; *see also* Pigmented macules on face
nonmelanoma criteria of, 171
Pigmented lesion, 184
atypical, 188
prospective monitoring, 183–186
regression of lesion, 185
Pigmented macules on face, 169; *see also* Lentigo maligna
actinic keratosis, 175
differential diagnosis of, 169
flat pigmented lesions on face, 170
flat seborrheic keratosis, 170
lichen planus–like keratosis, 173, 174
nonmelanoma criteria of pigmented actinic keratosis, 171
nonmelanoma criteria of solar lentigo, 171
pigmented actinic keratosis, 170, 171, 172, 173, 174
pigmented network, 175
pigment network in between follicular openings, 172
seborrheic keratosis, 171, 172, 173, 175
solar lentigo, 174, 175
suspicious lesions management, 176
Pili; *see also* Hair shaft deformities
annulati, 164
torti, 163–164
Pinkus, fibroepithelioma of, 92
Pityriasis lichenoides chronica (PLC), 123
Pityriasis lichenoides et varioliformis acuta (PLEVA), 123; *see also* Inflammatory skin diseases
Pityriasis rosea (PR), 115; *see also* Inflammatory skin diseases
Pityriasis rubra pilaris, 122, 123; *see also* Inflammatory skin diseases
Plantar melanoma, 57, 58; *see also* Melanoma
advanced, 54
early, 53
Plasma serum, extravasated, 6
PLC, *see* Pityriasis lichenoides chronica
PLEVA, *see* Pityriasis lichenoides et varioliformis acuta
Pohl-pinkus constrictions, 161; *see also* Hair shaft deformities
Poorly differentiated squamous cell carcinoma, 69
Porokeratosis, 120, 121; *see also* Inflammatory skin diseases
PR, *see* Pityriasis rosea
PRP, *see* Parallel ridge pattern

Prurigo nodularis, 123–124; *see also* Inflammatory skin diseases
Pseudomonilethrix, 161; *see also* Hair shaft deformities
Pseudonetwork, 50
Pseudonits, 132; *see also* Parasitoses
Psoriasis, 111; *see also* Inflammatory skin diseases
  Auspitz sign, 111, 112
  dermatoscopy in, 111
  lesion in patient under treatment with biologic agent, 113
  psoriatic balanitis, 112
  psoriatic lesion of scalp, 112
  psoriatic plaque, 112
  red globular rings pattern, 112
  scalp, 111–112
  thick white scales in palmoplantar, 112
Purpuric dermatoses, 122
Pyogenic granuloma, 81, 82; *see also* Vascular tumors

R

Recurrent nevus, 36; *see also* Nevus
Reed nevus, 30–31, 32, 177; *see also* Nevus
  homogenous pattern in, 178
  reticular pattern in, 178
Regrowing hairs, 144; *see also* Trichoscopy
Reticular nevus, 20; *see also* Nevus
Rosacea, 119; *see also* Inflammatory skin diseases
  associated demodicosis, 119, 120
  clinical image of, 120
  and discoid lupus erythematosus, 120
Rosettes, 13
  in actinic keratosis, 98

S

Sarcoidosis, 118; *see also* Granulomatous skin diseases
Sarcoma
  angiosarcoma, 108
  dermal, 70
  kaposi sarcoma, 107, 108
Scabies, 131, 132; *see also* Parasitoses
Scalp
  cellulitis, 159
  dissecting cellulitis of, 159
  nevus, 24, 25
  phthiriasis of, 132–133
Sclerodermiform, 91
Sclerosing nevus, 36; *see also* Nevus
Sebaceous hyperplasia, 84, 85; *see also* Adnexal tumors
Seborrheic keratosis (SK), 14, 42, 49, 171, 172, 173, 175; *see also* Epithelial skin tumors; Pigmented macules on face
  acanthotic type of, 78, 79
  capillary loops in common warts, 78
  cerebriform pattern, 78
  comedo-like openings, 78
  irritated, 78
  keratotic type, 79
  multiple milia-like cysts in, 77
  reticulated, 79
  sharp demarcation of borders, 78
Sebum, 3
Senile lentigo, *see* Solar lentigo
Shiny milia-like cysts, 12
SK, *see* Seborrheic keratosis
Skin cancer, keratinocyte, 96–104
SL, *see* Solar lentigo
Solar lentigo (SL), 49, 75, 76, 172, 173, 174, 175; *see also* Epithelial skin tumors; Pigmented macules on face
  nonmelanoma criteria of, 171
Spitz nevus, 29, 31–32; *see also* Nevus
Spitzoid-looking lesion, 176; *see also* Lesions
  atypical Spitz nevi, 179, 180
  dermatoscopic starburst pattern, 178
  dermatoscopic features, 177–181
  facts, 177
  management, 176–182
  nonpigmented Spitz nevus, 178
  pigmented Spitz nevus, 178, 179
  Spitz nevus, 180
  spitzoid melanoma, 179, 180, 181
Squamous cell carcinoma (SCC), 96, 100; *see also* Keratinocyte skin cancer
  amorphous white-yellow keratin mass, 101
  blood spots in keratin masses, 103
  dermatoscopic criteria of, 100
  developing as centrally ulcerated nodule, 101
  developing as indurated and ulcerated plaque, 101
  dotted and glomerular vessels in, 102
  hairpin vessels in, 102
  linear-irregular vessels in, 102
  moderately differentiated, 105
  poorly differentiated, 69, 103, 104
  progression from AK into invasive SCC, 104
  well-differentiated, 101–103
  white halos, 102
  white structureless areas in, 102
  white-yellow scales in, 101
Subcorneal and subungual hemorrhage, 81, 82, 83; *see also* Vascular tumors
Subungual
  hemorrhage, 54
  nevus, 28, 61
Subungual melanoma, 56; *see also* Melanoma
  advanced, 58
  congenital subungual nevus, 59
  dermatoscopic features, 59
  drug-induced melanonychia, 58
  Hutchinson sign, 57
  longitudinal melanonychia, 58, 59
  onychodystrophia, 58
  reactive pigmentation, 59
  subungual hemorrhage, 59, 60
  subungual lentigo, 59
Superficial
  basal cell carcinoma, 68, 91, 93
  small erosions, 12

T

Target
globules of congenital nevus, 24
network of congenital nevus, 23
Targetoid hemosiderotic nevus, 33, 34
Temporal triangular alopecia (TTA), 159–160; *see also* Trichoscopy in children
10-second rule in single lesions, 187–188
Terminal hairs, 143, 157; *see also* Trichoscopy
Tick bites, 139; *see also* Infectious skin diseases
Tinea capitis, 153; *see also* Noncicatricial alopecias
clinical presentation of, 153
coma hairs in, 153
corkscrew hairs in, 153
i-hairs in, 155
Morse-code hairs and i-hairs, 154
trichoscopic features of, 153
zig-zag hairs in, 154
Tinea corporis, 141; *see also* Infectious skin diseases
Total-body examination, 186–187
Traumatized nevus, 33, 34; *see also* Nevus
Trichoptilosis, 163; *see also* Hair shaft deformities
in trichotillomania, 151
Trichorrhexis; *see also* Hair shaft deformities
invaginata, 162, 163
nodosa, 161–162
Trichoschisis, 163; *see also* Hair shaft deformities
Trichoscopy, 143
alopecia, 144
characteristics of cicatricial alopecias, 160
hair shaft deformities, 161–164
noncicatricial alopecias, 144–154
normal hair shaft, 143
primary cicatricial alopecias, 154–159
regrowing hairs, 144
trichoscopic findings in temporal and occipital areas of scalp, 144
vellus hairs, 143, 144
Trichoscopy in children, 159; *see also* Trichoscopy
aplasia cutis, 160–161
loose anagen hair syndrome, 160
temporal triangular alopecia, 159–160
Trichotillomania, 151; *see also* Noncicatricial alopecias
black dots forming hair dust in, 152
coiled hairs and hook hairs, 152
flame hair in, 152
focal hemorrhage, 153
hook hair and V sign in, 152
trichoptilosis in, 151
tulip hair and flame hairs in, 152
V sign in, 152, 153
TTA, *see* Temporal triangular alopecia
Tumors; *see also* Benign nonmelanocytic skin tumors
adnexal, 84–85
common adnexal, 84–85
epithelial skin, 75
of fibrous tissue, 82–84
malignant vascular, 107–108
melanocytic nail, 28
vascular, 80–82
Tumors of fibrous tissue, 82; *see also* Benign nonmelanocytic skin tumors
dermatofibroma, 82–84
Twisted hairs, *see* Pili—torti
Two-step algorithm, 42, 46; *see also* Melanoma

U

Ugly duckling sign, 182
Urticarial vasculitis, 121; *see also* Inflammatory skin diseases

V

Vascular lacunes, sharply demarcated, 12
Vascular tumors, 80; *see also* Benign nonmelanocytic skin tumors
angiokeratoma, 81
cherry angioma, 80
malignant, 107–108
pyogenic granuloma, 81, 82
subcorneal and subungual hemorrhage, 81, 82, 83
Vellus hairs, 143, 144; *see also* Trichoscopy
Vessels, 2
as dots, 10
multiple, 10
Viral infections, 134; *see also* Infectious skin diseases
human papillomavirus, 136–139
molluscum contagiosum, 134–135
V sign, 152, 153; *see also* Trichotillomania
Vulvar nevus, 29; *see also* Nevus

W

Warts
genital, 136; *see also* Anogenital warts
palmoplantar, 137; *see also* Human papillomavirus
white-colored, 136
Wickham striae (WS), 113
WS, *see* Wickham striae

Y

Yellow clod sign, 113

Z

Zig-zag hairs, 154